AF478226

Evolution of Cancer

Evolution of Cancer

Shinichi Okuyama and Hitoshi Mishina

UNIVERSITY OF TOKYO PRESS

To my wife Junko and my late first wife Masako, and children, Yuriko, Izumi, Takashi, Jun, Midori and Shaw——SO
To my wife Hisako and children, Haruko, Hiroaki and Yoshiko—— HM

Contents

Foreword 1

Evolution of Cancer is the result of many years of hard work and deliberation by the two authors. Having known Drs. Okuyama and Mishina for many years as gifted researchers and clinical radiation oncologists, I was very glad to accept their request to write a foreword to this book.

As is usual with a book as unique as this one, I felt it difficult at first to follow the authors' ideas. However, I was eventually overwhelmed by their enthusiasm for incorporating evolutionary concepts into the treatment of cancer. It is not often that we see such a splendid melding of basic oncology with clinical research as has been achieved by the present authors.

As the death toll from cancer increased, the increased importance of cancer management became clear. First, surgical cancer intervention attracted oncologists, for the method literally implied "removal" of the cancer mass. There followed Roentgen's discovery of ionizing radiation, which provided us with a second potential means of cancer management, i.e., radiotherapy. This novel approach to radiation therapy of cancer, however, has long been hindered by the strong barrier of radioresistance. Radiotherapy is, in essence, a local chemotherapy. When the authors arrived at this notion, they had to define the origin of selective radiosensitivity. They assumed that cancer represents the status of having achieved anti-evolution, or a devolution from the mammalian norm. In such an archaic state, ionization density can be greater than the norm, handling of the resultant noxious products may be less effective, and the process of repair of DNA damage may be defective. The authors went further by searching for clues to the evolutionary implications of the process of carcinogenesis and cachectic status, and their successes resulted in this volume.

Modern molecular oncology seems to have promised development of the ultimate means to manage cancer cells in the near future. Nonetheless, the development of novel diagnostic methods in terms of tumor imaging and *in vitro* assay should also be encouraged in the interest of achieving evolutionary and endosymbiotic understanding of cancer cells as well as novel radiotherapeutic modifications.

I believe that this seemingly difficult concept will be warmly received by oncologists worldwide, and provide an important step forward toward the management of cancer, the disease of the twentieth century.

Masahiro Iio, M. D., Ph.D.
Professor and Chairman
Department of Radiology, Faculty of Medicine
The University of Tokyo

Foreword 2

I first became acquainted with Dr. Okuyama when he was a postgraduate medical student majoring in internal medicine at the Research Institute for Tuberculosis, Leprosy and Cancer, Tohoku University, Sendai. He would raise questions about the relative values of *in vivo* verification and *in vitro* demonstration for showing the effects of neutralizing antibodies to viruses and microorganisms; curious though these questions sometimes were, they did perhaps bring him to an understanding of the nature and meaning of model experiments. During these years, he had a thorough grounding in immunology, especially in ontogeny and the phylogeny of immune competence. Moving to the Department of Radiology and Nuclear Medicine of the same Institute, he devoted himself to cancer radiotherapy and to investigations into ways of increasing the therapeutic efficacy of radiotherapy and chemotherapy. This enquiry was still continued when he moved to Sendai's Tohoku Rosai Hospital, to the Department of Radiology. He had already learned that radiation damage to DNA can be repaired, and that bleomycin can have an important role in the repair process. Dr. Okuyama's subsequent work continued and developed these principles in the domain of chemotherapy, resulting in the theory of high-dose chemotherapy induction and small-dose perpetuation chemotherapy using, for example, combinations of cisplatin and bleomycin, large doses of bleomycin, or neocarzinostatin.

Although the term *biological response modifier* was coined elsewhere, it is in Japan that most substances belonging to this classificantion have been developed: OK-432, PSK, lentinan, and Bestatin. From the recognition that all of these substances are active in areas of archaic and quasi-specific, rather than truly specific, immunity came the important hypothesis that cancer itself should be regarded as the effect of loss of tissue specificity and devolution to the point of archaism. Current clinical achievements in Japan with these substances lend a great deal of credibility to this view.

All life bears within it its own evolutionary history, inscribed in the gene. This is just as true for neoplasms as for other cells. No less multifarious are cancer and leukemia and their originating and developmental processes. Molecular oncology is certainly throwing a great deal of light on individual carcinogenetic processes. Nevertheless, it still remains to discover the organization within the genome of the carcinogenetic sequence. Ultimately, of course, our interest is centered on the nature and organization of counteracting devices, such as anti-oncogenes, that have arisen in response to carcinogenetic insults, and their relevant structures and functions.

The authors started their investigations with the origin of the selective radiosensitivity of cancer, and arrived at the recognition that cancer status may represent *devolution* from the normal mammalian attainment, and that human carcinogenesis itself changes with advancing age in accordance with the phylogenetic order of evolution of life on earth. *The Evolution of Cancer* is thus both a basic oncogenic thesis and a classification of clinical therapeutic practice from an evolutionary point of view.

I found the authors' attempt to provide an integrated view of cancer impressive, and think they should be forgiven a slight practical dogmatism as long as they make no claims to infallibility.

Nakao Ishida, M. D., Ph.D.
Professor Emeritus, Tohoku University
Former President of Tohoku University

Foreword 3

Dr. Mishina and I used to work together at the Department of Radiology, Fukushima Medical College, Fukushima, where he was my associate professor. He was good at mathematics and mechanics, and we invented and patented several types of tomographic apparatus before he moved to Tohoku Rosai Hospital, Sendai, in 1962. We also engaged in radiotherapy of cancer patients, and we could not but realize how incurable many of their cases were. We experienced a case of malignant lymphoma which happened to regress following a course of acute bacterial infection of the tumor. Dr. Mishina was deeply impressed by that event, although we had no definite idea what mechanisms could have been involved. As soon as OK-432 (NSC-B116209), a viable streptococcal preparation, became clinically available, he was naturally absorbed by that agent, and developed a host of techniques for its optimal administration, for its therapeutic effectiveness was apparently dependent on the sites of the tumors and their metastases within the body and on the routing of its administration as well. At first, most scientists believed that OK-432 exerts its anticancer effects via specific immunity. However, later studies presented data in favor of nonspecific and, therefore, archaic forms of immunity. Dr. Mishina, together with Dr. Okuyama, discloses that "devolved cancer cells have to be counteracted by archaic or more primitive immune mechanisms." The probable importance of this type of logical acknowledgement of that modality of treatment cannot be overestimated.

I am greatly impressed by the authors' endeavor as clinicians to construct a logical strategy of anticancer techniques. They always had to begin with scarce clinical evidence, but were not infrequently successful in arriving at logical principles and appropriate applications. They frequently composed clinical model experiments as well as *in vitro* and *in vivo* studies, which will greatly benefit both clinicians and basic researchers.

Akira Matsukawa, M. D., Ph.D.
Professor Emeritus and Former Dean
Fukushima Medical College

Preface

The therapeutic difficulties we have encountered in the treatment of cancer patients are often so vexing that we sometimes despair of being of any use at all to such patients. Still, we cannot just wait in limbo for the development of a brilliant universal cancer medicine. The initial step may be to develop techniques of reinforcing and integrating the therapeutic effects of those anticancer treatments that are currently available: developing spatial and/or temporal concentration of drugs, taking advantage of the interactions of drug effects when given sequentially, applying radiation damage to DNA chemotherapeutically, and learning to biologically distinguish cancer cells in terms of superoxide dismutase and water content. At the same time, we can make adjustments in our way of thinking about cancer.

In our search for a means of adequately integrating the currently available anti-cancer treatments, in the absence of any singly curative agents, we discussed the effective applications of radiotherapy and scrutinized the possible underlying mechanisms. In the process, we eventually arrived at the recognition that cancer may represent a process of evolution in reverse—a sort of "devolution" from more highly developed to less developed forms. This concept made it easier to understand a host of principles of cancer diagnosis and therapy: angiographic delineation of tumors, rather specific deposition of radiogallium for tumor imaging, the well-known selective radiosensitivity of cancers, discovery of the anticancer effect of tetracyclines, and quasispecific immunotherapy. These notions can also support our attempt to biologically differentiate cancer cells from the normal mammalian cells and organs.

Cancer itself could in fact have evolved from archaic simpler forms to the more complex types. This concept, derived from an epidemiological analysis of age distribution of cancer incidence, was verified by analyzing cancer incidence in patients with Fanconi's anemia and in the population of

Nagasaki City 30 years after the detonation of an atomic bomb there. (On the other hand, cachexia appeared to be devolutionary in its incidence.)

These hypotheses linking cancer to evolution have practical applications in better analysis and comprehension of the natural history of carcinogenesis along the lines of the evolution of animal life, and may contribute to development of clinical techniques for preventing and treating cancer. Recent progress in molecular oncology definitely supports our evolutionary concepts.

Our original intention was to write a book on cancer diagnosis and therapy based on the devolutionary concept of cancer. However, Professor Toshio Kuroki of the Institute of Medical Science, University of Tokyo, advised us to include discussions of the evolutionary aspects of carcinogenesis. Ms. Etsuko Hamao, Editor at the University of Tokyo Press, encouraged us to write our book in English. We had the advice of the Press editors in rewriting the text in order to avoid redundancy and indirectness and to make it idiomatic. We are grateful to those who advised us, especially Dr. Sohei Kondo, Professor Emeritus, Osaka University, Osaka; Dr. Eugene P. Cronkite, Brookhaven National Laboratory, Upton, New York; and Dr. Harold L. Atkins, Professor, Department of Radiology, State University of New York at Stony Brook, Stony Brook, New York. We are indebted to the Eastern Leukenia Association, New York, the Laborers' Welfare Foundation (Rodo Fukushi Jigyodan), Tokyo, and Tohoku Rosai Hospital Clinical Research Foundation, Sendai, for supporting our research and publications.

I. EVOLUTION OF CANCER STRATEGIES AGAINST HOST HUMANS

Chapter 1

The Evolutionary Concept of Cancer

„Kampf dem Krebs. Krebs ist heilblar."
————*Wilhelm K. Roentgen*, Physics
(1845-1923)

Radiologists and radiotherapists, following Dr. Roentgen's injunction to fight and cure cancer (Fig. 1), have focused a great deal of attention on the relative selectivity of radiotherapeutic effects on malignancies. Irradiation of a tumor mass deep in the body may well eradicate the tumor without causing any severe reactions in overlying normal tissues such as the skin, muscles, or heart. This selective effect is achieved when the irradiated cancer cells receive enough energy to cause lethal damage to their DNA. The capacity of cancer cells for repair is generally less than that of normal cells (Yatani *et al*. 1983). During irradiation, radicals such as superoxide are generated when the electrons in water molecules are ejected by the incident radiation photons and are immediately captured by the oxygen anions. Cancer cells are deficient in superoxide dismutase, which disposes of superoxide radicals, and are therefore susceptible to these radicals (Oberley and Buettner 1979; Okuyama and Mishina 1981a). However, the intratumoral distribution of oxygen molecules is not always homogeneous, and the environment tends to be hypoxic.

The question of what causes the selective effect of radiation on cancer cells was the starting point for the current evolutionary concept of cancer (Okuyama and Mishina 1982a; 1984b; 1985a, c). We realized that we had long assumed that the water density of cancer cells and normal cells was identi-

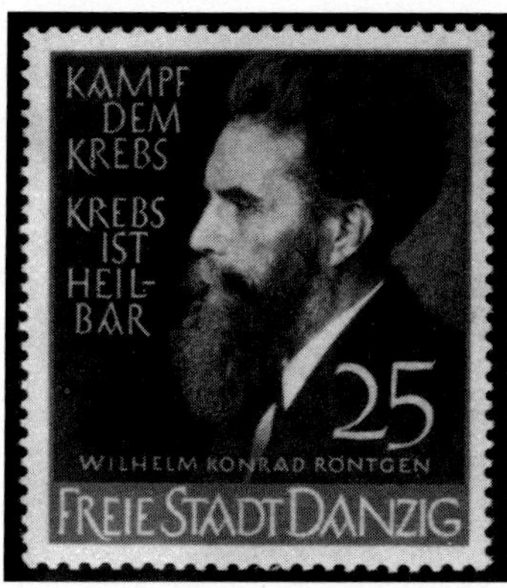

Fig. 1. "Fight cancer. Cancer is curable." The quoted is attributed to Roentgen.

cal. However, if there were a substantial difference between the two types of cells such that the water density was higher in cancer cells, greater radiotherapeutic effects could be expected in the cancer cells. We immediately looked for confirmation in the literature, where we found several relevant publications (Craig and Waterhouse 1957; Damadian 1971).

Continuous study of various attributes of cancer led us to develop an evolutionary concept of cancer (Fig. 2) (Okuyama and Mishina 1984b; 1985a). (1) The increased water density of cancer cells might be reminiscent of ancient life in the deep sea, where cells needed increased intracellular hydrostatic pressure to cope with the aquatic environment; (2) A hypoxic milieu in which the atmospheric oxygen concentration was lower than it is now could have kept the cells less dependent upon superoxide dismutase. (3) Primitive cells may have had a reduced capacity to repair ultraviolet (UV) damage to DNA. As the atmospheric oxygen concentrations increased, the UV rays from the sun could have excited the oxygen molecules, to generating ozone, which would have risen to form the ozone layer. This layer was capable of absorbing the UV rays and serving as an effective screen for life on earth. In other words, the cells then present had to protect themselves from UV irradiation either by sheltering themselves under a UV-proof screen or by acquiring the capacity to repair UV-induced DNA damage. Cancer cells seem to have

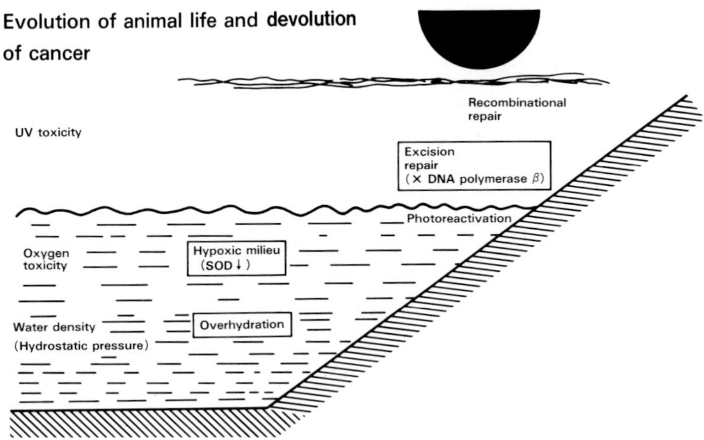

Fig. 2. Evolutionary concept of cancer. The three characteristics of cancer cells described in the text——increased hydrostatic pressure, hypoxia, and reduced capacity to repair damage from UV irradiation——indicate that cancer cells have reverted to the phylogenetic stage when animal life was conducted deep in the sea.

lost this capacity to an appreciable degree (Yatani *et al.* 1983).

As soon as our original evolutionary concept of cancer had been developed, we reviewed tumor angiograms. Tumor vessels revealed the abrupt development of fine arborescence from relatively large arterioles, in marked contrast to the gradual reduction in vascular diameter seen in normal vessels nourishing normal tissues. Tumors are thought to secrete tumor angiogenesis factor (TAF), or "angiogenin" (Folkman *et al.* 1971). This factor is capable of inducing capillary formation from host vessels. This abrupt, fine aroborescence seems to be a strategy by which cancer is able to secure for itself a hypoxic milieu, because the degree of reduction in vascular diameter is expected to guarantee an abrupt fall in blood pressure and a subsequent decrease in oxygen partial pressure among the numerous cancer cells. A characteristic of tumor vessels is their inability to mature into normal arterioles and venules (Algire and Chalkley 1945). Thus, in our evolutionary concept, cancer is thought to represent early stages of phylogeny rather than early stages of ontogeny.

In June 1986, we read of a similar concept by a pathologist (Setala 1984), who described cancer as a "devolution" to the pre-eukaryotic state. His hypothesis is firmly based on observations of chemical carcinogenesis in experimental animals. According to Setala, cancer devolution is "dry" rather than "wet," as we described it above. Carcinogenesis per se takes place at the *locus minoris resistentiae*, because of the endosymbiotic nature of mammalian cells (Margulis 1981).

The evolutionary concept of cancer may well be expanded to various aspects of oncology: (1) differences in the radiosensitivity of malignancies from different organ systems (Okuyama and Mishina 1985h); (2) tumor affinitive mechanisms of different tumor imaging agents (Okuyama and Mishina 1985d); and (3) the pathophysiological basis of cancer epidemiology, especially that ensuing from the atomic bombing (Okuyama and Mishina 1986b; 1987a; 1988a).

In this book, we look at cancer from an evoultionary point of view, with the hope that the concepts presented will have revolutionary implications.

Chapter 2

Evolutionary Epidemiology of Cancer

Prediction is one of the functions of science.
——*Bertrand Russell*, Mathematics and Philosophy (*1872-1970*)

Cancer epidemiology was once a purely descriptive science, with few attempts made to achieve biological analysis (Segi 1977; Segi *et al.* 1981). The present survey of published data on cancer incidence was undertaken to obtain evolutionary and biological insights into the nature of carcinogenesis. The motivation for this survey was provided by our observation that cancer itself may represent a state of evolutionary retrogression, or anti-evolution (Okuyama and Mishina 1984b; 1985d; 1986b; 1987a). Cancer cells seem to have regressed to a pre-eukaryotic state characterized by overhydration (Craig and Waterhouse 1957; Damadian 1971), a low level of superoxide dismutase (SOD) (Oberley and Buettner 1979; Okuyama and Mishina 1981a), and a decreased capacity for excision repair (Yatani *et al.* 1983).

The nonepithelial-epithelial tumor shift seems to be related to evolution (Okuyama and Mishina 1986b). Nature's experiments on carcinogenesis, as manifested in Fanconi's anemia, for example, have helped us decipher parts of the overall picture (Okuyama and Mishina 1987a). In the present work, special emphasis has been placed on elucidating the link between the human being as a mammal and carcinogenesis. Analyses of cancer incidence have indicated that the incidence is invariably lower in females than in males, and that human carcinogenesis seems to proceed in an evolutionary or phylogenetic sequence. Carcinogenesis may have had an evolutionary history of its own: a single change in DNA might have brought about the simplest forms of leukemia, which would then have forced the human host to respond with a series of defenses, resulting in the probable step-by-step evolution of carcinogenesis. The retroviral etiology of cancer seems to be the most novel carcinogenetic strategy, as the virus is known to be capable of taking advantage of the ultimate assembly of carcinogenetic information in the host species in the form of "proto-oncogenes." It is hoped that the present investigation into the evolutionary epidemiology of cancer will help to further research on the development of diagnostic techniques and facilitate a better understanding of the pathogenesis and pathophysiology of cancer.

Sources and Classification of Data

Cancer incidence data for the five-year period from 1973 through 1977 published by WHO (Waterhous *et al.* 1982) were used throughout these investigations. Data from Miyagi Prefecture, Japan (Waterhous *et al.* 1982), were used for comparison.

Evolutionary categorization of human organ systems as the basis of analysis   Human organ systems were categorized into four major classes (Okuyama and Mishina 1985h): (1) mammalian (breast, uterus, and prostate); (2) premammalian (homeothermic: lung and thyroid; poikilothermic: stomach, intestine, liver, and pancreas); (3) prevertebral (hemopoietic and connective tissues; nonepithelial tissues including brain, kidney, and bone; and (4) evolutionarily secured (testis and ovary). The gonads were so designated because their genetic cells have to be protected against damage to DNA. If damage occurs, the cells are quickly eliminated to conserve the integrity of the species (*horror autotoxicus*). As indicated by the dynamic changes in radiosensitivity of these cells (Prasad 1974), DNA repair that is prone to err is not permitted. The homeothermic organs are likely to have achieved full development during the Carboniferous Period, taking advantage of the increased atmospheric oxygen concentrations. These organs are thus related to energy expenditure, and include the respiratory system and thyroid gland. The digestive organs could have fully evolved prior to homeothermic life.

The stages of life have been divided into three periods: prereproductive, reproductive, and postreproductive (postmenopausal).

Cancer Incidence

Age distribution   As shown in Fig. 1, neoplasms are not limited to adulthood, but can occur as soon as early infancy. Although epithelial tumors were rare during infancy, their incidence rises exponentially in both males and females. The nonepithelial tumors, however, are more common than epithelial tumors during infancy and childhood, but are surpassed by epithelial tumors around the time of puberty. This transition has been designated the nonepithelial-epithelial tumor shift (Okuyama and Mishina 1986b; 1987a; 1988a).

Cancer incidence among mammalian and premammalian organ systems   A comparison was made between the populations of a Japanese prefecture (Miyagi) and the City of Los Angeles (Table 1). First of all, the cancer incidence in terms of world age-standardized rates (ASR) was greater in Los Angeles than in Japan. In Japan, tumors of the gastrointestinal system or the poikilothermic organs were the most prevalent, while those of the mammalian symbol organs——breast, uterus, and prostate——were much less common. In contrast, mammalian symbol neoplasms predominated in Los Angeles, while those of the digestive system were much less common. Cancers of the homeothermic organs were more frequent among Los Angelenos.

Age distribution of tumors in the evolutionarily secured organs Curves of the incidence of testicular tumors had three peaks, during the periods of prereproductiveness, reproductiveness, and postreproductiveness. Incidence curves of the ovarian cancers were biphasic, lacking the initial infantile or prereproductive peak. Thus, ovarian tumors were common during puberty and around menopause.

Age distribution of tumor incidence in the prevertebral symbol organs   Leukemias are representative of both nonepithelial and prevertebral tumors. Lymphatic leukemias were characterized by biphasic curves, prereproductive and postreproduc-

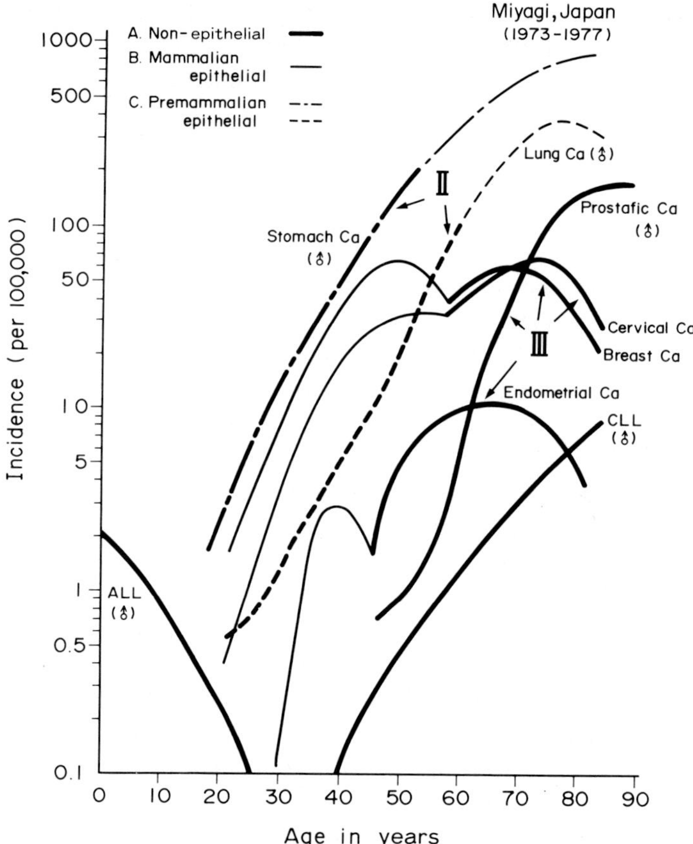

Fig. 1. Evolutionary profile of carcinogenesis. The incidence of carcinogenesis appears to progress with aging: (I) prevertebral (leukemias); (II) vertebral-premammalian symbol organs (stomach and lung cancers); and (III) vertebral-mammalian symbol organs [prostate, (male uterus), uterine endometrium, cervix uteri, and breast]. If the incidence rates were converted to probability values, the curves would show the probability of a man or woman of having tumors of various categories along the line of evolution.

tive, lacking the reproductive peak. The first curve consisted of the descending limb only, unlike the curves described above. The myeloid leukemias had three peaks, irrespective of the mother population.

Age distribution of cancers in the premammalian symbol organs: poikilothermic and homeothermic symbols With both lung and stomach cancers, the increases in cancer inci-

Table 1. Cancer incidence in terms of ASR world: Mammalian vs premammalian organs

			Miyagi	Osaka	LA, whites	LA, blacks
ASR world for all sites		(M)	208.9	204.9	287.3	321.6
		(F)	139.0	137.9	283.7	243.1
Mammalian		Prostate	(M)	4.6	2.3	44.3	79.1
	Breast and uterus	(F)	37.9	32.4	131.7	99.7
Pre-mammal-lian	Homeo-thermic	Lung, pharynx, and larynx	(M)	29.9	27.8	70.5	88.0
			(F)	10.6	10.2	25.9	22.2
	Poikilo-thermic	Esophagus, stomach, intestine, colorectum, liver, and pancreas	(M)	133.6	93.2	67.9	81.3
			(F)	83.8	59.6	48.5	58.6

dence with age were exponential. However, these curves appeared to reach a single peak and then drop off (Fig. 1). Each curve can therefore be expressed by a single function.

Age distribution of cancers in the mammalian symbol organs
While the curve for breast cancer from the Los Angeles population appeared monofunctional, that from Miyagi, Japan, was bifunctional. Close scrutiny of other curves, including those from the Los Angeles population, indicated that they were bifunctional. In the Miyagi population at least, the earlier peak covered the active period of reproduction, while the later one occurred during that following menopause (Fig. 1). Thus, the findings seem to suggest that breast cancers have two different pathogeneses, one directly related to reproductive periodicity and the other not. The endometrial cancers also formed two peaks, although they were more prevalent among the older group. In other words, endometrial tumors may be primarily a disease of the elderly. The curves for uterine cervical cancer were also bifunctional, indicating that the implications could be the same as those for breast and endometrial cancers.

The prostate may be a male homologue of the uterus (Hamilton *et al.* 1959). The cancer incidence curve for that organ was definitely monofunctional, peaking during the

later years, or the period of postreproductiveness (Fig. 1).
Rationale for evolutionary analysis of cancer incidence
The beginning of our evolutionary concept of cancer
emerged from analysis of the selective effectiveness of radiotherapy (Okuyama and Mishina 1984b; 1985c; 1985h). Cancer per se was thought to represent devolution or regression
beyond fetalism, along the lines of evolution of animal life:
(1) increased water density (Craig and Waterhouse 1957;
Damadian 1971), (2) reduced SOD (Oberley and Buettner
1979; Okuyama and Mishina 1981a), and (3) deficient excision repair (Yatani *et al.* 1983). These fragments of evidence
seemed to provide a basis for the evolutionary concept of cancer (Okuyama and Mishina 1984b) (Fig. 2, chapter 1): reversion to primitive life in the deep sea (high hydraulic pressure),
where the effects of UV and oxygen would have been low;
therefore, the demand for superoxide dismutase (SOD) and
excision repair of DNA damage could have been low. Higher
intracellular pressure can also be generated by increasing the
concentrations of cytoplasmic solutes. Conversely, the cytoplasmic pressure can be reduced through inclusion of
enough microorganelles, such as ribosomes and mitochondria.
Thus, carcinogenesis could well represent the retrogression
of once normal cells along the line of evolution. According to
our view (Okuyama and Mishina 1984b) and that of others
(Setala 1984; Kroon *et al.* 1985), the status of cancer may
imply derangement of cellular function as well as the degree
of "pre-eukaryotism": tetracyclines are capable of discrimi-
nating cancer cells from normal cells, killing the former selectively (Okuyama *et al.* 1984c; Okuyama *et al.* 1987a; van
Bogert *et al.* 1986).

A second rationale for our evolutionary analysis of the incidence of cancer is the circumstantial evidence that atmospheric oxygen concentrations varied greatly in the past
(Berkner and Marshall 1965), exerting a major influence on
the evolution of animals: (1) emergence of the ozone layers,
which enabled animals to emerge from the deep sea into shal-
low seas and waters, eventually moving onto land; (2) acquisition of Cu, ZnSOD to cope with constantly emerging intrinsic
active oxygen moieties, especially superoxide (Asada 1976);
and (3) occurrence of mammalian evolution under decreased

atmospheric oxygen concentrations towards the end of the Carboniferous Period, presumably allowing mammalian symbol organs such as the breast to elaborate less superoxide dismutase (Patterson 1978; Sykes *et al.* 1978).

Cancer incidence curves in the elucidation of the evolutionary significance of carcinogenesis in humans   Obviously, the cancer incidence curves shown here do not necessarily represent exact mathematical incidence functions. However, they at least approximate trends, and provide practical help in analyzing the evolutionary hypothesis, especially when their possible relationships to reproductiveness are taken into account, as will be seen below.

Biological implications of carcinogenesis in humans as suggested by the analysis of cancer incidence   One of the cardinal merits of the present investigation seems to be the discrimination of mammalian symbol organs from other premammalian organs in order to extract probable biological and evolutionary implications. In this regard, the following findings were useful: (1) that the nonepithelial-epithelial tumor shift is observed among both the Los Angeles and Japanese populations (Okuyama and Mishina 1986b); (2) that the Los Angelenos suffer mainly from tumors of the mammalian symbol organs and homeothermic organs, while the Japanese have more tumors of the homeothermic and poikilothermic organs; (3) that cancers of the female mammalian symbol organs form two peaks, one during the active reproductive period and the other during the postmenopausal, postreproductive period; (4) that cancers of the prostate, the male homologue of the uterus, appear to represent tumors of non-reproductiveness; and (5) that the gonadal tumors show generally low incidence rates, suggesting the probable presence of specific anticancer mechanisms. Thus, important biological significance may be attributed to the different incidences of cancer in different organ systems.

Probable evolutionary and phylogenetic implications of different cancer incidences in the respective organ systems   The process of ontogeny reflects the phylogenic sequence. This also seems to hold true for carcinogenesis with advancing aging. The incidence of neoplasms of organ systems of different phylogenetic order changes with aging: (1) leukemias (prevertebral) and tumors of the brain, kidney, and bone (vertebral-nonepithelial); (2) cancers of the gastrointestinal system (vertebral-epithelial-poikilothermic) and respiratory cancers (vertebral-epithelial-homeothermic); and, last, (3) cancers of the mammalian symbol organs, prostate, uterus, and breast. Thus, the sequence of change in incidence resembles that of phylogeny.

Cancers of the mammalian symbol organs during the active reproductive and postreproductive periods We took it for granted that cancers of the mammalian symbol organs occurring during the period of postreproductiveness fit the evolutionary hypthesis, because cancers of the prostate appear to be postreproductive, and because the same principle seems to apply to other mammalian symbol cancers, i.e., those of the breast, cervix, and endometrium. Table 2 summarizes the results of the analysis of cancer incidence in terms of the prereproductive, reproductive, and postreproductive periods. All types of cancers are present during the period of postreproductiveness. In the prereproductive period, positive results are seen only for cancer of the testis and leukemias. The incidence of tumors during the period of active reproductiveness varied: cancers of the prostate and lymphatic leukemias were not seen, while definite positive results were observed for cancers of the

Table 2. Cancer occurrence in terms of prereproductive, reproductive, and postreproductive periods

Organ systems				Pre-reprod.	Repro-ductive	Post-reprod.
Evolutionarily secured			Testis	Yes	Yes	Yes
			Ovary	No	Yes	Yes
Verte-bral	Mammalian symbol organs		Prostate	No	No	Yes
			Endo-metrium	No	(Yes)	Yes
			Cervix	No	Yes	Yes
			Breast	No	Yes	Yes
	Premam-malian	Homeo-thermic	Lung	No	Yes	Yes
		Poikilo-thermic	Stomach	No	Yes	Yes
Prevertebral			Leukemias			
			Lymphatic	Yes	No	Yes
			Myeloid	Yes	Yes	Yes

breast and uterine cervix, as mentioned earlier. Smaller rises were observed for cancers of the uterine endometrium, and we suspect that that function could have been a novel evolutionary emergence, as the disease is primarily a cancer of postmenopausal women (Robbins and Angell 1976). It is intriguing that cancer of the uterine endometrium is often preceded by a series of progressively abnormal cellular proliferations, which eventually lead to *in situ* carcinoma, as in the case of prostatic cancer. This deserves a critical investigation in terms of retrogressive expansion of the disease towards the younger generation: simple continuous expansion or an emergence of a novel disease from a different etiology and pathogenesis.

The mechanisms involved in these breast and cervical cancers are likely to be different from those of postmenopausal tumors, as indicated by evidence from retroviral etiology (zur Hausen 1982; Baird 1983), implicating recent amplification of a long-existent mechanism or emergence of a new mechanism as the result of retroviral infection, chemical contamination, or the influence of modern civilization. Sugano (1980) suggests that basic cancer be distinguished from variables in all organ systems. In the case of breast cancer, scirrhous carcinoma, which is prevalent among postmenopausal women, is a variable cancer. This appears to contradict the "evolutionarily orthodox" neoplasms listed under "postreproductiveness" in Table 2. We do not feel able to offer any further comments in this regard at the moment. Nonetheless, it seems sufficiently intriguing to note that attempts to induce carcinogenesis of the prostate with 1, 2-benz-pyrene were successful only when this chemical was administered to experimental animals with glandular regression and atrophy (Fingerhut and Veenema 1977), but not when it was given simultaneously with castration (Moore and Melchinonna 1937).

Cancer incidence among the premammalian, vertebral organs during the period of active reproductivity   In spite of the preceding discussion on mammalian symbol organs, carcinomas of the premammalian organ systems, as represented by those of the lung and stomach, may not be directly related to reproductive activity. Their exponential rises were steep and continuous, and there did not appear to be any appreciable troughs in the vicinity of the transition from the reproductive to postreproductive periods. Males in Los Angeles, both white and black, showed an increasing trend in the incidence of lung cancer during the periods of reproductiveness and postreproductiveness that was identical to that in Japanese males. This indicates an identical extrinsic factor rather than changes in racial intrinsic factors. The incidence rates of stomach cancer for both male and female Japanese in Japan were remarkably higher than those for Japanese in Los Angeles and Hawaii. The rates in mainland Japanese were further characterized by much earlier rises in the curves. These findings are also suggestive of the probable contribution of extrinsic factors like traditional diet as well as water-soluble trace elements in the soil. They may bear no relationship to reproductive activity. Nonetheless, Sugano's hypothesis (1980) of basic vs variable cancers may be of great help in deciphering the evolutionary context of cancers of the lung and stomach, i.e., the premammalian symbol organs.

Different histological types of cancer seem to prevail in different age groups. For example, the undifferentiated type of stomach cancer is more common in the young, while the differentiated type is widespread in the elderly. Among lung cancers, adenocarcinomas are found in the young, while squamous cell types predominate in the elderly. Sugano's criterion for the diagnosis of basic vs variable cancers seems to be statistical stability in terms of chronology and histology. This kind of discussion clearly contributes to our studies. The curve for Miyagi females, however, appears to form a depression between the ages of 50 and 55. Since a similar phenomenon seems to occur in Hawaian males, it may be preferable to abandon the idea of postreproductiveness as a criterion for designating evolutionary orthodox cancer. Rather, the fundamental concept of basic vs variable cancer seems more applicable to lung and stomach cancers. Thus, premammalian carcinomas can be categorized as belonging to the reproductive period, although they may not necessarily have any substantial correlation to reproduction. The evolutionary progression of carcinogenesis can best be described as follows: (1) leukemia, (2) premammalian epithelial tumors, and (3) mammalian epithelial tumors (Fig. 1). In explaining his model of clonal evolution in neoplasia, Nowell stated that human tumors with minimal chromosomal

change (diploid acute leukemia, chronic granulocytic leukemia) are considered to represent early stages in clonal evolution,
while human solid cancers, typically highly aneuploid, are to
be seen as occurring late in the developmental processs (1977).
We think further classification of the solid epithelial cancers is
required from an evolutionary point of view.

Cancer incidence among the prevertebral organ systems   Cells
of the hematopoietic organs are of prevertebral origin, and
their neoplasms were found to be prevalent during the early
periods of life. The lymphatic leukemias were both pre- and
postreproductive, while the non-lymphoid leukemias were tri-
phasic. Acute lymphocytic leukemia tends to occur in younger
children prior to involution of the thymus (Schimpff 1986), and
may be related to the establishment of the immune system.
The probable evolutionary implications of chromosomal breakage syndromes that are prone to develop leukemias have
already been discussed (Okuyama and Mishina 1987a). The
absence of lymphatic leukemias during the "reproductive
period" could be related to the maintained integrity of the
immune system during that period. The maintenance of this
integrity is vital to the host's defense against autoantigeniza-
tion and subsequent self destruction (*horror autotoxicus*)
(Okuyama and Mishina 1985h). The high sensitivity of lymphocytes to glucocorticoids (Fauci and Dale 1975) through
"apoptosis" (Kerr and Searle 1980) may have evolutionary
significance as well (Kobayashi 1980). The mechanism could
be useful in surveying abnormal lymphocytes that might
emerge from time to time and impinge upon the host cells
too.

*Cancer incidence among the evolutionarily secured organ
systems*   As discussed earlier, testicular tumors are encountered in all three periods. Curiously, however, the maximum incidence rates were similar in all three: about two per
100,000 population. Ovarian tumors were almost totally
absent during the prereproductive period. The gonads have
to be designed and constructed to conserve genetic information without error. Genetic material, therefore, has to be protected from the continuous emergence of intrinsic active oxygen molecules that takes place in homeothermic animals.
This may be especially true in mammalian species because of

the extraordinary paucity of offspring produced by one mammalian female during her life. As the generation of these oxygen radicals depends on the topical temperature and oxygen concentration, the critical organs have to be kept cooler and/or less vascularized. In the testis, these requirements are met by its externalization. Both the seminal plasma and testicle show superoxide dismutase activity (Johansson *et al.* 1986). While radiation damage to DNA is generally repairable, damaged testicular cells are not always repaired and have to be eliminated by the special process of apoptosis (Harrison 1975). Presumably, the constant flux caused by the sequential divisions of spermatogenesis also contributes to the dilution of abnormalities as suggested by the hypothesis that hindrance to the exfoliative flow of glandular epithelial cells facilitates the establishment of cancer cells (Fujita 1983; Takahashi and Seiji 1983). Thus, exfoliation may help to keep the incidence of cancer relatively low in the testis.

In the ovary, the hypoxic milieu seems to be generated by sequestering the germ cells in the avascular layers of follicular and granulosa cells (Bloom and Fawcett 1975; Burns 1979). The SOD content in the rat is not high compared with the liver, kidney, and adrenal (Peeters-Joris *et al.* 1975). That of human ovarian tumors is not especially high either (Sykes *et al.* 1978). The oocytes contain the so-called lampbrush chromosomal loops, which are condensed and surrounded by a dense sheath of ribonucleoprotein (Baker 1971). This would seem to render these cells radioresistant and resistant to radiomimetic insults such as superoxide radicals.

It seems necessary to consider the cardinal reason for the externalization of the testis as compared with the ovary. In the latter organ, meiosis of the oogonia is completed some time after birth, and they do not persist (Prasad 1974). The remaining primary and secondary oocytes are moderately radiosensitive. Spermatogonia in the testis, however, have to reside *in situ* as long as the biological demand for sperm persists. As these cells are highly radiosensitive, they are sensitive to superoxide radicals as well. Therefore, they have to be "refrigerated" through exteriorization that persists throughout life.

This evolutionary and physiological background may explain the relatively low incidence of testicular tumors throughout the entire age range: there is a hypoxic milieu throughout. In contrast, the ovary, which is within the body, is a natural target of active oxygen molecules because of the temperature, oxygenation, and hormonal changes. The higher incidence of cancer in the ovary after menopause would naturally ensue as the anticancer mechanisms in other organ systems disintegrate. Thus, except for the postreproductive period, these organs may well be secured evolutionarily and be less likely to develop cancers.

Cell kinetics in the evolutionary hypothesis of carcinogenesis
Whether or not it involves the proto-oncogenes, carcinogenesis seems to result from the disintegration of DNA whether it lies in a single proto-oncogene or a series of them. Our studies on carcinogenesis among patients with Fanconi's anemia who have two major abnormalities, SOD deficiency (Joenje *et al.* 1979; Yoshimitsu *et al.* 1983) and easy chromosomal breakage (Ahmed and Setlow 1978), were in good agreement with the conclusion (Okuyama and Mishina 1987a) that increased superoxide and other active oxygens (Scarpa *et al.* 1984) incur chromosomal breakage which may not be promptly repaired. This is not to say that the DNA lesions are always carcinogenetic. The age spread of cancer is remarkably wide: the average age of diagnosis of leukemia was $14.8\pm$ 6.5 years of age, hepatoma development, 18.5 ± 9.3, and carcinoma, 23.9 ± 6.8. Thus, the entire series of carcinogenetic events among the Fanconi's anemia patients was stochastic, and progressed through multiple steps.

The current theory of carcinogenesis indicates that core information resides in the DNA, whether it is intrinsic or extrinsic and whether or not any further enclosure and/or rearrangement of different genes is involved (Temin 1982; Land *et al.* 1983; Klein and Klein 1985). The concept of proto-oncogenes is functional as well as material, and their basic structures seem to have been preserved during evolution (Roussel *et al.* 1979; Sheiness and Bishop 1979; Persson *et al.* 1984). A host of mechanisms must be capable of activating the dormant proto-oncogenes as well as producing novel carcinogenetic information that might result from irradiation, intrinsic superoxide toxicity, or intrinsic or extrinsic chemi-

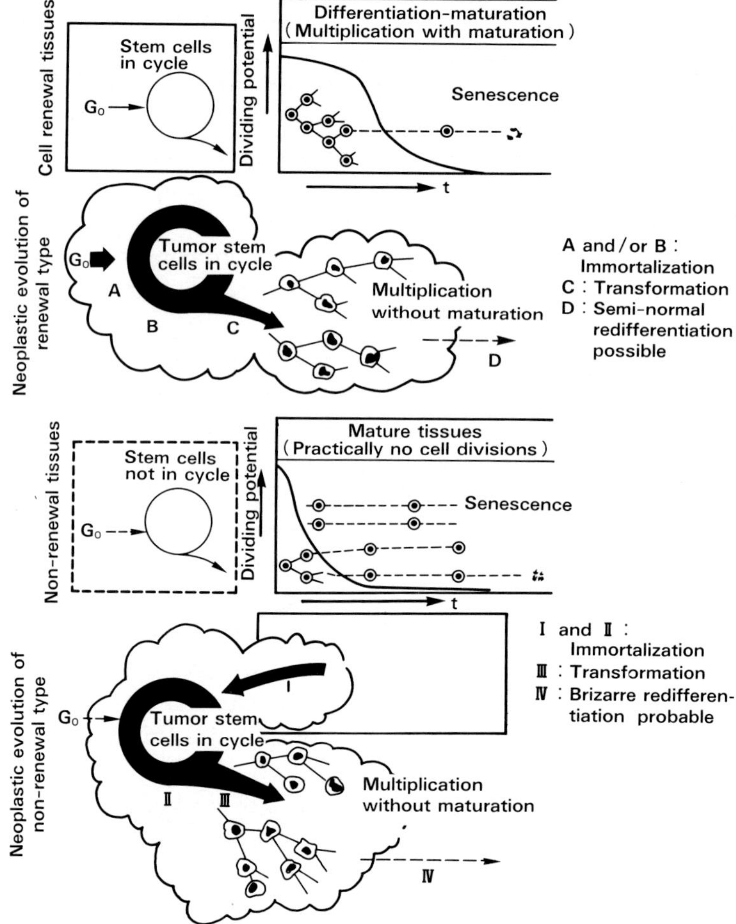

Fig. 2. Carcinogenesis in terms of cell renewal and nonrenewal types. The presence of cancer surges in the mammalian symbol organs even during postreproductiveness, especially in the prostate, seems to suggest the nonrenewal type of carcinogenesis. As the process is apparently controlled by the gene products of proto-oncogenes or new DNA carcinogenetic information, carcinogenesis per se would be dependent on the sensitivity of the receptors on the cancer candidate cells rather than the reality of renewal cell cycling.

cal insults.

As cancer cells are generated by dint of these changes in DNA, the next step in carcinogenesis may be to multiply endlessly and practice cancer manifestations such as contiguous invasion, distant metastasis, and production of cachexia through metabolic affection (cancer phanerosis). This sort of phanerosis is made possible by the production of relevant gene products. Therefore, certain DNA changes can result in the production of factors that might gear in G_0 cells to the cell cycle and/or G_1 cells to DNA synthesis, and result in eventual immortalization and transformation. The experimental carcinogenesis induced in the atrophic prostate by Fingerhut and Veenema (1977) seems to be one such example. If there were such an analogy in human carcinogenesis, most of the postreproductive cancers of the mammalian symbol organs would likely fall into this category (Fig. 2). Obviously, most carcinogenesis must involve active cell cycling in the systems of cell renewal, whether rapid or slow (Cairns 1975; Buick and Pollak 1984). Nonetheless, the results from the present cancer epidemiology indicate the need for reconcilation with the reversion type of carcinogenesis as well. Should such a mechanism bear any evolutionary significance, it would be that of mitigating against excessive survival after reproductiveness (Hirayama 1986). Nature may not be happy with the species' costs of prolonged survival. Thus, human cancer epidemiology can be regarded as having a multitude of evolutionary implications.

Chapter 3

Fanconi's Anemia as an Evolutionary Experiment on Carcinogenesis

> *As the fossils are to the earth's history, so are the genes to the evolutionary history of life.*
> ——*H. Kihara (1893-1976)*, Genetics

Malignancies appear particularly prone to develop in two major disease groups, one in which repair of DNA damage is impaired (xeroderma pigmentosum, Fanconi's anemia, and Bloom's syndrome) and the other in which immunologic competency is drastically compromised (Schwartz 1986). Fanconi's anemia is of special interest in terms of the carcinogenetic mechanisms involved, because the syndrome is characterized by two major molecular defects: a reduction in cellular superoxide dismutase (SOD) activity (Yoshimitsu *et al.* 1984; Scarpa *et al.* 1985) and defective repair of DNA damage (Ahmed and Setlow 1978). In the general population, childhood malignancies are characterized by the predominance of nonepithelial tumors like leukemias and tumors of the brain, kidney, and bone, whereas adult tumors are 90% epithelial, a phenomenon that has been called nonepithelial-epithelial tumor shift (Okuyama and Mishina 1986b). In contrast, chromosomal abnormalities like trisomy 21 that are firmly established by the time of birth facilitate the emergence of leukemias (Rosner and Lee 1972).

When immunological incompetence is involved, the resulting tumors are mainly leukemias and lymphomas (Kersey *et al.* 1974). Bloom's syndrome is intriguing because nonepithelial tumors predominate during early life but are replaced by cancers in adulthood (German *et al.* 1977). In Fanconi's anemia, however, cases of cancer are also reported, in spite of the chromosomal breakage (Dosik *et al.* 1970; Reed *et al.* 1983). Thus, more extensive epidemiological studies and comparison with other evolutionary carcinogenetic experiments are needed to obtain further insights. The results reported here suggest that the evolution sometimes betrays itself by abandoning the archaic anticancer defense lines that circumvent superoxide toxicity, repair damaged DNA, and provide immune surveillance, strategies which have been of distinct evolutionary significance.

Evolutionary categorization of organ systems   Epidemiological studies on cancer that are based on an evolutionary concept have often been more elucidating than conventional presentations (Okuyama and Mishina 1986b). In the evolutionary model, the human organ systems are categorized into epithelial, nonepithelial, and gonadal (evolutionarily secured). The nonepithelial group contains the hematopoietic system, bone, kidney, brain, and other connective tissues while the epithelial group includes the gastrointestinal system, hepatobiliary system, respiratory organs, and thyroid, and the breast, uterus, and prostate, which are the mammalian symbol organs.

Collection of cancer cases   A review of the literature from 1952 to 1987 revealed 85 cases of Fanconi's anemia accompanied by neoplasms. These were classified in accordance with their tumor categorization: leukemias, lymphomas, brain, kidney, and bone tumors (nonepithelial), and cancers (epithelial). The control data were based on males from Miyagi Prefecture, Japan, and covered the five-year period from 1973 through 1977, as reported in a WHO publication (Waterhous *et al.* 1982).

Analysis of cases   The 85 above-mentioned cases of Fanconi's anemia accompanied by neoplastic development were analyzed and found to be 45% nonepithelial and 55% epithelial (Table 1). Among the non-epithelial tumors, 43% were leukemic and 1% brain tumors. The average age at which the leukemias developed was 14.8 ± 6.5 years (40); for those with epithelial tumors, it was 18.5 ± 9.3 (30) for hepatomas and 23.9 ± 6.8 (15) for squamous cell carcinomas (Fig. 1). In most cases, development of hepatomas was related to prolonged administration of oxymetholone for the treatment of pancytopenia, especially anemia.

FANCONI'S ANEMIA

Table 1. Nature's evolutionary experiments on carcinogenesis

	Impaired DNA repair (28B.y.)	Decreased Cu, Zn–SOD (420M.y.)	Immunodeficiencies			Cancer incidence				
			T-cell (500M.y.)	B-cell (350M.y.)	L.N. (150M.y.)	Total	Nonepithelial			Epithelial
							Leuk.	Lymph.	BKB	
Males (0–14 y.o.)						0.008	46	3	24	13%
(Miyagi (15–24)	—	—	—	—	—	0.010	24	15	16	39%
Prefecture) (25–34)						0.024	10	5	9	62%
(35–79)						0.046	2	2	3	88%
Down's syndrome	Trisomy 21	(−)	(−)	(−)	(−)	3.7%	100%	—	—	—
Fanconi's anemia	(+)	(+)	(NK cell?)	(IgA?)	(−)	10+	43	—	1	55%
Xeroderma pigmentosum	(+)	(−)	(−)	(−)	(−)	44	—	—	—	‡ (Skin)
Bloom's syndrome	Chromosomal instability	(−)	(+)	(−)	(−)	18.3	46 (Early)	15	8	31% (Late)
Congenital X-linked (Bruton)	X-linked	—	(−)	(+)	(−)	0.7	83	17%	—	—
Severe combined immuno-deficiency	X-linked	—	(+)	(+)	(−)	2	33	67%	—	—
Common variable immuno-deficiency	—	—	(±)	(+)	(−)	8	10	56	4	29%
Wiskott-Aldrich syndrome	X-linked	—	(+)	(−)	(−)	12	13	79	8%	—
Ataxia telangiectasia	—	—	(+)	(+)	(−)	10+	21	62	10	11%
IgM deficiency	—	—	(−)	(+)	(−)		—	83	17%	—
IgA deficiency	—	—	(−)	(+)	(+)		—	15	16	69%
Duncan's syndrome	X-linked	—	(+)	(+)	(+)		—	‡	—	—
Acquired immunodeficiency syndrome (AIDS)	—	—	(+)	(−)	(+)	Ca.15%	8	58	25	8%

B.y., billion years; M.y., million years; L.N., lymph node; Leuk., leukemias; Lymph., lymphomas; BKB, brain, kidney, and bone; y.o., years old

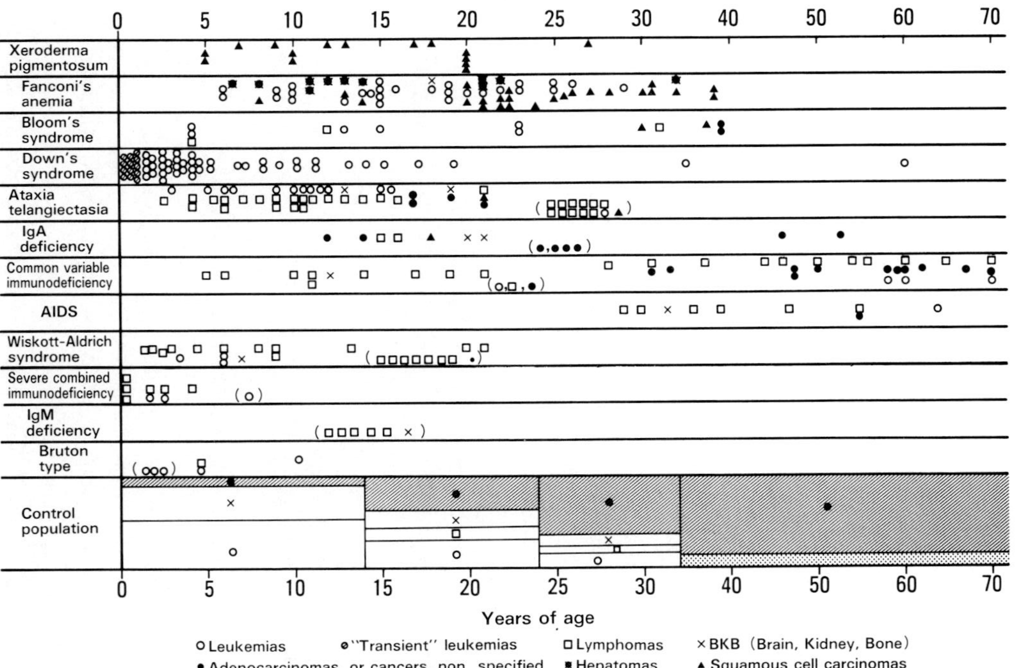

Fig. 1. Age distribution of neoplasms: An evolutionary experiment on carcinogenesis. The age distribution of Fanconi's anemia was studied and compared with other cancer-prone diseases and the control male population of Miyagi Prefecture, Japan. Different cancer-prone diseases have different patterns of neoplastic age distribution. There is a definite nonepithelial-epithelial tumor shift in the control population. The same phenomenon applies to Fanconi's anemia if we take into consideration the fact that hepatomas develop as a result of the prolonged administration of oxymetholone, iatrogenically, in an accelerated way. Chromosomal injuries to the proto-oncogenes or those creating novel "oncogenes" from chromosomal breakage would lead to leukemias and cancers, presumably in accordance with their number and/or combination: fewer for leukemias and more for cancers (Nowell 1976; Watson *et al.* 1987).

Evolutionary developments and experimentation   Cancer is a disease syndrome that results from the untoward expression of proto-oncogenes or the derangement and subsequent expression of any *de novo* abnormality (Cronkite 1974; Klein and Klein 1984). The capacity for excision repair of DNA damage developed as early as 2.8 billion years ago (Kondo 1978). The major defense mechanism, Cu,ZnSOD, is thought to have been acquired 420 million years ago (Asada 1976). T-cell evolution has been dated back 500 million years, while the emergence of B-cells and the constitution of lymph nodes occurred as late as 350 and 150 million years ago, respectively (Good *et al.* 1965). These biological acquisitions must have paralleled closely the physicochemical alterations on the earth: notably, the reduction of intensity of the ultraviolet rays reaching the earth as the atmospheric oxygen concentrations started rising (excision repair); maximal accumulation of the atmospheric oxygen concentration in the vicinity of the Carboniferous Period (Cu, ZnSOD) (Berkner and Marshall 1965; Asada 1976); the explosive increase in marine animal species with the acquisition of efficient photosynthesis of carbohydrates and resultant surplus nourishment (Nakamura 1983), demanding subtle species discrimination as well as self-nonself discrimination (T-cell evolution as the pisces propagated) (Good 1971); and further microbial and chemical contamination of the sea, necessitating humoral barriers surrounding the gastrointestinal tract by dint of B-cells and plasma cells (higher pisces) (Good *et al.* 1965; Nakamura 1983).

The evolution of the immunoglobulins seems to have taken place in the order IgM, IgG, IgA (Bellanti 1971). The evolution of the lymph nodes may have biological implications other than probable functional efficiency, as the event took place in the mammalians (Good *et al.* 1965). Any defects in these defense lines, should they happen to lead to carcinogenesis, can be regarded as evolutionary experiments on the merits of such selective and discrete functional aberrations.

Evolutionary carcinogenetic experiments in chromosomal breakage syndrome   As seen in Table 1, Down's syndrome is characterized by the development of acute leukemias in childhood (Rosner and Lee 1972) as well as the chromosomal abnormality trisomy 21. It is noteworthy that 21% of the cases of Rosner and Lee and 17% of the 276 cases in their review were diagnosed as having leukemia early in their infancy. Thus, the leukemia can be called "constitutional." Chromosome 21 seems to be closely related to hemoblastic proliferation (Mitelman 1985). According to the report, there were 11 cases of "constitutional" leukemias and two of leukemoid reactions, or "transient leukemias." Their chromosomal analysis revealed a variety of changes. Trisomy 21 by itself may not always be potent enough to maintain leukemic carcinogenesis, and either an intensification of the information on chromosome 21 or cooperation with chromosome 8 seems mandatory in most cases. The latter chromosome contains the c-*myc* proto-oncogene which might be responsible for the immortalization of target cells. The proto-oncogene(s) contained in chromosome 21 could be transforming rather than immortalizing and would therefore necessitate intensification through overdosing (double trisomy 21 or ring formation) or cooperation with the c-*myc* proto-oncogene on chromosome 8 or the *erb B* and/or *mos* proto-oncogenes on chromosome 7 through ring formation (Benedict *et al*. 1979; Testa *et al*. 1979; Hagemeijer *et al*. 1981; Heaton *et al*. 1981; Tricot *et al*. 1981; Debiec-Rychter *et al*. 1982; Kaneko *et al*. 1982; Alimena *et al*. 1985; Mitelman 1985). In Down's syndrome, evolution thus seems to have conducted a carcinogenetic experiment on chromosomal "disintegration" without any superimposing definite viral infections.

In xeroderma pigmentosum (XP) and Bloom's syndrome (BS), the chromosomal aberrations are not yet established at the time of birth; rather, they arise and accumulate with time. The DNA damage to be incurred may not be specifically targeted, and therefore the probability of hitting the necessary proto-oncogenes may not be sufficiently high. By 25 years of age, the DNA breakage in BS can induce leukemias, and after that, carcinomas (German *et al*. 1977). It is of special interest that these cancers were of gastrointestinal origin and that IgA deficiency is probable in BS (Pathak and Epstein 1971). In XP, however, skin cancers tend to emerge in young adults, while leukemias are not seen (Robbins *et al*. 1974; Takebe *et al*. 1977).

Evolutionary carcinogenetic experiments in the immune defective syndromes   In immunodeficiency syndromes as well, cancer incidence rates are increased (Table 1). However, the contribution of these syndromes to carcinogenesis appears to be indirect. Patients with Nezelof and DiGeorge syndromes ——purely isolated T-cell deficits——are likely to succumb to bacterial and viral infections before they develop malignancies. Further, they do not have "constitutional" or childhood tumors.

As shown in Fig. 1, carcinomas are confined to the older age categories; the nonepithelial tumors, to the younger generations. Secondly, there are no cases of leukemia in these categories excepting AT, one of the chromosomal breakage syndromes, and therefore, there are lymphomatous tumors only. Thirdly, the carcinomas are principally of the gastrointestinal tract. Lastly, what is common to these immunodeficiencies is the eventual IgA deficiency.

Can it simply be supposed that defective antiviral defense lines along the respiratory and gastrointestinal tracts in these patients brought about oncogenetic sequelae and that T-cells failed to reject newly arising tumor cells (Möller and Möller 1978)? As previously believed, lymphomatous oncogenesis could be related to the greater probability of infections and the resultant overwhelming antigenic insults (Kersey *et al.* 1973; Kaplan *et al.* 1987). In Wiskott-Aldrich syndrome, a severe combined immunodeficiency disease, IgM deficiency and Bruton type agammaglobulinemia, the tumors fall entirely within the nonepithelial categories occurring during the earliest periods of life. Thus, IgA deficiency in Bruton-type agammaglobulinemia may not be able to sustain these patients long enough for gastrointestinal carcinogenesis to develop. T-cell deficits are not necessarily directly carcinogenetic but may indirectly facilitate disease processes in such a way that the disease progresses along the evolutionary ladder of immunodeficiency. In other words, the secretory IgA barrier may be an anticarcinogenetic mechanism with evolutionary implications.

Humoral immunity is essential for defense against infections caused by leukemogenic viruses (Weiser *et al.* 1969) and probably for surveillance against cancer as well. Phylogenetically, IgM appeared with the advent of the cyclostomes, and IgA, with mammalian evolution (Bellanti 1971). The ontogeny of human IgM takes place during fetal life, and that of IgA, after birth (Bellanti 1971). IgM is confined to the circulating blood because of the size of its pentamer molecules. As the first antibody produced in response to an immunogen, its primary function is to fight against invading microorganisms. It does so even at low doses of the immunogen, in marked contrast to the IgG response (Hood *et al.* 1978; Weissman *et al.* 1978). IgA is a secretory antibody preferentially located in the gastrointestinal and respiratory tracts and the breast (Hood *et al.* 1978). It is interesting that in IgA deficiency the majority of carcinomas are limited to sites where IgA would be expected to be located: esophagus, stomach, colon, lung, and breast (Kersey *et al.* 1973). Discrete defects of single B-cell subpopulations, as in the case of IgA deficiency, would not necessarily be fatal to patients (Gatti and Good 1971), but would enable them to live longer while rendering them vulnerable to oncogenic viruses. IgA deficiency could be secondary to T-cell loss, as in the case of AT. Immunodeficiency would then develop later in life in those patients with the common variable immunodeficiency (Alexander and Good 1977). This scenario would explain the absence of leukemias during childhood and the staggered incidence of lymphomas and cancers over the entire range of adulthood.

Fanconi's anemia as an evolutionary carcinogenetic experiment
We initially expected FA to provide a re-creation of the non-epithelial-epithelial tumor shift observed in normal populations (Okuyama and Mishina 1986b). It is detectable in Fig. 1 if one eliminates incidence of hepatomas, which can largely be made iatrogenic with the therapeutic use of oxymetholone. The increased susceptibility of FA cells to carcinogenetic insults is well known (Todaro *et al.* 1966; Sasaki and Tonomura 1973), although it is not known whether the changes cause immortalization or transformation, or both. The third peculiarity of FA is the total absence of lymphomas. Fourth, epithelial tumors other than hepatomas were exclusively squamous cell carcinomas of the tongue, esophagus, or female external genitalia. Three papers have discussed the immunological status of FA patients, noting defects in cel-

lular immunity (Pedersen *et al.* 1977; Hersey *et al.* 1982) and the absence of IgA (Abels and Reed 1973). Thus, the premature surge in epithelial tumors in FA may be related to reduced immune surveillance by NK cells against emerging cancer cells or by IgA against viral invasions through the gastrointestinal and female genital tracts, because NK cells are greatly and rather selectively sensitive to radiation and therefore to superoxide radicals, and are thought to have evolved prior to T- and B-cells (Kumagai 1985). Thus, FA may embrace the most archaic carcinogenetic defects: (1) reduced Cu, ZnSOD, which would lead to increased DNA damage, (2) defective DNA repair, and, possibly, (3) defective NK cell immune surveillance or (4) IgA deficiency.

Implications of evolutionary carcinogenetic experiments
Carcinogenesis may be a complicated process involving genetic material and cellular proliferation on the one hand and

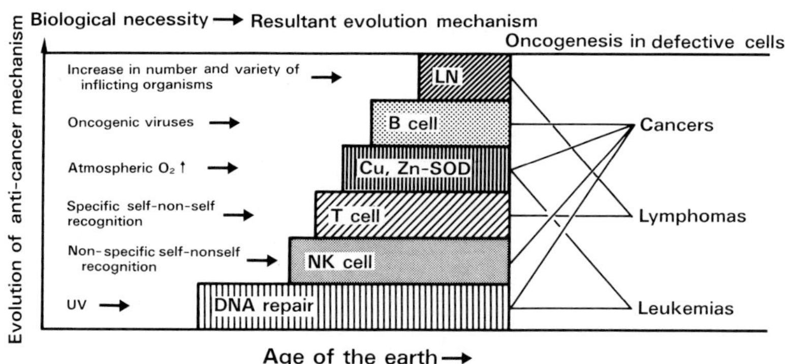

Fig. 2. Evolutionary stratification of anticancer mechanisms. As evolution progressed, a number of biological necessities could have led eventually to the acquisition of a host of defense mechanisms which were, however, not necessarily intended primarily to defend against carcinogenesis. Nonetheless, the resultant effects included those mitigating against cancer. The most primitive neoplasms could have been DNA disintegrative leukemias with multiple disintegrations. Lymphomas could be younger, resulting from continued, potent antigenic stimulation and reactive lymphoproliferation. The most recent neoplasms may be the lymphomas, the result of retroviral infections. They are recent in the sense that the oncogenic information is derived from humans or primates, animals high on the evolutionary ladder (Okuyama and Mishina 1988a).

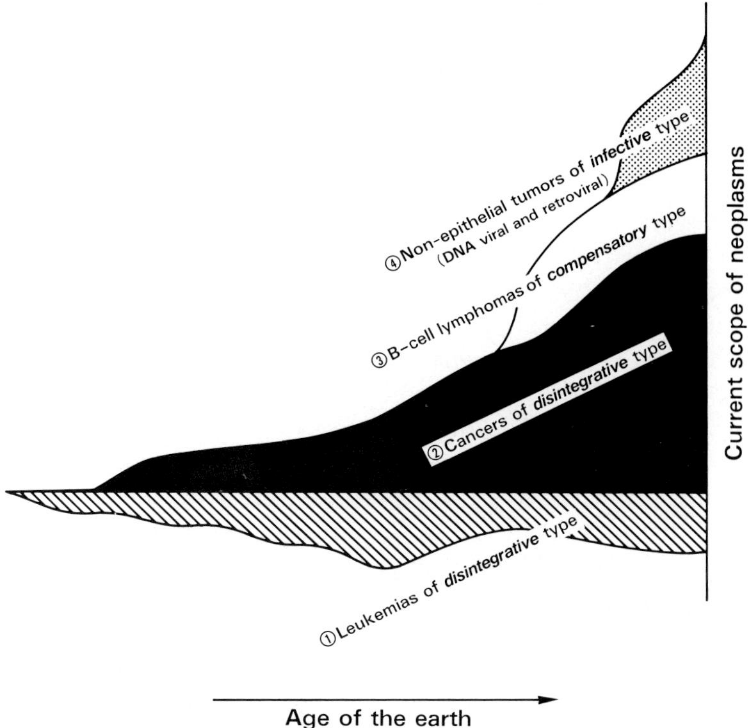

Fig. 3. Neoplastic evolution: a hypothesis based on the history of DNA damage and its repair (Ahmed and Setlow 1978; Asada 1976), evolution of the immune systems (Kumagai 1985), epidemiology of lymphomas (Schwartz 1986), neoplastic evolution in AIDS (Kaplan *et al.* 1987), and the evolutionary significance of Fanconi's anemia (discussed above). Leukemias resulting from unrepaired DNA damage, or the disintegrative type of tumor development, could have been the most archaic. Single immortalization frequently seems insufficient to induce leukemias, necessitating additional transformational events in solid tumors (Hanafusa *et al.* 1977). The retroviral infection-neoplastic conversion may be the newest, for the evolution of the retroviruses is the most recent (Okuyama and Mishina 1988a).

physical and biological intrusion on the other. In addition, aging is probably important. Chromosomal breakage syndromes and immunodeficiencies have proved helpful in clarifying human carcinogenesis, especially in trying to undo the conglomerates. The evolutionary anticancer strategy suggested in the present study involves (1) excision repair of damaged DNA, (2) efficient detoxification of superoxide dismutase (Cu, ZnSOD), and (3) IgA blocking of intruding viruses that may lead to DNA damage following invasion of respiratory and gastrointestinal barriers. All of these elements in the strategy have definite evolutionary dating of their own, as described above. Finally, (4) the lymphomatous transformation per se can be due to compensatory proliferation and subsequent malignant transformation in any of the clones of the remaining T- or B-cell lines (Kersey *et al.* 1974). However, viral transformation is also probable, in view of the scope of the oncogenous viruses and the definite antiviral repertoire of the immunoglobulins: IgM against viruses circulating in the peripheral blood, IgG against viral particles swarming in the interstitial space as well as in the blood, and IgA against viruses crossing the mucous membranes (Alexander and Good 1977). Viral oncogenesis may have triple evolutionary significance: (1) evolutionary preservation of the proto-oncogenes; (2) probable "recent" evolution of the viruses affecting human beings (Matthews 1983); and (3) retroviral infectivity across the species barrier (Gallo *et al.* 1977). The probable evolution of anticancer mechanisms thus seems clearer (Figs. 2 and 3).

Statistical studies cannot avoid being circumstantial. However, it is sincerely hoped that the present investigation will provide suggestions for many areas of cancer research. Further studies are obviously needed.

Chapter 4

Cancer Incidence in the Population of Nagasaki 30 Years after the Atomic Bombing

The incidence of radiation-induced cancer among atomic bomb survivors continues to be high 40 years after exposure, and much remains unknown about radiation carcinogenesis.
——I. Shigematsu and A. Kagan, Radiation Biology (*1986*)

Our study of the epidemiological aspects of cancer based on WHO data (Waterhous *et al.* 1982) showed a predominance of nonepithelial tumors in infancy and adolescence, and a predominance of epithelial tumors thereafter (nonepithelial-epithelial tumor shift) (Okuyama and Mishina 1986b). In hope of obtaining insight into the underlying evolutionary mechanisms, epidemiological studies were expanded to include the population of Nagasaki 30 years after the atomic bombing. In spite of probable dilution of the fraction of atomic bomb survivors, the investigation was considered valid because such radiation is penetrating and because its carcinogenetic manifestations would require a long time. The results indicated that the atomic bombing still influences that victim population.

Cancer incidence data for the five years from 1973 through 1977 published by WHO (Waterhous *et al.* 1982) were used throughout. Four Japanese populations were cited in the publication: the cities of Fukuoka and Nagasaki and the prefectures of Miyagi and Osaka. The population of each was as follows: Fukuoka, 2,056,064 males and 2,210,330 females; Miyagi, 960,245 males and 995,022 females; Nagasaki, 214,005 males and 236,189 females; and Osaka, 4,132,495 males and 4,146,430 females. A separate report put the number of atomic bomb survivors in the population of Nagasaki at 37.8%, 33,037 (33.4%) males and 48,964 (41.6%) females, all aged 25 years or above (Ikeda *et al.* 1986). No comparable data were available for Hiroshima.

Epidemiological studies of cancer based on an evolutionary concept may be more elucidating than those of the conventional presentations (Segi *et al.* 1981; Okuyama and Mishina 1985d; h; 1986b; 1987a). The evolutionary concept categorizes human organ systems into epithelial, nonepithelial, and gonadal (evolutionarily secured). The nonepithelial group comprises the hematopoietic system, brain, kidney, bone, and other connective tissues, while the epithelial group includes the gastrointestinal system and hepatobiliary systems, respiratory organs and thyroid, and the breast, uterus, and prostate, which are the mammalian symbol organs. The gonads are designated "evolutionarily secured," because gonadal cells require protection or ease of elimination when damaged in order to conserve the species. In principle, DNA repair that is prone to error is not permitted. Classification of mammalian vs pre-mammalian was also employed. The latter was again divided into the homeothermic and poiklothermic (Okuyama and Mishina 1985h). The homeothermic organs are those that could have fully evolved in order to take advantage of the increased atmospheric oxygen concentrations during the Carboniferous Period and therefore are related to energy expenditure. The respiratory system and thyroid gland (Kobayashi 1975) may be included here. Statistic analysis was carried out according to the method described elsewhere (Ipsen and Feigl 1970).

Cancer incidence in Japan 30 years after the atomic bombing
Cancer incidence rates which had already been corrected for standardized populations and annually averaged (ASR) were used, in addition to crude average annual incidence (Table 1). Although crude incidence varied widely among populations, ASR world for the control populations of Fukuoka, Miyagi, and Osaka appeared consistent, ranging from 202 to 209 in males, while that for Nagasaki was as high as 309. In females, the values were much lower, but the trends were identical.

Changes in age-standardized cancer incidence 30 years after the atomic bombing   Table 2 shows significantly higher cancer incidence rates for Nagasaki 30 years after the atomic bombing compared with the control populations. The difference

Table 1. Crude average annual cancer incidence in Japan (1973–1977) and ASR world (age-standardized rates)

		Nagasaki	Fukuoka	Miyagi	Osaka
Males	Average	0.28%	0.08%	0.206%	0.16%
	ASR*	301.9	201.9	208.9	204.9
Females	Average	0.24%	0.07%	0.154%	0.138%
	ASR*	216.1	143.9	139.0	137.9

* ASR per 100,000 population.

Table 2. Age distribution of the age-standardized cancer incidence 30 years after atomic bombing (1973–1977)

	Males		Females	
Age group	Nagasaki	Miyagi	Nagasaki	Miyagi
0——14	79.0	20.8	49.3	23.9
15——24	42.4	21.9	35.7	24.3
25——34	86.1	50.0	142.1*	79.5
35——79	9791.3	6967.2	7460.7**	4045.9

* Includes *in situ* cancer of the cervix uteri (Total uterine cancer ASR were 14.6 for Nagasaki and 5.6 for Miyagi.)

** The respective values were 704.8 for Nagasaki and 333.7 for Miyagi.

was apparent at all age levels in both sexes. There was no discrimination between nonepithelial and epithelial tumors in terms of the higher cancer incidence in the Nagasaki population. However, when the relative incidence was calculated and compared, the incidence of nonepithelial tumors was higher in Nagasaki than Miyagi. The nonepithelial-epthelial tumor shift took place in Nagasaki, as it did in the control populations. In females, the shift took place 10 years earlier in Nagasaki than in Miyagi Prefecture. The incidence of leukemia was much higher in all age groups, regardless of sex. The incidence appeared greater with advancing age in males who had passed middle age, whereas they were parallel in females. Lymphosarcomas and multiple myelomas seemed to be responsible for the higher incidence in males.

Relative cancer incidence according to evolutionary status

In spite of the merits of ASR in elucidating the influence of culture (Okuyama and Mishina 1988b), when cancer incidences in terms of ASR Japan were compared between organ groups with different evolutionary implications—that is, the mammalian symbol organs and the homeothermic and poikilothermic organs—the cancer distribution was identical in Nagasaki and other control populations, although the ASR values were significantly greater in Nagasaki. When the rates for the individual female mammalian symbol organs were compared, noteworthy distinctions appeared. There were significant increases in uterine cervical cancers and choriocarcinomas, although definite conclusions cannot be found for cervical cancers because of the inclusion of carcinomas *in situ* (Table 3). Higher incidences for cervical cancers were observed in both the reproductive and postmenopausal periods, not unlike the control populations. With choriocarcinomas, however, the data for Nagasaki revealed two peaks that were higher and appeared earlier than those of the control populations (Fig. 1).

Discussion   This was not a direct survey of atomic bomb survivors. The residual radiation morbidity of the original victim population of Nagasaki has been diluted by the influx and outflow of people during the past 30 years as well as by deaths of the survivors from other etiologies. It should also be noted that persistent, low-dose radiation could have been possible from the contaminated air, water, and soil even among those who were not in the city at the time of the bombing. Nonetheless, we thought a survey such as this was indispensable to determine how whole-body exposure to atomic bomb radiation, fallout, or activation radiation would affect

Table 3. Cancer incidence in the population of Nagasaki 30 years after the atomic bombing (1973–1977) compared with control populations: Statistical analysis of individual mammalian symbol organs

| High incidence of | Significance of Nagasaki data vis-à-vis | | | |
| | Miyagi | | Osaka | |
	Male	Female	Male	Female
Non-epithelial	Yes*	Yes*	Yes*	Yes*
Breast cancer		No		No
Cervical cancer		Yes*,**		No
Ovarian cancer		No		No
Choriocarcinoma		No		Yes*

  * Statistically significant at p < 0.01.

** Nagasaki data includes carcinoma *in situ*.

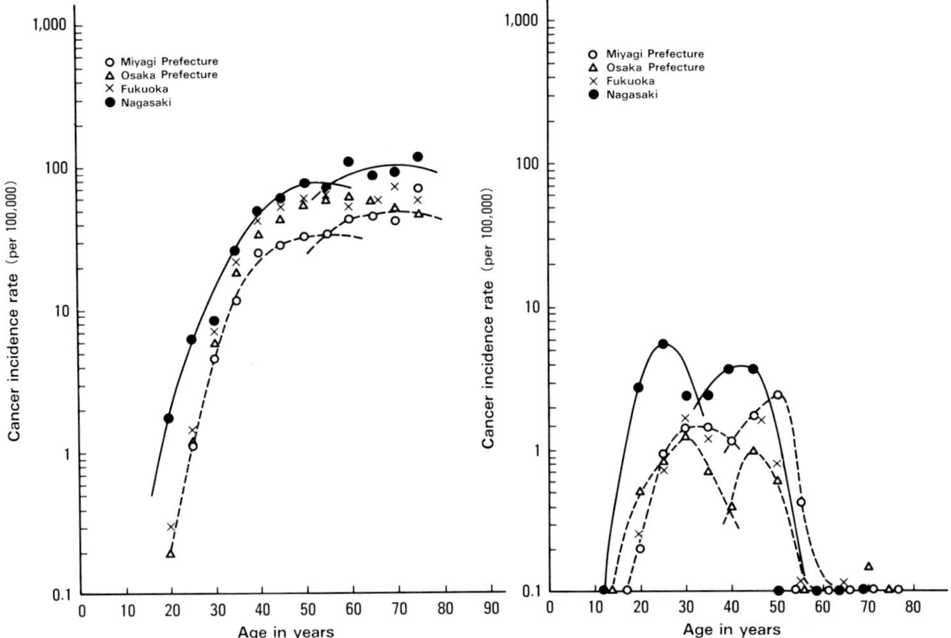

Fig. 1. Age spread of cancer incidence of the mammalian symbol organs.

A. Uterine cervical cancer. As was the case with the controls, there were 2 peaks of higher incidence in Nagasaki, one during the period of active reproductiveness, and the other during postre-productiveness. The incidence in Nagasaki was significantly higher than in Miyagi controls (p<0.01). Undisputable contribution to the heights from inclusion of *in situ* cancers seemed probable. The transitional values from other controls may be suggestive of contribution of other factors such as viral etiologies, too. Thus, the radiation did not appear to affect the incidence pattern of cervical cancer.

B. Uterine choriocarcinoma. The incidence curves were bi-peaked as in the controls. The peaks were definitely higher than any of them (p<0.01). However, they apparently shifted leftward, suggesting possible accumulation of DNA damage in that population.

the cancer incidence in terms of the evolutionary concept of cancer. Topical irradiation did not appear sufficient in this regard. Unfortunately, we were unable to locate integrated statistics of the cancer incidence of Nagasaki and Hiroshima (Shigematsu and Kagan 1986).

In spite of the possible limitations of epidemiological surveys (Travis 1975), the present analysis of cancer morbidity data for Nagasaki even 30 years after the bombing yielded the following results: (1) the age evolution of neoplasms was significantly higher than in the controls; (2) the higher incidence of nonepithelial tumors was due to the increased incidence of lymphosarcomas and multiple myelomas; (3) among the mammalian symbol organs, the incidence of uterine cervical cancers was higher; (4) among the evolutionarily secured organs, there was a higher incidence of choriocarcinomas, although the epidemiological significance of this is unclear (Bracken *et al.* 1984); (5) in females, the nonepithelial-epithelial tumor shift took place 10 years earlier in the population of Nagasaki than in that of Miyagi Prefecture. Whether these findings are directly related to the atomic bombing and what their implications are for the evolutionary concept of cancer will require further investigation.

The incidence of human cancer, as described elsewhere (Okuyama and Mishina 1988b), shows the following dynamic and evolutionary characteristics. (1) A phenomenon of nonepithelial-epithelial tumor shift takes place with advancing age. (2) Cancers of the mammalian symbol organs and those of homeothermic evolution are more prevalent in the United States than in Japan, while the reverse is true for cancers of poikilothermic evolution. (3) Cancers of the breast and uterus, the female mammalian symbol organs, are prevalent in two distinct age groups, active reproductive and postreproductive, while prostatic cancers are prevalent only in the period of postreproductiveness. (4) Cancers of the premammalian organs show incidence curves characterized by exponential growth beyond the age of 30 years.

The present investigation was primarily intended to clarify if and how radiation per se affects the processes of carcinogenesis. The atomic bombing of Hirohsima and Nagasaki could have served that purpose if adequate statistics had been available. According to available descriptions, the incidence of cancer is definitely higher in the population of Nagasaki than in three control Japanese populations. While increases in cancer were roughly dose-dependent, it is noteworthy that both the relative and absolute risks of oncogenesis among the survivors were "paradoxically" greater in the 0-9—rad group than the 100+rad group. Taking into account the fact that at the time of the bombing there were no definite curative regimens for most epithelial cancers, the time of death could be translated into the approximate time of diagnosis. In this way, data on comparison of age at death could be understood to mean that the shortest latency for the clinical emergence of neoplasms was determined by the age of the survivors at the time of exposure rather than the radiation dosage; that is, the older the age at exposure, the shorter the latency (Kato 1986). Taking into account the data of excess incidence/10^6 PYR for selected neoplasms (Kato 1986; Monzen and Wakabayashi 1986) and data on the incidence of leukemia among survivors (Ichimaru *et al.* 1986), a hypothetical incidence function schema can be constructed (Fig. 2). The above-mentioned paradoxical dose response could probably be resolved by taking the time factor into account. Critical data for the first

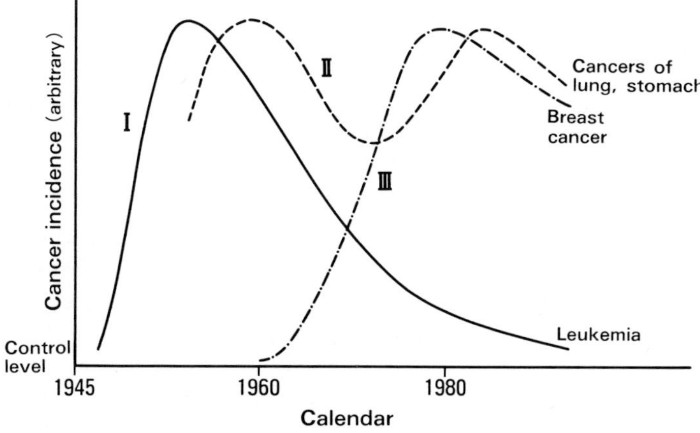

Fig. 2. Neoplastic development in the population of Nagasaki City following the atomic bombing. The curves are based on the data of Ichimaru et al. for leukemia (1986) and Kato (1986) and Monzen and Wakabayashi (1986) for epithelial tumors. The non-epithelial-epithelial tumor shift seems to have taken place in the case of chronological evolution of radiation carcinogenesis. Cancers of the mammalian symbol organs looked as if they had represented a cohort migration of the reproductive people until they submerged into those of the postreproductivephase.

surges in the incidence of cancer are permanently lost, presumably because of the difficulty of collecting data under the
circumstances. The data of our analysis may, therefore, represent the latter parts of the function curves.

Leukemia rates among nonexposed Nagasaki residents are
reported to have risen after 1958, while those of survivors
exposed in the vicinity of the hypocenter peaked between
1950 and 1951, according to a survey covering 1945-1965
(Itoga 1965). This finding may be consistent with the present
population-based data 30 years later. The problem of how the
carcinogenetic effects of atomic radiation could have spread
throughout the population will be discussed below.

DNA damage, whether as the result of the potency of oncogene products (immortalizing factors (i) (Hanafusa *et al.*
1977)) and/or sensitivity of rapidly renewing systems, would
certainly lead to oncogenesis among the nonepithelial organs.
For example, the single activation of c-*myc* is probable in leukemias and neuroblastomas. This seems to be the case with
the leukemias of Fanconi's anemia, in which both Cu,
ZnSOD deficiency (Yoshimitsu *et al.* 1984) and defective
DNA repair (Ahmed and Setlow 1978) cooperate to increase
the probability of oncogenic activation and/or formation of
new oncogenic DNA changes (leukemias of the disintegrative
type) (Fig. 3 in Chapter 3). For oncogenesis of the epithelial
systems, transforming factors (t) have to be generated along
with immortalization (Hanafusa *et al.* 1977; Land *et al.* 1983;
Ruley 1983), and there can be other barriers to the eventual
clinical emergence (cancer phanerosis) of such "cancer babies."

To return to the atomic radiation oncogenesis scheme,
curves I and II in Fig. 2 could have resulted as i or $i+t$ took
place in the high exposure groups. The first peaks of group
II must have receded by 1959 for the above-mentioned para-
dox to be explained. The second peaks would result from $i+t$
and aging. The curve for breast cancer (III) did not show the
first peak, presumably because of the breast's lack of sensitivity to carcinogenetic stimuli prior to puberty and after menopause. As soon as the candidate fraction of the population
arrived at puberty and reproductiveness, the curve started
rising. This trend may resemble a cohort labeling of erythrocytes with radioiron in which labeled cells emerge from

the bone marrow, circulate in the peripheral blood, and eventually disappear with senescence. By the same token, it could be predicted that prostatic cancer would also present a cohort of increased incidence. The data for ovarian tumors revealed a type-III curve (Tokuoka 1986), although no data were available for testicular tumors. A higher incidence in cases of chronic lymphocytic leukemia, chronic myeloid leukemia, lymphosarcoma, and multiple myeloma is known to occur toward the end of curve I. This has to be the case with those people exposed to lower doses of radiation, and synergism with aging cannot be excluded. We suspect that these curves possess some evolutionary significance, as will be discussed soon.

We have already presented the idea of classifying the organ systems into categories that reflect evolutionary change (Okuyama and Mishina 1984a; 1985h). Table 4 shows how well the curves fit the evolutionary categorization of organ systems. Radiation carcinogenesis following the atomic bombing thus seems to reiterate the phylogenetic sequence of different organ systems.

Choriocarcinoma may constitute a distinct neoplastic category because it is a graft-versus-host reaction of fetal cells (usually male) against those of the mother. Radiation damage to DNA is generally repairable. In the testis, however, damaged cells may not always be repaired and need to be eliminated by the special process of apoptosis (Harrison 1975). DNA lesions produced in the spermatids may not be repaired.

Table 4. Evolutionary fitting of atomic bomb radiation carcinogenesis: A hypothetical model

Evolutionary age			Symbol organs	Fitting curves
Evolutionarily secured			Testis and ovary	III (Ovary)
Verte- bral	Mammalian symbols		Prostate, breast, and uterus	III
	Premam- malian	Homeothermic	Thyroid and respiratory system	II
		Poikilothermic	Digestive tract	II
			Brain, kidney, and bone	(I)
Prevertebral			Hematopoietic	I

However, abrogation of such lesions, if fertilization takes place, can be obtained either through repair by enzymes of the ovum or through abortion by the time of implantation (Prasad 1974). Because choriocarcinoma is essentially a disease resulting from oncogenic gene expression (Sarkar *et al.* 1986) on the part of the fetus, an analysis of its incidence could have offered a sensitive indicator of the radiation effects of the atomic bombing. Because both c-*myc* and c-*ras* are activated and expressed, two-step carcinogenesis involving $i+t$ is probable. As reported earlier (Ujeno 1985), choriocarinoma may occur even with very low levels of radiation, and its oncogenesis is one of the repair-defective, "disintegrative" types (Sheppard *et al.* 1985), like that of Fanconi's anemia (Okuyama and Mishina 1987a).

Choriocarcinoma may thus be a tumor of the evolutionarily secured organs. How it was affected by atomic radiation remains unknown, and its curves cannot be categorized. However, it may be feasible to make the following conjecture. In males, it affects those in the reproductive age range at the time of exposure. At high doses, permanent sterility ensues; at low doses, transient sterility because of apoptosis of the spermatids and glandular atrophy are likely. When transient sterility recovers, DNA damage is probable. If this damage remains unrepaired at the time of fertilization, a host of abnormalities are likely (Sheppard *et al.* 1985). In females, the reproductive age range may be the sole limiting factor insofar as the incidence curves are concerned. Thus, morbidity would not accumulate beyond certain limits, and the curves would taper thereafter.

The contribution of the background radiation cannot always be determined. The doses absorbed by the testicles at the time of the explosion in Nagasaki were estimated to be 6870 rad at 500 m, 852 rad at 1000 m, 109 at 1500 m, and 13 rad at 2000 m from the hypocenter (Hashizume *et al.* 1974). The residual radioactivity 60 days later was 0.3 mR per hour at the hypocenter and 0.03 at most within 1000 m. Therefore, the estimated exposure for a man entering the hypocenter one hour after the explosion and standing there for infinity would be 1.4 R at most. The fallout of fission products occurred predominantly in the Nishiyama district of Nagasaki,

3 km east of the hypocenter (Pace and Smith 1946). The residual radioactivity 60 days later was 1.0 mR per hour at most. Thus, a similar estimate of exposure would have been 10 R at most (Arakawa 1968). Nonetheless, measurable radioactivity could have emanated as a result of thermal neutron activation of the rocks and soil, for example, 122 kev gamma rays from Eu-152, whose half-life is 13 years (Maruyama 1986). The background radioactivity in the Nagasaki area, however, seems to have decayed sufficiently by the time a nationwide survey on radioactivity was carried out between 1968 and 1977: it was 8.8 ± 0.8 micro R per hour, completely within the national average range (7.4-10.6) (Abe *et al.* 1969).

Candidates for cancer may thus include not only those directly surviving the atomic bomb and those who entered the city immediately thereafter, but also those who lived in the city for some time after the bombing and were exposed to the high background radiation; those whose parent or parents were exposed to radiation in one way or another may also be candidates, as described above (Itoga 1965). Circumstantial evidence seems to indicate that chromosomal aberrations eventually result in untoward oncogene expression and induce choriocarcinomas (Sugimori *et al.* 1978; Sarkar *et al.* 1986). A hypothetical curve for choriocarcinoma would thus be likely to resemble that for breast cancer (III).

The sequence of oncogenesis resulting from atomic radiation seems to have followed the evolutionary stratification suggested for Fanconi's anemia (Okuyama and Mishina 1987 a; 1988a) but in an accelerated way. Atomic radiation may not have generated any novel carcinogenetic mechanisms, or any new and bizarre types of leukemias. The sequence of events, however, seems to apparently adhere to the law of biochemical evolution of Horowitz (1945): the evolution of the basic syntheses proceeds in a stepwise manner, involving one mutation at a time, but the order of attainment of individual steps was in the reverse direction from that in which synthesis proceeds in the chain; thus, the ultimate synthesis was the first to be acquired in the course of evolution, the penultimate step next, and so on. If it is accepted that the most important component of carcinogenesis is DNA change, then the type of carcinogenesis resulting from the disintegration of DNA could have been the initial process. Thus, the most primitive neoplasms in terms of biology could have been leukemias of DNA disintegration. The means to repair DNA by excision was acquired as long ago as 2.8 billion years (Kondo 1978), and defective DNA repair and other chromosome breakage syndromes give rise to leukemias (Schwartz 1986; Okuyama and Mishina 1987a) (Fig. 3 in Chapter 3).

The second category of neoplasms could have been solid epithelial tumors of the disintegrative type involving multiple disintegrations. The NK cell could have been developed in response to such neoplasms (Kumagai 1985). Cellular and humoral immunities have been traced back some 400 million years (Good *et al.* 1965). These mechanisms, however, could have contributed to lymphomatogenesis as the result of potent and continued antigenic stimulation followed by reactive lymphoproliferation. The most recent neoplasms may be lymphomas resulting from retroviral infections. These are recent in the sense that the oncogenic information is derived from humans or primates, animals high on the evolutionary ladder (Gallo *et al.* 1977; Matthews 1983; Kaplan *et al.* 1987). Needless to say, a multitude of mechanisms, both promoting and attacking carcinogenesis, have evolved and been stratified in the interim (Okuyama and Mishina 1987a; 1988a). Thus, the application of Horowitz's law to the science of carcinogenesis may be borne out.

Nevertheless, there seem to be definite epidemiological differences between atomic bomb radiation carcinogenesis and normal carcinogenesis, and probably in terms of changes in oncogene levels. In Fig. 2, curve I (leukemias) shows a peak 10 years after the atomic bombing. Curve III (breast cancer) peaks at the 25th year after the detonation. Curve II (cancers of the lung and stomach) has two peaks: normal, age-related cancer incidence, and incidence relative to the atomic bombing (Monzen and Wakabayashi 1986). The second is more than 10 years ahead of the first, indicating that an acceleration of carcinogenesis is probable in the exposed population. Taking advantage of cell cycle time estimates for human colonic cells (24 hr, Lipkin *et al.* 1962) and normoblasts (16.5 hr, Bond *et al.* 1958), the numbers of cell cyclings were approximated for curves I and II. The results were identical for the two: 5475 cell cyclings for leukemias in 10 years, and the same for cancers of the lung and stomach in 15 years.

There are three major devices for prevention of carcinogenesis in cell renewal systems (Cairns 1975): (1) segregation and protection of the parental DNA; (2) reduction of the number of stem cells; and (3) compartmentalization of cells to restrain the opportunities for competition between cells. At the time of exposure to the atomic bomb radiation, the stem cell pool size in the exposed individual was not necessarily increased. If the intestine is irradiated experimentally, the compartmentalization is broken up, and groups of cells containing stem cells are induced to migrate (Tsubouchi and Matsuzawa 1973), presumably in search of a hypoxic milieu (Okuyama *et al.* 1988). If carcinogenesis necessitates priming and processing of mutants, radiation from the atomic bombing could have produced all or some changes in the DNA in the cell renewal systems at the time of exposure, and that it damaged the programs for appropriate compartmentalization of cells, thus promoting cancer phanerosis. The time required for processing a priming mutation through immortalization, transformation, and cancer phanerosis may be dependent on the number of cell cyclings. The observed acceleration may therefore be ascribed to this type of damage to the DNA strands, and possibly to defective compartmentalization as well.

Mass exposure to radiation is a constant threat worldwide, as clearly seen in the power plant accident that occurred in Chernobyl, USSR, in 1986. Although regrettable, such incidents of mass exposure are likely to provide data to supplement the Nagasaki curves and further test the evolutionary concept of cancer.

Chapter 5

Carcinogenesis in Evolution

> *Human tumors with minimal chromo-*
> *some change (diploid acute leukemia,*
> *chronic granulocytic leukemia) are con-*
> *sidered to be early in clonal evolution;*
> *human solid cancers, typically highly*
> *aneuploid, are viewed as late in the*
> *developmental process.*
> ——*P. C. Nowell*, Pathology, *1976*

Is Carcinogenesis Evolving?

Our answer to the question of whether carcinogenesis is still evolving is yes. To pose this question at the outset may appear somewhat extreme. Nonetheless, it is relevant in discussing cancer as an evolutionary process. Sugano has proposed two distinct categories of cancers, basic and variable (1980). The latter denotes those cancers whose incidence fluctuates with differences in sociological and environmental background. Although Sugano did not discuss the possibility that modern chemical carcinogenesis might have evolutionary implications, we strongly suspect that this may be the case.

We based our epidemiological analysis of cancer incidence on natural populations, selected disease populations (Fanconi's anemia), and the population of a city on which the atomic bomb was dropped (Nagasaki) (Okuyama and Mishina 1987a; 1988a, b).

The concept of carcinogenesis in evolution implies that earlier carcinogenetic processes could have been quite different from the contemporary ones, and that the future evolution of carcinogenesis may be quite different from the present. Thus, the carcinogenesis itself may be in the process of evolution. A body of evidence, ranging from direct to circumstantial, supports this notion. First, there could have been major changes in agents capable of inducing neoplasms: radiation itself could have changed from time to time as the earth's natural radiation sources decayed and cosmic radiation fluctuated. Potentially carcinogenetic chemical contaminants could also have changed from time to time. The appearance or acquisition of proto-oncogenes and the contribution to carcinogenesis of retroviruses may be included here because they are not necessarily too archaic (Matthews 1983).

Second, as evolution progressed, the DNA content of animal cells increased, providing a greater repertoire for mechanisms to evolve to handle noxious effectors. Third, the present eukaryotic cell is a composite, presumably resulting from endosymbiosis (Margulis 1981), and carcinogenesis may be a sort of dyscrasia in the syntax of this symbiosis (Setala 1984). Fourth, a wide range of mechanisms to help eliminate cancer cells could have evolved step by step. In other words, carcinogenesis is essentially a nuclear or cellular core disease, one with which the nucleus must have long struggled, taking full advantage of available genetic materials. Thus, cancer is better understood as a dynamic process still in evolution rather than an established and perfected one.

Evolutionary experiments on carcinogenesis have produced Down's syndrome, Fanconi's anemia, xeroderma pigmentosum, Bloom's syndrome, ataxia telangiectasia, primary immunodeficiency diseases, common variable unclassified immunodeficiency, and acquired immunodeficiency syndrome.

A host of diseases exist in which the patients are prone to develop malignancies. Most of them arise as the result of genetic or chromosomal deviations, but acquired forms are also possible. Analysis of such diseases may help in deciphering portions of the mechanisms of carcinogenesis.

Descriptions of Cancer-Prone Diseases

Concise but relevant descriptions of the cancer-prone diseases are given below:

Down's syndrome   This is a clinical syndrome caused by the chromosomal abnormality known as trisomy 21, which results from a mutation that may take place during the meiotic formation of the ovum (Robbins and Cotran 1979). Children who have this disorder are liable to develop acute leukemias.

Fanconi's anemia   This is a congenital disease characterized by anemia, renal rickets, and growth retardation. Development of a variety of neoplasms has been reported, mostly leukemias (Ruddon 1981). It is an autosomal recessive disorder whose chromosomes display excessive fragility in cell culture. Reduced Cu, ZnSOD activity in the blood cells has been reported (Yoshimitsu *et al.* 1984; Scarpa *et al.* 1985). Defective repair of DNA damage is also well-known (Ahmed and Setlow 1978; Izakovic *et al.* 1985): namely, defective transport of enzymes functioning in DNA repair from cytoplasm to nucleus. There seems to be a direct correlation between cause and effect in these two pathologies.

Xeroderma pigmentosum   This syndrome is characterized by extreme sensitivity of the skin to sunlight or ultraviolet light (UV), and death is usually due to skin cancer. While the normal skin cells are able to repair UV damage to DNA by cut-and-patch repair (excision repair), those from patients with xeroderma pigmentosum cannot perform this repair and apparently lack UV-specific endonuclease. It is an autosomal recessive syndrome. Responsible mutations may occur at any one of at least seven different chromosomal sites (King and Stansfield 1985).

Bloom's syndrome   This is also an autosomal recessive syndrome characterized by sun-sensitive telangiectatic erythema of the face, short stature, defective immunity, and excessive chromosomal fragility in cell culture. Patients commonly develop leukemias, but other forms of malignancy have also been reported (German *et al.* 1977).

Ataxia telangiectasia   This syndrome is characterized by cerebellar ataxia and frequent respiratory infections. It is an autosomal recessive disease with defects in both cellular and humoral immunity. In early life the immune system appears normal; beginning around the fifth year of life, the patients develop a progressive immune deficiency that is characterized by defective cellular immunity and, often, by a total lack of IgA (and sometimes IgE) (Hood *et al.* 1978). Increased chromosomal fragility is also to be seen in cell culture because of the defective ability to repair DNA damage. Over 10% of the patients develop malignancy, mainly involving the lymphoid tissue (Kersey *et al.* 1973; Schwartz 1986). It should be noted that patients suffer from both chromosomal breakage syndrome and immunodeficiencies.

Primary immunodeficiency diseases This is a composite group of immunodeficiency diseases that has T- and B-cell bifunctional deficiency as its common feature (Schwartz 1986). The group includes infantile X-linked Bruton's agammaglobulinemia, severe combined immunodeficiency disease, and Wiskott-Aldrich syndrome. Wiskott-Aldrich syndrome, however, is characterized by a progressive loss of T-cell functions.

Common, variable unclassified immunodeficiency (acquired hypogammaglobulinemia) This is an acquired form of immunodeficiency whose origin is unknown. The onset is usually between 15 and 35 years, and it affects both males and females. Patients have symptoms of recurrent infection and are usually found to have detectable, but very low, levels of total immunoglobulin. Although T-cell numbers and function are usually normal, some patients have T-cell defects, probably those of suppressor T-cells, which may grow severer as the disease progesses (Golub 1987).

Acquired immunodeficiency syndrome (AIDS) This is a retroviral infection (HTLV-III) that induces immunodeficiency as a result of T-cell exhaustion. It has been proposed that the helper cell subset is selectively involved (Klatzmann *et al.* 1984; Laurence *et al* 1984). Neoplastic complications, mostly lymphomas, have recently been noted (Kaplan *et al.* 1987). The retroviral acquisition is thought to be a recent one, however (Matthews 1983).

Fanconi's Anemia as an Evolutionary Experiment on Carcinogenesis (Okuyama and Mishina 1987a)

To facilitate the present discussion, it seems useful to study the carcinogenetic mechanisms of Fanconi's anemia.

Fanconi's anemia is a congenital disease characterized by anemia, renal rickets, and growth retardation. Development of a variety of neoplasms, mainly leukemias, has been reported. The disease carries two fundamental defects: reduced cuprozinc superoxide dismutase (Cu, ZnSOD) (Joenje *et al.* 1979; Yoshimitsu *et al.* 1984; Scarpa *et al.* 1985) and defective DNA repair (Ahmed and Setlow 1978). These primary defects would lead to secondary changes that are prone to encourage carcinogenesis along with the development of anemia, renal damage, and growth retardation. This model mimics radiation carcinogenesis in that superoxide radicals are also "incisive." In the case of Fanconi's anemia, however, the DNA damage is further amplified because of the reduced capacity for repair. Epidemiologic analysis of neoplasms in this syndrome (Okuyama and Mishina 1987a) revealed that their age distribution was 14.5 ± 6.7 years for leukemias; 18.5 ± 9.3 years for hepatomas, and 23.8 ± 6.9 years for squamous cell carcinomas. Thus, the nonepithelial-epithelial tumor shift is observed in Fanconi's anemia. The development of hepatomas may be a manifestation of prolonged exposure to oxymetholone, an anabolic steroid for the treatment of intractable anemias. It is definitely iatrogenic. The phenomenon may be representative of chemical carcinogenesis in the presence of defective DNA repair.

Undoubtedly, neoplastic formation itself is a genetic disorder, and may start with changes in the genes and chromosomes. However, it should be noted that surveillance against emerging tumors is not necessarily a direct sequel of the genetic disorder. This appears to be the case with Fanconi's anemia: NK cells are remarkably sensitive to radiation (Kumagai 1985) and, therefore, to superoxide radicals, which flood as a result of reduced Cu, ZnSOD. T- and B-cell depletion followed by hypogammaglobulinemias may ensue in time. The latter would likely result in a loss of barriers against the oncogenic viruses in the respiratory and gastrointestinal tracts and genitalia. The tumors seen among patients with Fanconi's anemia are almost entirely limited to squamous cell types occurring in the oropharyngoesophagus and vulvovagina. This supports the ease of access by the oncogenetic viruses. In the normal state, the susceptible target tissues are designed to lose their cells through desquamation. Carcinomas may result when this mechanism of cell loss is disordered in one way or another, as in stomach cancer and amelanotic melanoma (Fujita 1983; Takahashi and Seiji 1983).

One way to elucidate the evolution of carcinogenesis may be to take into account the dating of each pro- and anticancer mechanism. Table 1 in Chapter 3 lists the dates for the emergence of the anticancer mechanisms (Okuyama and Mishina 1987a).

The evolutionary chronology of these mechanisms seems to have been well established. Radiation effects on DNA are of prime importance, and life forms acquired the ability to treat the constantly emerging breaks in double-stranded DNA by excision repair some 2.8 billion years ago, making this one of the oldest mechanisms (Kondo 1972). Because the concept of cancer is applicable only to multicellular organisms, actual cancers may not have afflicted unicellular organisms, even in the presence of this type of defect in DNA repair. Cu, ZnSOD dates back 420 million years (Asada 1976). The acquisition of this enzyme could have been vital for land animals, especially when the atmospheric oxygen concentrations increased dramatically during the Carboniferous Period. The evolution of NK cells may also be quite old (Kumagai 1985). Primitive T-cells could have emerged among species of lamprey 500 million years ago, B-cells among the sharks about 350 million years ago, and lymph nodes in the mammalian animals 150 million years ago (Good *et al.* 1965; 1971). T-cell deficiencies imply defective function in that category of lymphocytes, but may suggest that B-cells, their counterparts, have been reciprocally forced to proliferate against viral or bacterial stimulation. This may also occur in any complementary subpopulation of T- or B-cells.

For our purposes, it is important to concentrate on the leukemias and cancers that may be "natural" neoplasms of Fanconi's anemia. The primary defects are defective DNA repair and deficient Cu, ZnSOD, leading to hypersuperoxidemia or topical increases in superoxide concentrations. According to the theorem of Nowell (1971) and the statement of Watson *et al.* (1987), leukemias initially result in a decreased number of oncogenic DNA changes. When the number becomes greater, the probability of developing cancers may also be increased. NK cell deficiency, which is secondary to hypersuperoxidemia, lessens the effectiveness of cancer surveillance. IgA deficiency is also a secondary event, one that probably leads to defective barriers against viral invasions, and would therefore encourage viral carcinogenesis. Hepatomagenesis resulting from the prolonged administration of oxymetholone may also be dependent upon the primary defect of DNA repair. Thus, the pro- and anticancer carcinogenetic mechanisms may be stratified according to evolution, as will be discussed in greater detail below.

Other Evolutionary Experiments on Carcinogenesis

Having studied the particular case of Fanconi's anemia, we may proceed with other cancer-prone diseases. Although the study of cancer incidence appears complicated, this can be overcome by categorizing disorders according to chromosomal or immune defects (Table 1; Fig. 1). Among the chromosomal aberration syndromes, leukemias predominate during childhood, while cancers emerge in adulthood, except for xeroderma pigmentosum, in which the DNA-damaging insult is sunlight and the target organ is the superficial skin; the organs deep in the body are therefore likely to be exempted. There are definitely no lymphomas.

The status of immunity is divided into three categories: T, B and Nil immunity. T immunity is intended to imply the preservation of T-cell immunity (cellular immunity) and defective B-cell immunity. In the case of Nil immunity, both T- and B-cell immunities are defective, but may vary in degree from one case to another. Among the immune deficiencies, however, cancers occur in the pure T immunity category but not in the pure B category (Fig. 1). Conversely, lymphomas occur in the B immunity category but not in the pure T type. Leukemias are common to both forms, but are confined to childhood. Their leukemogenetic significance will be discussed below. Thus, we may tentatively conclude that the emergence of cancer is influenced by T immunity, while that of lymphomas is influenced by the B type.

In the Nil immunity category, both cancers and lymphomas are seen. This obvious contradiction can be overcome by assuming (1) that there are residual subsets of competent B- or T-cell components or (2) that one of the two is the primary defect and the other arises secondarily with time.

Table 1. Categories of cancer-prone disorders

Category	Pathology	Chronology	Clinical syndrome	Malignancies
Chromosome aberrations	Chromosomal mutation	Trisomy 21	Down's syndrome (Infants/children)	Acute leukemias
	Chromosamal breakage	Defective DNA repair (2800 m. yr.)*	Xeroderma pigmentosum	Cancers (skin)
			Bloom's syndrome	Leukemias (early) Cancers (late)
	Deficient SOD	(420 m. yr.)* plus defective DNA repair	Fanconi's anemia	Leukemias (early) Cancers (late)
Immune deficiencies	*Nil* immunity	(No *T*, no *B*)	Severe combined**	Leukemias, mostly lymphomas
			Common variable***	Lymphomas, less cancers
			Ataxia telangiectasia	Leukemias, mostly lymphomas
	T immunity	(*T*, no *B*)	Bruton's agammaglobuli-nemia (infants)	Mostly leukemias
			IgA deficiency (adolescents and adults)	Cancers
	B immunity	(No *T*, but *B*)	Wiskott-Aldrich syndrome	Lymphomas
		(350 m. yr.)*	AIDS	Lymphomas

*   Estimated time of evolution in millions of years.

**   Severe combined immunodeficiency.

***   Common variable immunodeficiency.

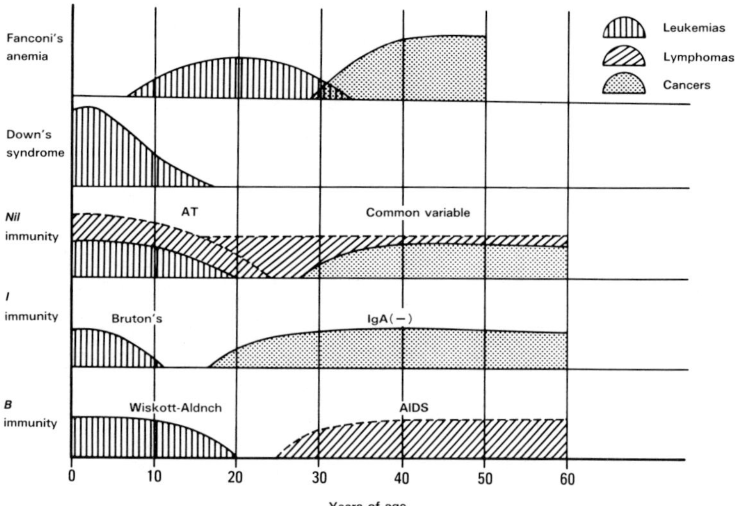

Fig. 1. Cancer-prone diseases in relation to different modes of immune status: *Nil,* or selective *T* or *B* immunity. The immune deficiencies, either defective *B* or *T*, during infancy and childhood invariably induce leukemias. Carcinogenesis in later life appears to result from defects in *B* immunity, while lymphomatous processes develop from defects in *T* immunity. In other words, leukemogenesis may be related to defects in the maintenance of DNA integrity, as surmised from Fanconi's anemia or Down's syndrome (disintegrative type). Defects in *B* immunity would facilitate invasion of the oncogenic viruses. Persistent antigenic stimulation and compensatory clonal lymphoid proliferation in *B* immunity may be related to lymphomagenesis.

In the case of ataxia telangiectasia, both types of immunity are intact for the first few years of life. Cellular immunity deteoriates first, followed by humoral immunity. This consecutive loss of different types of immunity is clearly reflected in the transition from lymphomas to cancers. The common variable immunodeficiencies are characterized by depletion of the suppressor T-cell subset (Golub 1987). The primary function of the suppressor T-cells is nonspecific, as well as specific, suppression of immune reactions. The nonspecific subsets of such cells are to disappear in the course of time. Premature disappearance is known to be closely related to the spontaneous development of autoimmune diseases such as autoimmune hemolytic anemia of New Zealand black mice. The lymphomatous transformation may be due to compensatory proliferation and subsequent malignant transformation in any of the clones of the remaining B-cell lineages (Kersey *et al.* 1974). (3) A third assumption is transformation of the oncogenous viruses, and the definite antiviral repertoire of the immunoglobulins: IgM against those viruses circulating in the peripheral blood, IgG against viral particles swarming in the interstitial space as well as in the blood, and IgA against those intruding across the mucous membrane (Alexander and Good 1977). Thus, B-cells may be strongly involved in the pathogenesis of cancers and lymphomas in terms of barriers against the oncogenic viruses and lymphoproliferative responses to compensate for the defective B-cell subsets.

Childhood leukemias are common to most of the syndromes of chromosomal breakage and immunodeficiency. Although it is included in the immunodeficiency group, ataxia telangiectasia is characterized by defective DNA repair and is therefore one of the chromosomal breakage syndromes. Bruton's congenital agammaglobulinemia and Wiskott-Aldrich syndrome are both X-linked and limited to boys. The X chromosomes contain the *ras* proto-oncogene, although it may be an inactive pseudogene (Sugiyama *et al.* 1985). We do not know if or how this type of proto-oncogene is activated. Nevertheless, the high incidence of malignancy (0.7% for Bruton's agammaglobulinemia and 12% for Wiskott-Aldrich syndrome) may support the X-chromosome hypothesis.

Although cancers first appeared to be limited to *T* immunity, closer examination seems to suggest that they arise when both *B* and *T* immunity are lost—to be exact, as soon as extensive and/or thorough T-cell depletion is attained (Fig. 1). In other words, cancers arise when the aforementioned immunological barriers against oncogenic viral intrusion have disintegrated and surveillance mechanisms, including NK cells, are lost.

Deciphering Evolutionary Carcinogenetic Experiments: Stratification and Chronology of Neoplasms

In Fanconi's anemia, the emergence of leukemias was seen to precede that of cancers. The primary carcinogenetic defects appeared to be reduced Cu, ZnSOD and deficient DNA repair. The reduction in the number of NK cells and IgA deficiency that occurred in later life were thought to be secondary sequelae. Leukemias appear in children, cancers in adults (Okuyama and Mishina 1987a). Nowell suggested that the leukemogenetic change in the chromosome may be smaller than that for the development of solid cancers (1976). There is a nonepithelial-epithelial tumor shift (Okuyama and Mishina 1986b). Thus, a scheme of carcinogenetic stratification can be formed (Fig. 2 in Chapter 3).

An obvious implication of the above is that evolution could have initially developed the ability to repair DNA to alleviate the carcinogenetic burden of ultraviolet rays. Although primarily intended to circumvent genetic damage, this mechanism, which is so vital for the preservation of species integrity, could have also helped in overcoming the untoward carcinogenetic effects of X- and gamma-rays and carcinogenetic chemicals. It may therefore be one of the fundamental anticancer mechanisms to have evolved during the earlier periods of primitive life and to have been preserved throughout the long history of evolution.

The immunological defense lines seem to have evolved comparatively recently. From the carcinogenetic point of view, they could help prevent or control some of the viral and bacterial infections responsible for neoplastic development, as suggested in the preceding chapter on cancer epidemiology. T-cell deficiencies are likely to permit B-cells to undergo lymphomatous transformation. *B* immunity puts up barriers against viral and bacterial infections that are liable to affect the genetic information of the infected cells, leading to oncogenesis, or to entice antigenic stimulation of the relevant clones of lymphocytes appropriate to the degree of lymphomatous transformation. The primary immunodeficiency diseases are limited in number. Victims of AIDS, however, are increasing in number, and the eventual development of neoplasms would certainly be a consideration unless adequate anti-AIDS therapies are developed. Leukemic development seems to be closely related to the integrity of chromosomes. However, it is not yet clear to what extent immunological cancer surveillance is in action here, in the sense that the host is constantly capable of detecting and eliminating the newly emerging aberrant cells.

Not all changes, however, initiate carcinogenetic processes. Those effectors incurring DNA damage are superoxide or other radicals, chemicals, or oncogenetic gene products. The damage has to be selected or targeted, segregated and secured, and adequately amplified before the eventual effects of immortalization and/or transformation of the affected lineages of cells are put into force. Viral infections are capable of endowing such immortalizing and transforming properties to the cells under selected circumstances and of advancing them through processes of carcinogenesis. Immunodeficiency states would thus promote the advancement of cells rendered carcinogenetic by radiation, chemical contamination, or viral infection.

Active oxygen moieties, especially superoxide anions, may have been a constant menace to oxidative life on earth, but Fe- and MnSOD molecules were apparently competent enough to detoxify them in pre-eukaryotic life. Nonetheless, DNA damage was inevitable, and the evolution of repair systems mandatory. The chromosomal breakage syndromes are characterized by defects in these repair systems. Fanconi's anemia is certainly stigmatized by this kind of defect. When the atmospheric oxygen concentration started to rise steeply around the Carboniferous Period, the evolution and acquisition of Cu, ZnSOD by the pre-eukaryotic cells took place in response, a property that was rapidly propagated throughout the eukaryotes as well, presumably through the process of endosymbiosis. Those with Fanconi's anemia suffer from pancytopenia, at least as the result of superoxide toxicity of the hematopoietic stem cells. When the DNA damage is segregated in such a way as to activate leukemogenic proto-oncogenes, leukemias may evolve. Lymphoid cells are also superoxide-sensitive, and clonal depletions could lead to viral and bacterial infections, then contribute to the activation of proto-oncogenes and defective cancer surveillance. Cu, ZnSOD is capable of helping to reduce intracellular and intercellular concentrations of superoxide and peroxide radicals because it also acts as a catalase on both moieties of radicals (Asada 1976).

Another evolutionary feature of the immune system provides additional clarification of carcinogenesis, similar to that suggested by the study of Fanconi's anemia (Okuyama and Mishina 1987a). In natural immunological surveillance against cancer, NK cells keep track of newly emerging cancer cells and eliminate them as soon as they arise. NK cells are extremely radiosensitive and, therefore, superoxide-sensitive.

Similar immunological defenses are applicable to other cancer-prone immunodeficiencies. In selective B immunity or T-cell deficiency, the integrity of the immunological system can be disorganized to the extent that appropriate antiviral immune antigenization fails to take place, causing patients to succumb to viral lymphomatous development or develop lymphomas of the hyperstimulation types if they survive the viral infection, as in the case of Duncan's syndrome, in which the Epstein-Barr virus is involved (Purtilo 1977), and AIDS (Kaplan *et al.* 1987). Circumstantial evidence that viruses can be involved in lymphomagenesis of the primary and secondary immunodeficiencies is discussed elsewhere (Little and Longo 1985). In preteen children, i.e., before full maturation of the thymus-dependent lymphoid cells, the viral infections that lead to non-Hodgkin's lymphomas can spread throughout the extranodal lymphatic tissues along the gastrointestinal tract, presumably as the virus invades and penetrates that organ.

We have just seen that carcinogenetic processes per se are evolutionarily and possibly strategically stratified. Each of the effective anticancer mechanisms that have evolved must have arisen from obvious biological necessity: defense against ultraviolet rays and possibly X- and gamma-rays, defense against diverse intruders, and detoxification of active oxygen molecules, especially after the advent of the Carboniferous Period, when the atmospheric oxygen concentrations rose so steeply. Any combination of defects in these anti-cancer mechanisms may result in oncogenesis in the course of time.

We can generalize by stating that these neoplasms must have evaded or penetrated these lines of defense in spite of abnormalities in the DNA itself and gene products such as tumor-specific antigens. Evolutionary experiments on carcinogenesis thus seem helpful in providing insights into carcinogenetic mechanisms: (1) childhood leukemias resulting from chromosomal breakage ("disintegrative" type); (2) adult cancers of the disintegrative type; (3) lymphomas of the "compensatory type"; and (4) leukemias, lymphomas, and cancers of the "infective type." The evolutionary chronology of these neoplasms is likely to have been in the order 1-4 (Okuyama and Mishina 1988a).

Neoplastic Evolution of Cell Renewal and Non-Renewable Types

As already emphasized, research on carcinogenesis can be approached by analyzing cancer incidences among general or selected populations, i.e., those that underwent atomic bombing or have cancer-prone diseases. We have learned that the general rule of nonepithelial-epithelial tumor shift with advancing age seems to be closely related to the ontogeny of immune competence. We have also distinguished the mammalian and premammalian epithelial tumors. Cancers of the female mammalian symbol organs were found to have a biphasic curve, with peaks in the period of active reproduction and after menopause. In the male, prostatic cancers show a peak in the latter age group, with no corresponding peak during the period of active reproduction. Thirdly, cancers of the lung and stomach, both representing the premammalian stage, show a steep rise from youth to old age. The different curves for different types of cancers may imply different pathogeneses. Generally speaking, the initial carcinogenetic changes in the stem cells can be perpetuated within the stem cell line, while similar alterations in the differentiated cells that will eventually exfoliate may not be "carcinogenetic" (Cronkite 1974; Cairns 1981). Changes that initiate immortalization and transformation are "infective" or "disintegrative."

This section will discuss whether DNA changes that take

place among such cells that have already ceased to multiply and are committed to full maturation and differentiation are still capable of causing the cells to revert back into cell cycle and enticing further immortalization and transformation, as suggested in the epidemiology of prostatic cancer.

Tissue Classification according to Mitotic Prospects or Capacity for Cell Renewal

After birth, not all somatic cells are in cell cycle. They can be classified into three different cell systems: (1) rapid cell renewal systems consisting of intermitotic cells and fixed postmitotic cells; (2) slow renewal systems consisting of those reverting postmitotic cells; and (3) nonrenewal systems consisting of fixed postmitotic cells (Rubin and Casarette 1968). This classification was originally employed to study the radiosensitivity of tissues, but it may deserve a second look.

Although incomplete, the data shown in Table 2 encourage our hypothetical distinctions of nonepithelial vs epithelial, vertebral vs prevertebral, and mammalian vs premammalian. The cell cycle time for the normoblast is as short as 16.5 hours

Table 2. Evolutionary implications of cell cycle times *in vivo* for normal human tissue cells

	Organ system	Cell cycle time	Reference
Verte-bral	Mammalian symbols		
	Vagina during estrus	(25 hr)	Thrasher *et al.* (1967)
	during diestrus	(72 hr)	
	Premammalian		
	Colonic	24 hr	Lipkin *et al.* (1962)
	Renal	24 hr	Westerveld *et al.* (1971)
Prevertebral			
	Normoblast	16.5 hr	Bond *et al.* (1958)
	Fibroblast	30 hr	Zosimovska *et al.* (1956)

1) The incidence of fibrosarcoma is insignificant in comparison with neoplasms of other organs.

2) The short cell cycle time for the normoblasts can be explained by probable adaptation to the hyperoxic environment of the circulating blood: The erythrocytes can be lost at greater rates than used in a hypoxic milieu.

N.B. Data in parentheses (Thrasher *et al.* 1967) are for the mouse.

(Bond *et al.* 1959). Although the data are for the mouse, the vaginal epithelium has a cell cycle time of 25 hours during estrus and 72 hours during diestrus (Thrasher *et al.* 1967). The prevalence of nonepithelial tumors during the earliest period of life and cancers of the mammalian symbol organs during the period of reproductiveness may be related to their respective active periods of cell proliferation either *a priori* or with periodicity. Conversely, tumors of the fibrous tissue would be much less likely to emerge. Whether their cell cycles are rapid or slow, these organs and tissues would yield to carcinogenesis of the cell renewal type. Although we do not have any cytokinetic confirmations, mammalian cancers that occur after menopause may, in principle, lack normal cell renewal because of postmenopausal atrophy. The situation may be the same with prostatic cancer as well. Attempts to induce carcinogenesis of the prostate with 1, 2-benz-pyrene were successful only when the chemical was administered to experimental animals with glandular regression and atrophy (Fingerhut and Veenema 1977), but not when it was given simultaneously with castration (Moore and MacMahon 1937). Thus, carcinogenesis of the nonrenewal type seems probable. In the slow renewal systems, G_0 cells shift to G_1 and subsequently follow the cell cycle through DNA synthesis, G_2, and mitosis. The transition or re-entry of G_0 cells into the cell cycle requires intracellular accumulation of cAMP for a limited period of time (Kuroki *et al.* 1982). The key substances capable of commencing the chain reactions may be EGF or cholera toxins for the epidermal cells (Kuroki 1981; Nakamura 1985). In the experimental induction of prostatic cancer, cells in the atrophic prostate gland can be in G_1 for prolonged or indefinite periods of time. There must be factors or substances capable of pulling these cells back into the cell cycle and forcing them to multiply indefinitely, for example, one or two of the oncogene products or aberrant tyrosine kinases. Although it does not necessarily support our hypothesis, the following statement has been made: "Although not perfectly correlated, cancers tend to arise in cells that continue to proliferate in adult life" (Watson *et al.* 1987). Further research needs to be carried out along these lines.

The evolutionary significance of such "reverting" carcinogenesis may be to promote and accelerate the efficient extinction of the elderly. This may constitute a challenge to aging that aims at renovation by a rapid evolution.

Propensity of Spontaneous Tumor Regression of the Nonepithelial Type

The induction of cancer redifferentiation can be an attractive, elegant means of treatment. The procedure has been shown to be feasible in the treatment of acute myeloid leukemias (Fibach *et al.* 1973; Sachs 1978; Housset *et al.* 1982). With solid tumors, it is thought to be impracticable (Matsuzawa 1981). Nonetheless, it is potentially practicable. Tumor redifferentiation is induced when bestatin is administered to breast cancer patients along with appropriate sex hormones (Okuyama and Mishina 1984a; c; 1985b; Okuyama *et al.* 1983 d; 1985b). Histologically, the peculiar property of piling up is lost, and the cells resume aligning themselves. That is, contact inhibition is ever present. There is a case for the possible return of the glandular secretory function. It seems worthwhile mentioning that those leukemias might "redifferentiate" on exposure to corticosteroids, which are by no means unphysiological. The collected cases of spontaneous regression of cancer (Everson and Cole 1966) have been rearranged according to our evolutionary calendar (Table 3). The table clearly indicates that the majority of recorded cases of spontaneous regression are of nonepithelial tumors. Because of probable acquisition of novel antigenicity, those of mammalian cancers could have been eliminated spontaneously. *Horror autotoxicus* could have made every effort to eliminate tumors arising in the gonads. Those tumors emerging during youth and through middle age, e.g., cancers of the lung and stomach, would not succumb even to the toughest immune surveillance. We may therefore conjecture that there is definite discrimination of nonepithelial tumors, presumably related to the mode of carcinogenesis along the line of cell renewal functions. As briefly suggested by Nowell (1976), this could involve quantitative changes in the chromosome, the ease of inducing chromosomal change, or some other factor. It is possible that human leukemogenesis and non-epithelial tumorigenesis can be achieved through changes in single proto-oncogenes, e.g., N-

Table 3. Collected cases of spontaneous regression of cancer: Nature's evolutionary experiment on *reverse* carcinogenesis [Everson and Cole (1960) as revised according to our hypothesis]

Category	Organ system	No. cases	% distribution
Evolutionarily secured	Testis	7	
	Ovary	7	
	Choriocarcinoma	19	20% *in toto*
Mammalian symbols	Breast	6	
	Uterus	4	
	Bladder	13	10% *in toto*
Homeothermic	Thyroid	1	
	Larynx	1	
	Lung	1	0% *in toto*
Poikilothermic	Tongue	1	
	Stomach	4	
	Liver	2	
	Colorectum	7	
	Pancreas	1	10% *in toto*
	Neuroblastoma	29	
	Malignant melanoma	19	
	Hypernephroma	31	
	Bone	8	
Prevertebral	Soft tissue sarcoma	11	60% *in toto*

ras and N-*myc* for neuroblastoma and leukemia. Thus, carcinogenesis may be simpler in prevertebral organ systems, and more complicated in more highly evolved systems.

Multistep Hypothesis of Carcinogenesis: Immortalization, Transformation, and Cancer Phanerosis

A third factor in neoplastic evolution is based on the discrimination of immortalization and transformation. Immortalization denotes unending proliferation and existence of cells, while transformation refers to their tumor formation. This distinction was first hypothesized by Hanafusa's group (Kawai *et al.* 1977; Hanafusa *et al.* 1977), who differentiated it from morphological and functional alterations, or transformational events. These processes of immortalization and transformation can be substantiated (Land *et al.* 1983; Ruley 1983). The induction of immortalization can be expedited when target cells are already in cell cycle, an observation that is true of most of tumors (Donner *et al.* 1982). However, expansion of

Table 4. Multistep carcinogenesis: Genetics of immortalization and transformation

Proto-oncogenes/oncogenes	Gene procucts/action sites
I. Immortalization genes	
myc, src	*i* proteins/nuclear matrix
Polyoma large T antigen	
Adenovirus Ela	
Host-cellular immortalization genes	
II. Transformation genes	
Ha-*ras*	*t* proteins/inner surface
N-*ras*	of the plasma membrane
Polyoma middle T antigen	
Adenovirus Elb	
Host cellular transformation genes	

the proto-oncogene theory and the hypothesis of immortalization vs transformation indicates that cells that are out of cell cycle may also be stimulated by the same mechanisms. This is especially likely when cancers of the prostate and endometrium in the elderly are considered, for these organs can be atrophic when the process of carcinogenesis takes place. In addition, proto-oncogenes are ubiquitous, and the probability of inducing point mutations in the DNA molecules of cells out of cell cycle is not necessarily negligible. The mutations are sometimes such that these postmitotic cells are stimulated to endless, uncontrolled proliferation. Radiation is an agent that can damage DNA, eventually leading to mutational consequences. Similar carcinogenic effects can be generated when chromosomal aberrations such as deletion, translocation, and cross-over take place. The genetic abnormalities that are thus induced and eventually become responsible for carcinogenesis may reside in the proto-oncogenes. This category of cancers can be designated "disintegrative" because of the loss of genetic integrity. Representative proto-oncogenes with potential immortalizing or transforming capability are listed in Table 4 (Abrams *et al.* 1982; Rassoulzadegan *et al.* 1982; 1983; Willingham *et al.* 1980; Newbold and Overell 1983; Land *et al.* 1983). Their possible pathways of activation are shown schematically in Fig. 2.

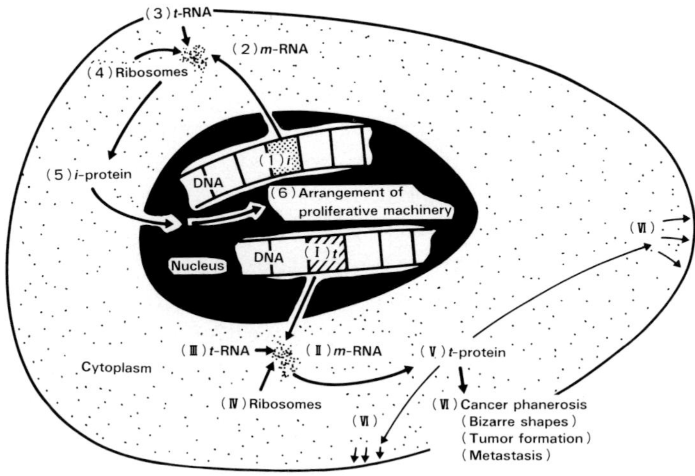

Fig. 2. Carcinogenesis in terms of immortalizing and transforming genes, and their respective active protein products in the cell. The immortalizing oncogene (i) in the nucleus eventually produces i protein, which induces derangement of the proliferative machinery toward endless multiplication. The transforming gene likewise produces t proteins that cause the cell to assume cancer cell morphology and other cancer attributes (cancer phanerosis). The entire scope of the t proteins can be multiplex, and their acquisition proceeds step by step (Nowell 1976; Watson *et al.* 1987). In addition, the multistep carcinogenetic processes could easily have incorporated a host of suppressor genes, to elaborate relevant s proteins (Klein and Klein 1985; Klein 1987).

Cancer Phanerosis as a Consequence of Immortalization and Transformation

Carcinogenesis is a complex, multistep process. Once the initial two steps of immortalization and transformation have exerted their effects in terms of molecular biology, a third step the manifestation of cancer occurs. To avoid possible confusion, the term "cancer phanerosis" is employed here. This term is intended to cover the observable, and frequently measurable, morphological, biochemical, and functional changes in candidate human cells, e.g., mass formation, contiguous invasions, and metastasis. Retroviruses and DNA viruses have the potential to induce immortalization and/or transformation (Table 4). In addition, there may be other "ill-defined" cellular oncogenes of either category (Newbold and Overell 1983). The changes involved may include any untoward activation of the proto-oncogenes that might result from point mutations due to radiation or chemical insult, DNA rearrangement, gene amplification, chromosomal translocations, or viral infection (Klein and Klein 1985; Klein 1987). These changes may well take place in nonrenewable cell types as well. In expressing their genes, they would lead to the production of specific functional proteins, i proteins, that would be localized in the nucleus and induce the immortalization of host cells, and t proteins that would be harbored in the inner surface of the plasma membrane and be capable of inducing transformation and cancer phanerosis (Fig. 2).

In rodents, at least, these two sets of oncogenes appear sufficient to induce cancer phanerosis of developing palpable tumors and submission of recipient animals when they are allowed to co-transfect cells *in vitro*; the resultant transformed cells are harvested for transplantation onto appropriate recipient animals (Kawai *et al.* 1977; Hanafusa *et al.* 1977). These experimental animal demonstrations can be applied to human beings, at least with regard to nonepithelial tumors arising in the early periods of life, as has already been suggested. For instance, in selected cases of acute leukemias, lymphomas, renal tumors, and neuroblastomas, activation of N-*myc* alone may be sufficient to evoke and maintain the pathology. It seems natural that the tumors should regress spontaneously as soon as the oncogene ceases to be activated, for whatever reason. The evolutionary age of the primary organ systems is of prime importance in such cases. The newer the organ system, the greater the structural and functional information, and the more complex and potent the protective mechanisms. This would hold true for organs ranging from the nonepithelial to the homeothermic. Carcinogenesis among the premammalian organ systems may therefore have to overcome this protective barrier by the multistep mechanisms suggested earlier. The resulting protection, however, would be endangered as soon as the sex hormones started to act on the mammalian organs.

The host patient has two or three lines of defense. The first, anticancer immunity, is based on circumstantial evidence from cancer epidemiology. This immunity is not necessarily aimed at cancer cells, but may not always be potent enough for effective immune surveillance. The discovery of an increasing number of tumor markers, which are being used for diagnosis and therapeutic monitoring, is such circumstantial evidence. Presumably, this kind of defense could have been provided as an anti-oncogene mechanism (Klein and Klein 1985; Klein 1987). Next, the oncogenes themselves may have strategically endeavored to reinforce their carcinogenetic capability by enclosure: HTLV-I virus, for example, produces multitudes of proteins that would eventually contribute to viral propagation (Nagashima *et al.* 1986).

There are 46 human chromosomes. In observing the proto-oncogenes on the chromosome map, we cannot but notice that sibling proto-oncogenes are distributed throughout several different chromosomes. The *myc*'s are located in chromosomes 2 and 8, and the *ras*'s, in chromosomes 1, 6, 11, 12, and X (Sugiyama *et al.* 1985). Why have the proto-oncogenes been scattered among the different chromosomes? Our instinctive answer at the moment is that this phenomenon is the third protective mechanism, one that harnesses the proto-oncogenes. It would therefore have profound evolutionary significance.

The fourth category of anticancer mechanism is related to cellular and tissue devices for cancer cell elimination and will be discussed later.

Nonviral Carcinogenesis

It is not impossible that all neoplasms will be found to arise as a result of one or more viral infections. Proof of this, however, awaits future studies. Nevertheless, there are cancer patients whose carcinogenesis appears to be closely related to exposure, at one time or another in their life, to certain amounts of radiation or chemicals. From the evolutionary point of view, nonviral (radiation and chemical) carcinogenesis may be much more archaic than the viral etiologies: radiation and potentially carcinogenetic chemicals could have existed prior to the emergence of life, whereas viruses could have appeared well after the advent of corresponding host animals.

The retroviruses, especially, have turned oncogenic rather recently by acquiring proto-oncogenes from normal host cells (Matthews 1983). Thus, nonviral carcinogenesis bears important evolutionary significance.

Evolutionary Features of Radiation Carcinogenesis

What is the role played by radiation in human history? The atomic bombing of Hiroshima and Nagasaki does not appear to have seeded any appreciable number of inheritable aberrations in the population (Neel *et al.* 1986). Nevertheless, our analysis has shown indisputable carcinogenetic effects in the victim population of Nagasaki as long as 30 years after the bombing (Okuyama and Mishina 1988a). We did not estimate the probable fraction of survivors present in the population during the study period. Considering the actual dilution resulting from A-bomb survivors leaving the city and other nonvictims entering it, the observed rates of cancer incidence may be cause for alarm. This observation must be confronted in one way or another.

The most conspicuous feature of the carcinogenesis related to atomic bombing appears to be evolutionary: the neoplastic sequelae started with leukemias, were followed by tumors of the stomach and lung, and finally were succeeded by tumors of the mammalian symbol organs. This sequence of neoplastic development appears to reflect the evolutionary history of animal life. We were initially perplexed by the complexity of atomic bomb radiation carcinogenesis, and the probable importance of this type of modelling cannot be overemphasized, especially in the light of the Chernobyl accident in 1986 and its probable neoplastic sequelae.

Most carcinogenetic mutations arise in the newly formed DNA strands of renewing cells during DNA synthesis, but not in the parental DNA strands (Cairns 1975). This segregative mechanism is one of the conspicuous evolutionary devices contributing to a reduction in the rate at which carcinogenetic mutations emerge. In the case of radiation carcinogenesis, mutations are induced on the parental DNA strands: both single and double strand breaks are inducible by irradiation. Thus, one of the evolutionary barriers is easily overcome by radiation.

Notwithstanding, evolution seems to have created a host of defenses against radiation carcinogenesis: (1) Most human genetic abnormalities are recessive traits that become phanerous only when the chromosomes are recessive homozygotes. (2) Most radiation-induced DNA lesions are repairable. (3) The DNA lesions occurring in testicular cells are not likely to be repaired, and these cells are apt to be lost through a particular process of cell death called apoptosis (Harrison 1975). In addition, DNA lesions produced in the spermatids are not repaired. Abrogation of such lesions, should fertilization take place, can be attained by either the repair enzymes of the ovum (Generoso *et al.* 1979) or abortion prior to implantation (Edmonds *et al.* 1982). (4) The human primordial oocytes residing in the peripheral circumference of the ovary contain "lampbrush chromosome loops" which are condensed and surrounded by a dense sheath of ribonucleoprotein (Fig. 3), making them radioresistant (Baker 1971). (5) Grave or fatal abnormalities may be deleted because the fetus cannot sustain life; they are therefore apt to be removed before birth. (6) Cancer may arise as the result of chromosomal aberrations in the somatic cells, whose number far surpasses that of the gonads. Thus, several lines of defense seem to have been designed to protect the human species from radiation; nevertheless, these are not sufficient to protect every survivor.

From the evolutionary point of view, radiation seems to have several important implications. Radiation events themselves are primarily nondiscriminating, and can act either advantagenously or disadvantageously, although most of them are harmful. In the long run, radiation helped to generate life in the primitive seas as it ionized water and other materials, causing the synthesis of a host of substances of biological significance, such as amino acids, although the primitive seas were reductive and could have contained insufficient molecular oxygen to actively propagate these ionizing effects. Radiation also promoted mutations. This may have been of limited significance until the advent of oxic atmospheres, where active oxygen molecules would have been abundant along the radiation pathways. As chemical reactions were promoted, so was the radiation damage to the

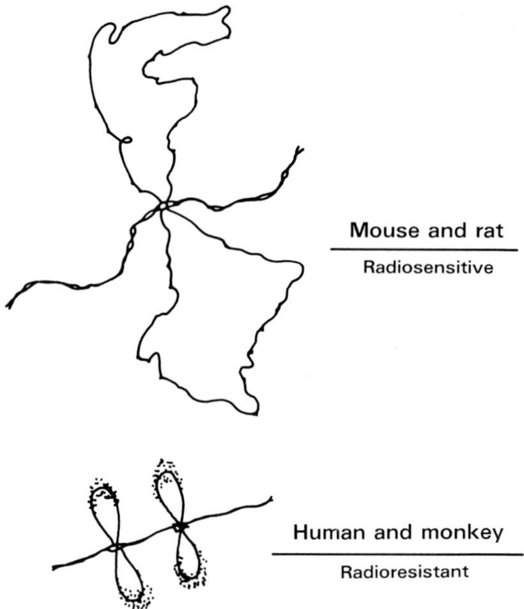

Fig. 3. The "lampbrush loop" for radioprotection of primate oocytes. This type of protection is not seen in rodents (Baker 1971). In terms of biological time, one day in the mouse corresponds to one month in the human (Makinodan 1977). Because the lifespan of primates is longer than that of rodents, the probability of DNA damage has to be reduced as much as possible. This would be the evolutionary meaning of the device.

genetic information, enticing *horror autotoxicus* (Kimball *et al.* 1976). Superoxid dismutase (SOD) seems to have been intended to cope with these active oxygen molecules (Asada 1976). The "rapid evolution" or induction of SOD and other enzymes that might be suited to the manipulation and detoxication of such toxic molecules is still observable among contemporary mammals (Cairns 1981); The acquisition of different capacities for the repair of DNA damage also has a long history of evolution: (1) the photoreactivation of ultraviolet damage, then (2) excision repair, (3) recombination repair, and most recently, (4) DNA redundancy (Kondo 1972). Thus, life seems to have struggled effectively with radiation.

Radiation Carcinogenesis as a Sequel to Abnormal Genes and/ or Untoward Expression of Proto-oncogenes

Why are the human DNAs packed separately in 46 chromosomes ? A logical classification and arrangement seems to be evidenced in the case of the sex chromosomes. The chromosomal mapping of the known oncogenes does not, however, inspire confidence in such a logical classification. Nature could have intentionally dissected and dispersed the oncogenes among the different chromosomes to reduce the probability of their association and resultant untoward activation. For example, a number of cell lines derived from Burkitt's lymphomas (BL) have a high frequency of translocation between chromosomes 8 and 14. Less frequent translocations occur between chromosomes 8 and 2, and 8 and 22. The human cellular oncogene *c-myc* is located on chromosome 8. The heavy chain immunoglobulin gene is located on chromosome 14, and the light chain kappa- and lambda-genes on chromosomes 2 and 22, respectively. The translocation between chromosomes 8 and 14 in BL translocates the *c-myc* proto-oncogene from chromosome 8 to the immunoglobulin region on chromosome 14 (Klein and Klein 1985). Nature has deliberately developed capping devices to suppress the inherited retinoblastoma genes: retinoblastomas arise as soon as the suppressive segments (*Rb*) are removed (Watson *et al*. 1987). Conversely, the chromosomes can be dissected in Fanconi's syndrome as a result of SOD and repair enzyme deficiencies. B lymphocytes are highly sensitive to radiation and the increased superoxide anions resulting from the SOD deficiency. The latter may encourage the emergence of leukemic cells by failing to block viral infections. Leukemic cells could also emerge should chromosomal defects happen to permit untoward activation and expression of leukemic proto-oncogenes. Chronic myelocytic leukemias are known to be an accumulation of chromosomal aberrations (Goldman 1986) that are targeted onto selected chromosomes (Huret *et al*. 1986). Similar changes certainly take place in the case of radiation damage to chromosomes, resulting in rearrangement, fragmentation, loss, exchange, translocation, and so on, eventually leading to *de novo* or untoward expression of oncogenes and carcinogenesis.

Further understanding of the process leading to carcinogenesis awaits future studies.

Evolutionary Aspects of Chemical Carcinogenesis

If we accept the concept that radiation effects are themselves chemocarcinogenetic, as discussed earlier, there are no essential conceptual differences in the understanding of carcinogenesis caused by chemicals except that the eventual effector substances could be generated through a paradoxical pathway also having an evolutionary history: the liver microsomal drug-metabolizing system (Goldstein *et al.* 1974). Alkylating agents such as cyclophosphamide, bleomycin, and cisplatin are radiomimetics, and they are capable of inducing double-strand breaks (Okuyama and Mishina 1980).

The oxidative metabolism of many drugs, including steroid hormones, is mediated by enzymes located in the microsomal fraction of mammalian liver, which consists of fragments of endoplasmic reticulum. The microsomes contain cytochrome P–450, which acts as the terminal oxidase for a variety of oxidative reactions undergone by drugs. The same situation applies not only to liver microsomes but also to those of the adrenal cortex, intestinal mucosa, and kidney. The primary purpose of the system is undoubtedly the detoxication of toxic substances. However, what would happen to the host if the chemical reactions led to the production of toxic substances as the result of the oxidation? This paradoxical situation occurs with most chemical carcinogens.

Chemical carcinogens may have been present even in the primitive seas, and the life forms existing then would have had to cope with them in one way or another. Figure 4 shows that there were several forms of P–450 enzymes (Sogawa 1986). Evolution was required to produce these endogenous metabolites in response to exogenous toxins. Bacterial P–450s were established during the pre-eukaryotic periods, and the steroidal types appeared as soon as the eukaryotes evolved, because steroids such as cholesterol are apparently indispensable to the formation of the flexible, dynamic membranes of these cells (Margulis 1981). The distinct evolution of the P–450s that deal with potentially carcinogenetic hydrocarbons seems to have taken place when the mammalians emerged

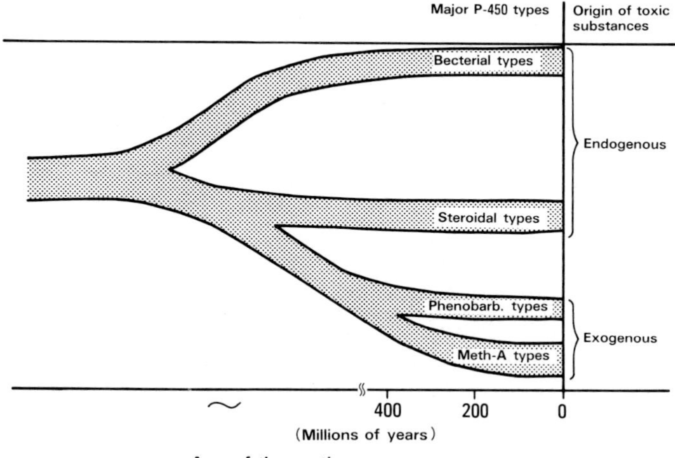

Fig. 4. Evolution of the drug-metabolizing system. There are four major enzyme types of P–450: bacterial and steroidal types for endogenous toxic substances, and phenobarbital and methyl-cholanthrene types for toxic substances of exogenous origin (Sogawa 1986). The latter types are of rather recent origin, but nonetheless far antedate modern civilization. Thus, chemical carcinogenesis may be the most recent, although its carcinogenetic mechanism of disintegration is one of the most archaic. Further evolution will be necessary to cope with current chemical carcinogens, unless we are able to develop adequate techniques of prophylaxis and decontamination (Modified from Sogawa, 1986).

and when atmospheric oxygen tension increased during the Carboniferous Period. Thus, chemical carcinogenesis may also have evolutionary significance.

Setala hypothesized a different process of carcinogenesis based on his experiments on chemical carcinogenesis (1984). It is intriguing that cancers may ensue when the *locus minoris* of symbiotic structures like the mitochondria is disordered. The end result is "devolution towards an ancient nucleated pre-eukaryotic level." We arrived independently at a similar anti-evolutionary concept of cancer. Based mainly on radiological evidence, we hypothesized that cancer develops to a state of increased water content, decreased SOD content, and defective excision repair (Okuyama and Mishina 1984b). The changes are thought to be characteristic of aquatic life, hidden and secure from life-threatening oxygen radicals and ultraviolet rays. In contrast to our hypothesis, Setala's cancer cells would lose water as a result of carcinogenesis. Nonetheless, his hypothesis should also be given due attention.

Harnessing the Emergence of Cancer *in vivo*

In spite of the progress of modern clinical oncology, the basic oncological sciences, and especially molecular biology, the entire phenomenon of carcinogenesis seems to remain shrouded in mystery, with occasional transparencies here and there. As shown elsewhere, taking an evolutionary view of the harnessing of carcinogenesis may again shed some light. There are several evolutionary categories that relate to the harnessing of carcinogenesis: DNA molecular, cellular, organic, and systemic. These will be discussed briefly below. They may also be suggestive of immediate clinical principles of anticancer therapy.

DNA Molecular Harnessing

Carcinogenesis may be genetically initiated in at least two ways: by the activation of the proto-oncogene(s) that have been present *a priori*, and by the disintegration of portions of DNA, possibly resulting in the *de novo* emergence of carcinogenetic information. The latter is a sequel of DNA damage from irradiation, chemical reactions, or improper repair. The net effect of irradiation is free radical toxicity, and the role of Cu,ZnSOD, which was acquired some 420 million years ago during the Carboniferous Period, cannot be overemphasized in the prevention of cancer. Many chemical reactions in the body produce free radicals, especially superoxide radicals that can be detoxified by Cu, ZnSOD. Therefore, Cu, ZnSOD contributes to the prevention of cancer. The distribution of SOD activity throughout the body appears to vary from organ to organ, yet it may follow a rule of evolutionary significance, as surmised from clinical data (Sykes *et al.* 1978; Okuyama and Mishina 1985h): atmospheric oxygen could have increased with the increasing age of the earth, culminating around the Carboniferous Period, when the atmospheric concentration of oxygen was such that it was possible for large animals to live on land (homeothermic life). At the same time, Cu, ZnSOD was acquired to alleviate possible damage from oxygen toxicity. Oxygen toxicity may be one of the most archaic forms of carcinogenesis, one that could have existed long before the separation of plant and animal phyla: the genes coded for excision repair are present in both phyla, and those of the mammalians have recently been shown to be largely homologous to those of yeast (van Duin et al. 1986). Excision repair is estimated to have been acquired 2.8 billion years ago (Kondo 1973).

The proto-oncogenes of most mammalian species have

Table 5. Similarity of amino acid sequences of *ras* proto-oncogene products

The results seem to suggest that similarity may exist among the original *ras* proto-oncogenes (Fukui 1985). Thus, this genetic information can be essential to life, and 6 conserved from species to species, and from generation to generation.

```
H-ras:  1~ 40:            MTEYKLVVVGAGGVGKSALTIQLIQNHFVDEYDPTIEDSY
SPRAS:  1~ 45:       MRSTYLREYKLVVVGDGGVGKSALTIQLIQSHFVDEYDPTIEDSY
YRAS1:  1~ 47: MQGNKSTIREYKIVVVGGGGVGKSALTIQFIQSYFVDGYDPTIEDSY
YRAS2:  1~ 47: MPLNKSNIREYKLVVVGGGGVGKSALTIQLTQSHFVDEYDPTIEDSY

H-ras: 41~ 87: RKQVVIDGETCLLDILDTAGQEEYSAMRDQYMRTGEGFLCVFAINNT
SPRAS: 46~ 92: RKKCEIDGEGALLDVLDTAGQEEYSAMREQYMRTGEGFLLVYNITSR
YRAS1: 48~ 94: RKQVVIDDKVSILDILDTAGQEEYSAMREQYMRTGEGFLLVYSVTSR
YRAS2: 48~ 94: RKQVVIDDEVSILDILDTAGQEEYSAMREQYMRNGEGFLLVYSITSK

H-ras: 88~133: KSFEDIHQYREQIKRVKDSDDVPMVLVGNKCDLAARTVESRQ-AQDL
SPRAS: 93~139: SSFDEISTFYQQILRVKDKDTFPVVLVANKCDLEAERVVSRREGEQL
YRAS1: 95~141: NSFDELLSIYQQIQRVKDSDYIPVVVVGNKLDLENERQVSYEDGLRL
YRAS2: 95~141: SSLDELMTYYQQILRVKDTDYVPIVVVGNKSDLENEKVVSYQDGLNM

H-ras:134~180: ARSYGIPYIETSAKTRQGVEDAFYTLVREIRQHKLRKLNPPDESGPG
SPRAS:140~186: AKSMHCLYVETSAKLRLNVEEAFYSLVRTIRRYNKSEEKGFQNKQAV
YRAS1:142~188: AKQLDAPFLETSAKQAINVDEAFYSLIRLVRDDGGKYNSMNRQLDNT
YRAS2:142~188: AKQMDAPFLETSAKQAINVEEAFYTLARLVRDEGGKYNKTLTENDNS

H-ras:181~185: CMSCK----------------------------------------
SPRAS:187~214: QIAQVPASTAKRASAVNNSKTEDEVSTK------------------.
YRAS1:189~235: NEIRDSELTSSATADIEKKNNGSYVLDNSLTNAGTGSSSKSAVNHNG
YRAS2:189~235: KQTSQDTKGSGANSVPRNSGGHRKMSNAANGKNVNSSTTVVNARNAS

H-ras:185~185: ---------------------------------------------
SPRAS:214~214: ---------------------------------------------
YRAS1:236~282: ETTKRTDEKNYVNQNNNNEGNTKYSSNGNGNRSDISRGNQNNALNSR
YRAS2:236~282: IESKTGLAGNEATNGKTQTVRTNIDNSTGQAGQANAQSANTVNNRVN

H-ras:186~189: -----------------------------------------CVLS
SPRAS:215~219: ----------------------------------------CCVIC
YRAS1:283~309: SKNSAEPNKNSSANARKEY-----------------SGGCCIIC
YRAS2:283~322: VNSKAGQVSNAKQARKQQAAPGGNTSEASKSGSGGCCIIS
```

been shown to be homologous to those of yeast (Table 5). There is also homology between avians and vertebrates (Sheiness and Bishop 1979) and primates and humans (Fig. 5) (Gallo *et al.* 1977). These proto-oncogenes may have been assigned one or two functions other than oncogenesis: *sis* for PDGF (platelet-derived growth factor; *erb B* for receptors for EGF (epithelial growth factor) (Waterfield 1986). In other words, their oncogenetic acquisition may be a disintegration secondary to insults from irradiation and chemical carcinogens. For instance, point mutations in the codons of proto-oncogenes are reported to result in their activation (Table 6) (Yuasa 1985). Thus, carcinogenesis through proto-oncogene activation may produce special, definite variants of the disintegrative type of cancer. This type may be slightly newer than the other type of disintegrative carcinogenesis. Nevertheless, the harnessing mechanism is repair of the DNA damage, especially excision repair.

Repair may take place in intermitotic cells. However, it

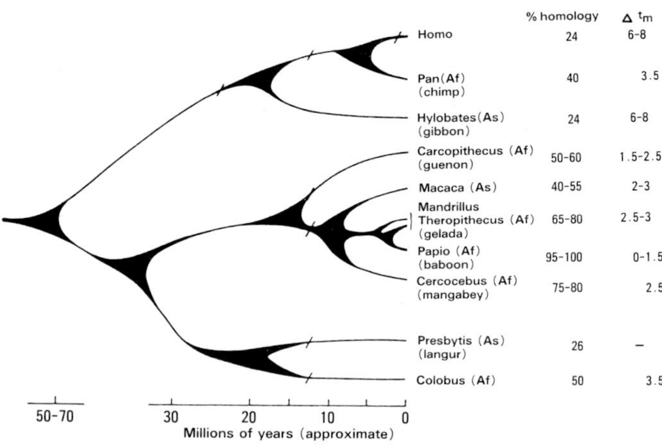

Fig. 5. Phylogenetic comparison of sequence homology of baboon virogenes in primates. Percent homology is determined by percent of ^{125}I-labeled BaEV RNA hybridized to DNA from a particular primate, normalized to percent RNA hybridized to DNA from baboons. t_m was the difference between t_m (midpoint of thermal transition) of hybrids formed with BaEV RNA and DNA of a particular primate and that of hybrids formed with BaEV RNA and DNA from baboons (Gallo *et al.* 1977). The comparison indicates conservation of the virogenes across the species barrier.

Table 6. Point mutations in *ras* transforming genes in humans

Transforming gene	Tumor	Codon	Base change	Amino acid change
H–*ras*				
T24	Bladder cancer	12	G → T	Gly → Val
Hs 242	Lung cancer	61	A → T	Gln → Leu
SK–2	Melanoma	61	A → T	Gln → Leu
Hs 0578T	Mammary cancer	12	G → A	Gly → Asp
K–*ras*				
Calu–1	Lung cancer	12	G → T	Gln → Gys
SW–480	Colon cancer	12	G → T	Gly → Val
PR 371	Lung cancer	12	G → T	Gly → Cys
PR 310	Lung cancer	61	A → T	Gln → His
N–*ras*				
SK–N–SH	Neuroblastoma	61	C → A	Gln → Lys
SW–1271	Lung cancer	61	A → G	Gln → Arg
HT 1080	Fibrosarcoma	61	C → A	Gln → Lys
PA 1	Teratoma	12	G → A	Gly → Asp

Bases: A=adenine; C=cytosine; G=guanine; and T=thymine.
Amino acids: Gly=glycine; Gln=glutamine; Arg=arginine; Asp=aspartae; Cys=cystein; Glu=glutamic acid; His=histidine; Leu=leucine; Lys=lysine; and Val=valine. (Reproduced from Yuasa, 1985)

would be more efficient if the problem cells were in cell cycle because they progress through the S phase of DNA synthesis. Conversely, cells in the S phase are usually the most radio-resistant (Watanabe 1982). In the ovary, oocytes are protected from radiation damage by special protein surrounding the DNA, the "lampbrush" loop (Fig. 3) (Baker 1971). With spermatids, the repair of DNA damage may be further accomplished with the help of repair enzymes in the partner ovum (Generoso *et al.* 1979).

The evolutionary hypothesis of nonepithelial-epithelial tumor shift should be recalled here. This hypothesis postulates that the oncogenetic mechanisms for these nonepithelial tumors are much simpler and/or the number of steps in carcinogenesis is fewer than in the epithelial tumors. Nowell suggested many years ago that human tumors with minimal chromosomal change (diploid acute leukemia, chronic granulocytic leukemia) are early in clonal evolution, while human solid cancers, typically highly aneuploid, are late in the developmental process (1976). Based on cancer incidence data, most leukemias are believed to result from the accumulation of two to four specific mutations within a single cell, while carcinomas may require anywhere from two to six or seven (Watson *et al.* 1987). Thus, host animals may be protected against carcinogenesis by at least two to seven anti-oncogene or mutation barriers.

Oncogenic retroviral infection constitutes one of the newest modes of carcinogenesis in the sense that the retroviruses are of very recent origin: the retroviruses related to *homo sapiens* could have emerged together with human beings (Matthews 1983). Retroviral infection is imported by oncogenes. It is a "genetic" disorder, but its prevention may be achieved by specific antiviral immunity through vaccination in the near future. Intervention is being carried out by discouraging breastfeeding by mothers who have been shown to be carriers of retroviruses like HTLV (Ando *et al.* 1986).

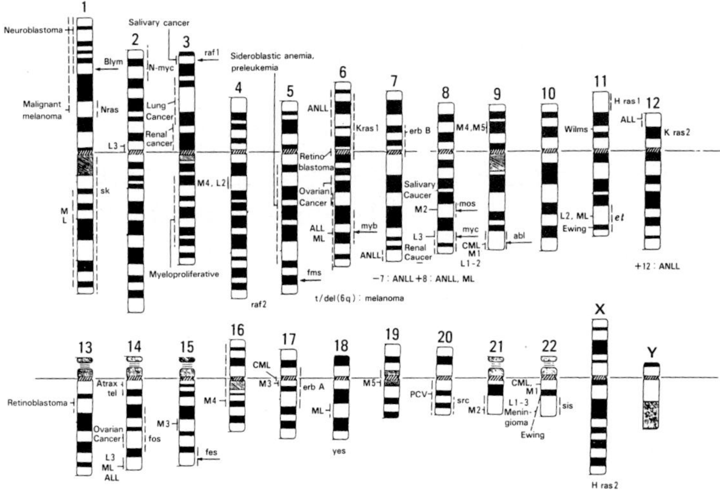

Fig. 6. Widespread distribution of proto-oncogenes and breakpoints in specific chromosome rearrangements: a probable deliberate anticancer device of nature. The design seems to discourage untoward activation of the proto-oncogenes. Conversely, deletion, translocation, and rearrangement of portions of the chromosomes would facilitate their activation (Sugiyama *et al.* 1985). This type of protective mechanism could have evolved together with the preservation of the proto-oncogenes.

Chromosomal Harnessing of Carcinogenesis

The first chromosomal mechanism for harnessing carcinogenesis is the duplication of genetic information, which obviously has definite advantages for the preservation of that information. A special mechanism of protection, segregation, and preservation of the master DNA strands is also probable (Cairns 1975).

The next mechanism is the separation and distribution of the candidate proto-oncogenes among a larger number of chromosomes (Fig. 6). The same principle can be further expanded by spacing the individual codons or groups of codons in the functional gene units (Fig. 7) (Waterfield 1985). Table 7 lists the neoplasms known for consistent chromosomal defects. Among them, retinoblastoma deserves special comment. Mutations at *Rb-1* are recessive, and their effect may arise through removal of the corresponding normal allele or homozygosity. Recessive mutations that predispose to cancer may be common to many different forms of neo-

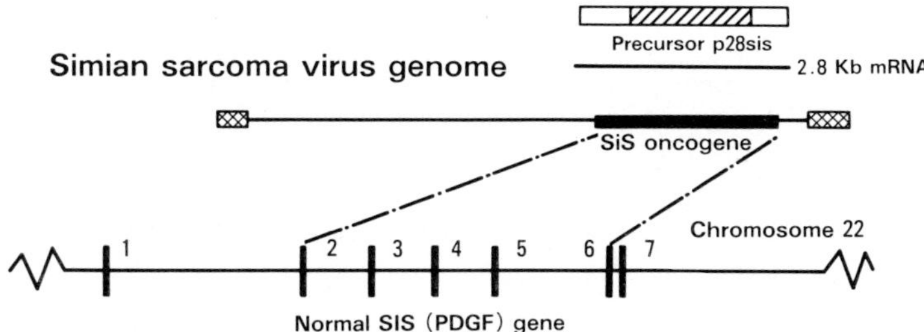

Fig. 7. Molecular anatomy of the *sis* genes. The structures are represented as lines which indicate nucleic acid or protein sequences. The solid bars or boxes are coding sequences of the genes. The crosshatched areas are virus LTRs (long terminal repeats) and the shaded regions are biologically active peptides (Waterfield 1986). The normal *sis* (PDGF) gene consists of several informative codons that are separated and spaced by the noninformative ones. This design may well reduce the probability of untoward activation of this information, or expose the process of sequential activation to surveillance, should such a mechanism exist. Conversely, an efficient way of making use of the information would be to put everything close together with appropriate spacing, as in the case of the *sis* oncogene. This is one of the intrachromosomal harnessing mechanisms.

Table 7. Neoplasms with a known consistent chromosome defect

Disease	Chromosome defect	Breakpoints or deletion
Leukemias		
Chronic myelogenous leukemia	t (9;22)	9q34.1 and 22q11.21
Acute nonlymphocytic leukemia		
M1	t (9;22)	9q34.1 and 22q11.21
M2	t (8; 21)	8q22.1 and 21q22.3
M3	t (15; 17)	15q22 and 17q11.2
M4	inv 16	p13.2 and q22
M4, M5	t (9; 11)	9p22 and 11q23
M1, M2, M4, M5, M6	del 5q	5q22q23
	del 7q	7q33q36
	+8	
Chronic lymphocytic leukemia	+12	
	t (11;14)	11q13 and 14q32
Acute lymphocytic leukemia		
L1–L2	t (9; 22)	9q34.1 and 22q11.21
L2	t (4; 11)	4q21 and 11q23
L3	t (8; 14)	8q24.13 and 14q32.33
Lymphomas		
Burkitt's, small noncleaved cell (non-Burkitt), large-cell immunoblastic	t (8; 14)	8q24.13 and 14q32.33
Follicular small cleaved, follicular mixed, and follicular large cell	t (14; 18)	14q32.3 and 18q21.3
Small-cell lymphocytic	+12	
Small-cell lymphocytic, transformed to diffuse large cell	t (11; 14)	11q13 and 14q32
Carcinomas		
Neuroblastoma, disseminated	del 1p	1p31p36
Small-cell lung carcinoma	del 3p	3p14p23
Papillary cystadenocarcinoma of ovary	t (6;14)	6q21 and 14q24
Constitutional retinoblastoma	del 13q	13q14.13
Retinoblastoma	del 13q	13q14
Aniridia-Wilms' tumor	del 11p	11p13
Wilms' tumor	del 11p	11p13
Benign Solid Tumors		
Mixed parotid gland tumor	t (3; 8)	3p25 and 8q21
Meningioma	−22	22

(Watson *et al.* 1987)

plasms (Watson *et al.* 1987). In other words, one or two key chromosomal safeguards may have evolved to prevent untoward activation of the proto-oncogenes (Ohno 1971).

Cellular and Organic Harnessing of Carcinogenesis

Cellular and organic harnessing of carcinogenesis consists of a system of mechanisms that provides topical eradication of abnormal cells that emerge as a result of oncogenic changes in the DNA and chromosomes.

The probable harnessing mechanisms for each organ are listed in Table 8. Many of these devices are self-explanatory. The basic principle of harnessing carcinogenesis at the organ level is rapid cell renewal accompanied by effective cellular exfoliation. The small intestine, for example, is an organ of rapid renewal and exfoliation that is seldom associated with primary malignancies.

Nature has provided three major ways of diminishing the

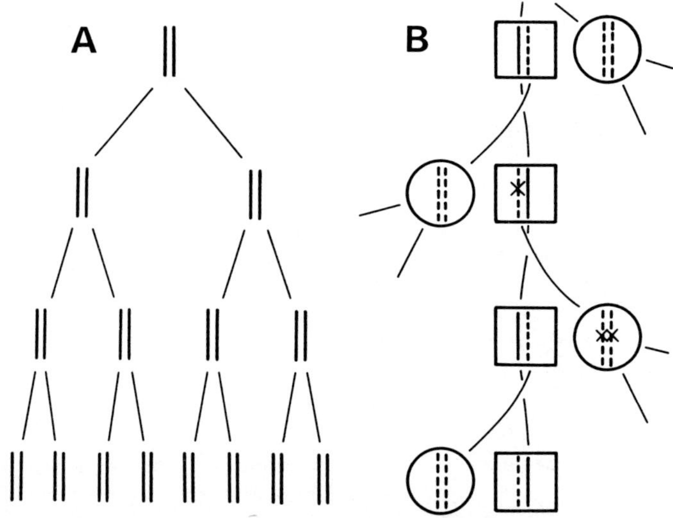

Fig. 8. The lineage of DNA undergoing semi-conservative replication. A. The segregation of a mutation, X, that arose as a copying error during duplication. B. Rearrangement of this lineage to fit the observation that parental strands segregate alternately to the right and left of the plane. Stem cells (—) keep the same parental DNA strands through successive cycles (Cairns 1975).

Table 8. Harnessing carcinogenesis through elimination of abnormalities *in vivo*

	Organ	Mode of elimination	Failing mechanism or predispositon
Evolutiona- rily secured	Testis	Exteriorization* Apoptosis	Orchism (seminoma)
	Ovary	Lampbrush loop (oocytes)* Graafian follicle*	
Mammalian symbol	Breast Cervix Endo- metrium	Cyclic growth and exfoliation	Hyperestrogenism and hypergonado- tropinism; viral dur- ing reproductiveness
	Prostate	——	Hypergonado- tropinism
Homeo- thermic	Lung Thyroid	—— ——	Squamous metaplasia ——
	Skin	Desquamation	Loss of polarity (a- melanotic melanoma)
Poililo- thermic	Stomach	Exfoliation Apoptosis	Atrophic gastritis Intestinal metaplasia "Closed loops" Post-ulcer cancer
	Liver Small intestine	Slow renewal Exfoliation	Retrovirus (HB) Practically no "closed loops"
	Colon	Exfoliation Colonic transit Gallbladder	Cholecystectomy and gallstones
	Brain	Blood-brain barrier* On-demand activity* Prostaglandin D_2	No BBB (meningioma)
	Kidney Bone	Cyclic activity* Growth and remodeling	
Prevertebral	Blood cells (Leukemias)	Maturation, senes- cence, and ex- foliation	Failed maturation (acute forms; CML) Failed senescence (CLL)
	(Lymphomas)	Maturation and senescence Apoptosis	Persistent stimulation

 * Devices that prevent the genesis of DNA damage.

rate at which mutants accumulate (Cairns 1975): (1) restrict-ing the number of stem cells; (2) adopting a special pattern of segregation of DNA strands to conserve the old strands (Fig. 8); and (3) compartmentalizing cells to facilitate exfolia-tion or desquamation. The mechanism of segregative conser-vation helps to exclude mutations arising in the new DNA strands during DNA synthesis.

When the mechanisms of exfoliation or desquamation are deranged in one way or another, cancerous foci may emerge. Abnormal cells lose their power of orientation as a result of loss of polarity, i.e., the ability of the cell to direct itself toward the direction from which oxygen and nutrients come, or conversely, in a cancer cell, to be able to sense the direc-tion of hypoxia and hyponutrition. This confusion of polarity may lead to retrograde procession of the abnormal cells. In the amelanotic melanomas, the cells would not advance toward the outer layers of the skin, but would move deep into the skin without exfoliating (Takahashi and Seiji 1983). In stomach cancer, a closed-loop mechanism would hold can-cer cells in the epithelium and prevent exfoliation (Fig. 9) (Fujita 1983). The surrounding soft tissue may also lose com-partmentalization capacity as the result of irradiation (Tsu-bouchi and Matsuzawa 1972). Thus, geography is important in the prevention of cancer phanerosis.

This principle, but in functional terms, may also apply to maturation and senescence as they constitute portions of cell renewal. Cells from acute forms of leukemia can be induced to "differentiate," eventually terminating themselves; there-fore, they could have defective maturational mechanisms (Sachs 1978). In contrast, cells from chronic lymphocytic leu-kemia (CLL) are "mature," yet they would not die off, in spite of their expected normal life span, and would accumu-late in the circulatory system. This could be one of the main reasons for the success of extracorporeal irradiation of blood in treating CLL. Although extracorporeal irradiation kills cir-culating CLL cells, it does not induce any compensatory in-crease in cellular proliferation in the CLL stem cell pool (Cronkite 1967; Schiffer 1968). Apoptosis originally implied the death of single cells within a solid organ, especially at the end of their normal life span (Lennox and Lennox 1986).

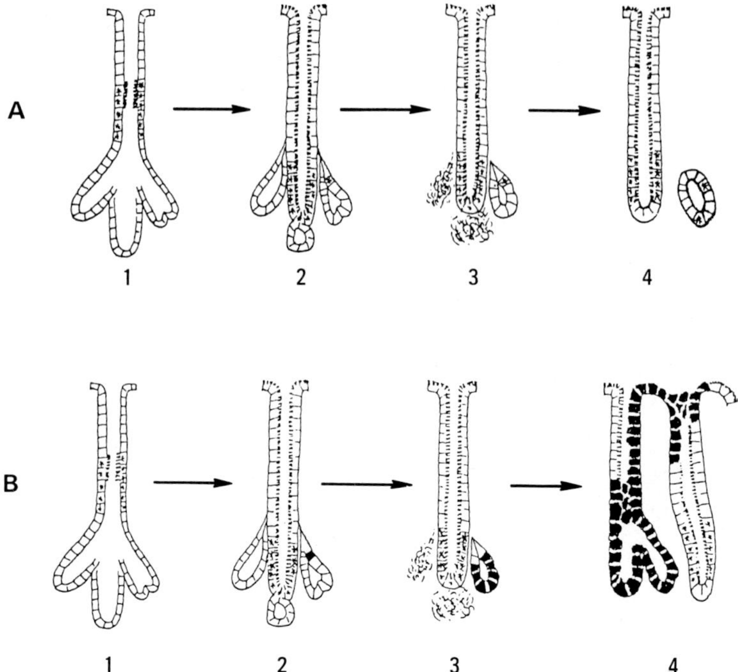

Fig. 9. Intestinal metaplasia as a carcinogenetic mechanism in the stomach. Stomach cancers may arise as a result of intestinal metaplasia. A. Natural progression of intestinal metaplasia in the human stomach. The epithelium of the intestinal metaplasia is shown with the brush border. It starts at the height of the generative cell zone and propagates upwards (1), and then slowly downwards (2). As the metaplasia progresses, the surplus glandular branches exfoliate. Those embedded in the depths of the mucosa are likely to be retained as blind glandular fragments (3). Most of the latter disappear. However, should they contain generative cells, they would persist and continue to grow, forming microcysts (4). This is a closed-loop mechanism. B. Transformation of the intestinal metaplasia into adenocarcinoma. If a cancer cell appears in the metaplasia (1), it will propagate and establish itself as a solid cancer when it is retained in a microcyst without exfoliation (Fujita 1983). Thus, exfoliation may be one of the natural harnessing mechanisms of the renewing systems which can be annihilated by the closed-loop mechanism.

However, the use of this word is being expanded. According to Kerr and Searle (1980), apoptosis occurs in neoplasms following anticancer chemotherapy or irradiation, and following treatment with corticosteroids or even hyperthermia to 43°C (Kerr and Searle 1980). Apoptosis takes place in two distinct phases (Fig. 10). In the first phase, the cells condense and bud to produce many membrane-enclosed apoptotic bodies. In the second, these bodies are phagocytosed and digested by nearby tissue cells. This occurs in normal tissues, for example, in the formation of interdigital clefts during embryogenesis. The process may be physiological with the corticosteroids in the sense that they enable the host animal to adapt to acute emergencies requiring a supply of energy at the cost

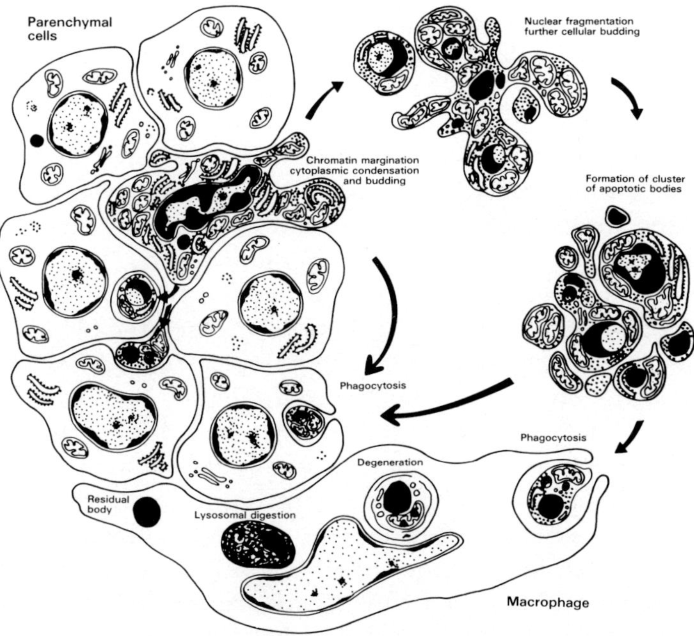

Fig. 10. Apoptosis as a means of harnessing carcinogenesis. The processes of apoptosis have been described (Kerr and Searle 1980). Untoward hypersecretion of corticosteroids during stress may contribute to the apoptosis of sensitive cell populations such as lymphocytes and testicular cells, and help to harness carcinogenesis in such sensitive cell populations.

of host cells such as lymphocytes, as well as prompting glycolysis (Kobayashi 1980): The target cells are destroyed and phagocytosed. This phenomenon thus has evolutionary implications.

Prostaglandin D_2 deserves special comment here. This substance appears to be ubiquitous in the brain. It is a neuromodular, and depolarizes cells (Shimizu *et al.* 1979). In terms of clinical biology, it is capable of affecting cells by modifying the cellular membrane charge. It can reduce the capacity of cancer cells to metastasize (Stringfellow and Fitzpatrick 1979; Fitzpatrick and Stringfellow 1979), and may induce redifferentiation of cancer cells (Okuyama and Mishina 1985f, g; Okuyama *et al.* 1985b). The same mechanism must be activated in the control of carcinogenesis in the central nervous system, where the tumor incidence is as low as 1.0 to 4.1 ASR (age-adjusted standard rates) World for Japanese males, as compared with the incidence of stomach cancer as high as 75 to 88 ASR World (Waterhous *et al.* 1982).

The higher the temperature, the greater the internal energy of molecules, the greater the probability of chemical reactions, and the greater the number of free radicals generated. The organs that hold vital genetic information, such as the testis and ovary, have to be protected from such radicals. The testis is exteriorized, in spite of the greater likelihood of trauma, to secure efficient cooling of the organ. In the ovary, the ova are encased in layers of follicular cells to prevent direct contact with the well-oxygenated blood and avoid assaults by free radicals, such as superoxide anions, and other chemical insults. Similar but more highly compromised devices are feasible in other organ systems. The blood-brain barrier, on-demand activity of the brain, and cyclic activation of the renal parenchyma can thus be accounted for. Studies on experimental animals indicate that SOD activities are low in these organs (Peeters-Joris *et al.* 1975; Peskin *et al.* 1977). Conversely, untoward activation of proto-oncogenes may occur in the generation of meningiomas because of the absence of such barriers to the meninx.

The carcinogenetic potential of bile acids may be evaded by the relatively rapid colonic transit of fecal material through the aid of "fibers." This effect can be offset by chole-cystectomy and/or cholelithiasis (Narisawa 1983).

The slow cell renewal of the liver may be an important factor in harnessing hepatomagenesis from HLV, for the latter is a weak oncogene whose infection would take many years to establish hepatomas.

Thus, evolution seems to have deliberately developed a set of cellular and organic devices to counteract the menace of carcinogenesis, however inadequate they might be.

Evolutionary Age of Neoplasms

Once we accept that the different anticancer mechanisms emerged and evolved at different times in evolutionary history, it is natural to speculate on the possible discrimination of neoplasms in terms of evolutionary age. Figure 3 in Chapter 3 shows the probable evolution of different types of neoplasms: disintegrative, compensatory, and infective. As was noted earlier, this categorization reflects the history of mechanisms for repairing DNA damage on the chromosomes, the evolution of the immune systems, and the assumption that viruses have their origins in the DNA molecules of their respective hosts and that the retroviruses are therefore the most recent. The disintegrative type of neoplasms, the oldest type, can be expanded to include cancers resulting from chemical carcinogens as well as radiation. As evolution proceeds, so is carcinogenesis itself likely to proceed, whatever the inducing agents and amplifying mechanisms.

Chapter 6

Cancer as a Metabolic Host: Devolution of Cancer in Biochemistry and Cachexia

> *The evolution of the basic syntheses pro-*
> *ceeded in a stepwise manner, involving*
> *one mutation at a time, but the order of*
> *attainment of individual steps—in the*
> *reverse direction from that in which the*
> *synthesis proceeds in the chain.*
> ——*H. N. Horowitz*, Biochemistry,
> 1945

Cancer cells seem to proliferate rapidly, have a high-pitched metabolism, and, through exploitation of the host, lead to cachexia. As reported elsewhere (Baserga 1965), it has long been assumed that cancer cells proliferate more rapidly than normal cells. Clinical observation shows that cancer patients may die even in the absence of overt malnutrition or cachexia, especially after the advent of intravenous hyperalimentation. This is true even in the absence of any appreciable infections or hemorrhagic episodes. In an experimental setting, ascites hepatoma cells have been shown to survive and proliferate under practical anoxia (Okuyama and Mishina 1985a; Okuyama *et al.* 1988). The cell cycle times of cancers are much longer than those of normal cell renewal systems (Sasaki *et al.* 1981). Finally, cancer cells are more vulnerable to oxygen toxicity (Oberley and Buettner 1979; Okuyama and Mishina 1981a). To reconcile these contradictions, one extreme can be taken as the norm, the other as a variant. Another way of handling the problem may be to take an evolutionary perspective.

Hypoxic Milieu as the Primary Cancer Environment

An interesting experiment was performed in the mouse (Denekampf *et al.* 1983): a tumor was subcutaneously transplanted in such a way that occlusion of its nourishing artery for as long as 18 hours eventually led to its complete sterilization. The tumor cells survived up to eight hours of occlusion (Fig. 1). Table 1 shows the data from gas and glucose analyses of ascites hepatoma cells *in vivo* during the phase of exponential growth (Okuyama and Mishina 1985d; Okuyama *et al.* 1988). Cancer cells *may* survive and proliferate under anoxia, in the absence of glucose, and during the log phase of rapid cellular proliferation. Cancer cells are sensitive to free-radical toxicity: cell kill from superoxide toxicity has been induced by inactivating superoxide dismutase (Cu, ZnSOD) with D-penicillamine (Okuyama and Mishina 1981a). Most tumor angiographic patterns seem to be in good agreement with these observations. As seen in Fig. 2, the tumor vascula-

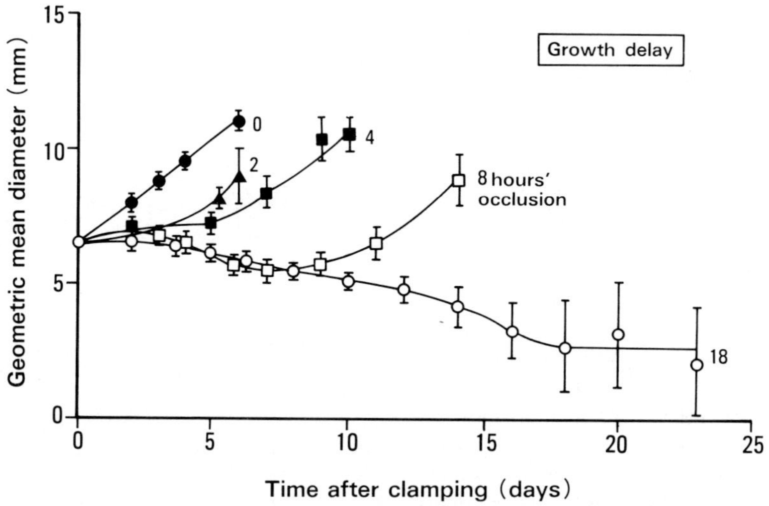

Fig. 1. Cancer as a hypoxic, hyponutritious, metabolic host (1): Vascular occlusion and tumor cell death. Growth curves for subcutaneous tumors measured *in situ* after no treatment (●) or after the specified period of vascular occlusion. Occlusion for 2hr (▲), 4 hr (■), 8hr (□) and 18hr (○). Clamping for periods of up to 8 hr induced a delay in tumor growth. Longer periods induced permanent disappearance of some of the treated tumors (Denekampf *et al.* 1983). It should be emphasized that the relevant vascular system is definitely effective in sterilizing the transplanted tumor when occluded, and that the cancer cells could still survive up to 8 hr. Such morbid cells are thus potentially capable of surviving the hypoxic milieu (see Table 1).

Table 1. Exponential growth of AH109A cells *in vivo*. In the peritoneum, the cells were grown under hypoxia to anoxia and hyponutrition. The ascites were aspirated on days 3 and 4 of transplantation when the cancer cells grew exponentially.

	pH	pCO_2	pO_2	Glucose	MDA
Blood	7.3±0.1	53.0±18.5	43.4±15.0	120±14	2.0±0
	(6)	(6)	(6)	(3)	(2)
Ascites	6.8±0.1	111.4±19.8	0.35±0.25	2.5±0.7	1.8±0.1
	(4)	(4)	(4)	(2)	(2)

♯) mmHg (pCO_2, pO_2), ♯2) mg/dl (glucose), ♯3) mcg/ml (MDA). (Okuyama *et al.* 1988d).

Figures in parentheses are the numbers of rats employed.

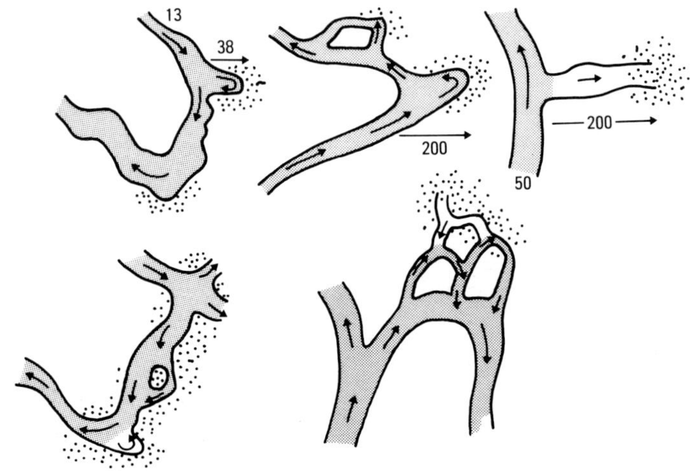

Fig. 2. Cancer as a hypoxic, hyponutritious, metabolic host (2): Tumor neovascularization (1). The cancer cells surrounding the host capillaries appear to entice budding of the vascular sprouts (neovascularization) (Yamaura 1971; Denekampf and Hobson 1982). The responsible factor(s) is known as TAF (tumor angiogenesis factor) (Folkman *et al.* 1971) or angiogenenin (Fett *et al.* 1985; Strydom *et al.* 1985; Kurachi *et al.* 1985). However, these tumor vessels will not mature into arterioles or venules (Algire and Chalkley 1945). (by courtsey of the author, Yamaura 1971)

ture is formed from the host capillaries by tumor angiogenesis factor (TAF) (Yamaura and Sato 1973; Folkman *et al.* 1971; Langer *et al.* 1980; Fett *et al.* 1985; Strydom *et al.* 1985; Kurachi *et al.* 1985). Tumor vasculature is characterized by abrupt sprouting and arborescence of numerous fine

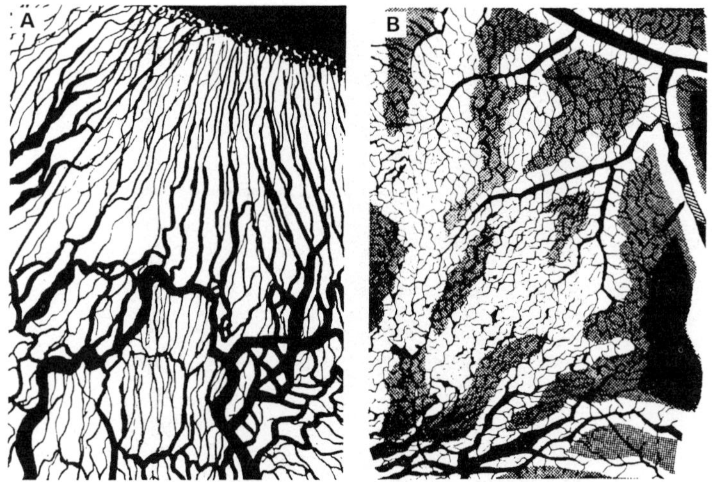

Fig. 3. Cancer as a hypoxic, hyponutritious, metabolic host (3): Tumor neovascularization (2). A. Normal capillary growth in response to tissue injury in the center. B. Cancerous capillary growth in response to tissue injury. Abrupt, fine, short arborescence is conspicuous (Yamaura 1971). This type of vascular change could cause the blood pressure to drop precipitously (Suwa *et al.* 1963).

vessels (Fig. 3) (Yamaura 1971). The factor, however, is not capable of allowing the vessels to mature into larger arterioles or venules (Algire and Chalkley 1945). A second factor may also be elaborated by the tumor to transform the larger vessels into less prominent ones. Figure 4 shows that the vasculature nourishing a hepatoma is characterized by an abrupt, proliferative outburst of fine arborescence. This design is well suited to reducing the blood pressure. Although the study in question was performed on normal arteries and arterioles, the reduction in the vasculature from 100 μm to 10 μm in diameter would be an efficient means causing the blood pressure to fall (Suwa *et al.* 1963).

Yet another mechanism appears to induce reduction in blood pressure in the tumor: the medial loss of elasticity (Fig. 5) (Suzuki *et al.* 1987). The arterial media of a normal host liver consist of numerous smooth muscle cells and scanty elastic fibers. However, as they approach the cancer, the media become thinner by losing the muscle cells, and in the actual vicinity of the tumor they are completely replaced by collage-

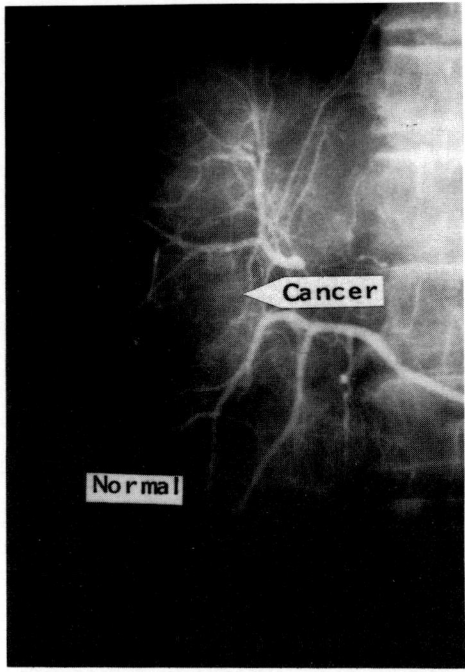

Fig. 4. Cancer as a hypoxic, hyponutritious, metabolic host (4): A. Tumor angiography in a patient with hepatoma. Abrupt, fine arborescence could effectively induce the required hypoxic microenvironment. B. Other attributes of tumor angiography, tumor stain, blood pooling, and spiral tortuosity may result from extraordinarily slowed traverse of the contrast media, trapping of the media in areas of central necrosis, and pressure from the surrounding tissue, respectively. Thus, angiographic diagnosis itself may have an evolutionary basis.

nous fibers, with practically no muscle cells remaining in the arterioles. The thinning appears most striking at vascular radii of 100 μm. This type of change may be brought about by factors such as toxohormone (Nakahara and Fukuoka 1961).

These mechanisms would help to more evenly distribute both oxygen and nutrients among the enormous number of cells. A hypoxic milieu would thus be secured in which the tumor cells would enjoy an environment containing fewer active oxygen molecules like superoxide radicals, to which tumor cells are so sensitive (Cole *et al.* 1972; Oberley and

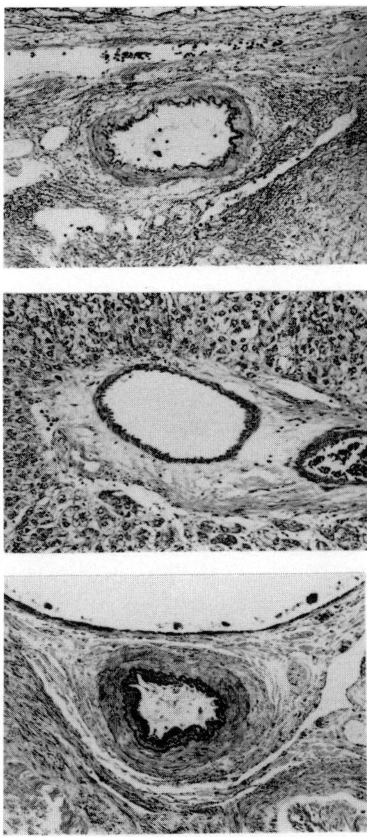

Fig. 5. Cancer as a hypoxic, hyponutritious, metabolic host (5): Hepatic arterioles, about 50 μm in radius, with differently developed muscular layers. Elastic-Goldner stain. A. An arteriole in a normal liver equipped with fully developed media. B. Lean muscular layer in a "tumor vessel" found in a nodule of hepatocellular carcinoma. C. A tumor-feeding hepatic arteriole in the vicinity of the tumor; the media appear thinner than in the normal control. Thus, host arterioles could have modified themselves in the presence of cancer (Suzuki *et al.* 1987). The probable contribution of TAF (angiogenin) and/or other humoral factors from the tumor should be considered along with any mechanical, hemodynamic feedback effects. Replacement of the media with collagenous tissue may imply that the medial content of SOD is less than normal in cancer patients as a result of the remote effect of cancer or toxohormone (Leuthauser *et al.* 1984) and that the resultant superoxide damage to the media could have been followed by collagenous replacement, as in the case of closure of the ductus arteriosus of Botallo (Frazer and Brady 1978).

Buettner 1979; Okuyama and Mishina 1981a; Urbach 1956). This kind of environment would be of crucial importance in preserving the genetic integrity of DNA, especially when the population itself contains "stem cells," but not the differentiated cells that eventually die off. Such an environment would also provide a peaceful milieu in which host agents like hormones would not cause any turmoil. Thus, cancer cells could obtain a hermitage for themselves.

The liability of malignant transformation of benign tumors is well-known. One of the greatest differences between malignant and normal cells is the former's loss of sensitivity to the direction from which oxygen and nutrients arrive, a kind of loss of polarity or escape from the effects of polarity. As shown in Fig. 6, the tumor cells at the brink of malignant transformation move out of their expected positions (Okuyama *et al.* 1988), possibly migrating toward areas where the oxygen tension is greatly reduced and which would therefore provide shelters from superoxide anions and other active oxygen moieties. Such cells may cluster as they migrate, forming tumorous nodules in secure, hypoxic areas of lowered toxicity (Tsubouchi and Matsuzawa 1973).

In contrast to the above, the SOD activity of leukemic cells is reported to be greatly increased (Yamanaka *et al.* 1979). This contradiction may be nothing but a whimsical variation, or the change may represent something important: recent evolutionary adaptation following the acute rise in atmospheric oxygen. The leukemic cells would have had to adapt to the oxic status of the circulating hyperoxic blood as they traversed the body by increasing SOD activity. This type of adaptation is well explained by the shortened cell cycle time (16.5 hr for normoblast, Bond *et al.* 1958) as compared with that for fibroblast (30 hr, Zosimovska *et al.* 1956). The intratumoral distribution of oxygen, however, may also be highly nonhomogeneous (Cole *et al.* 1983), and this type of adaptation may have taken place in cancer cells as quickly as it did in normal mammalian cells (Kimball *et al.* 1977).

Cancer Metabolism under Hypoxia

Hypoxic life is common in a host of animals (Hochachka

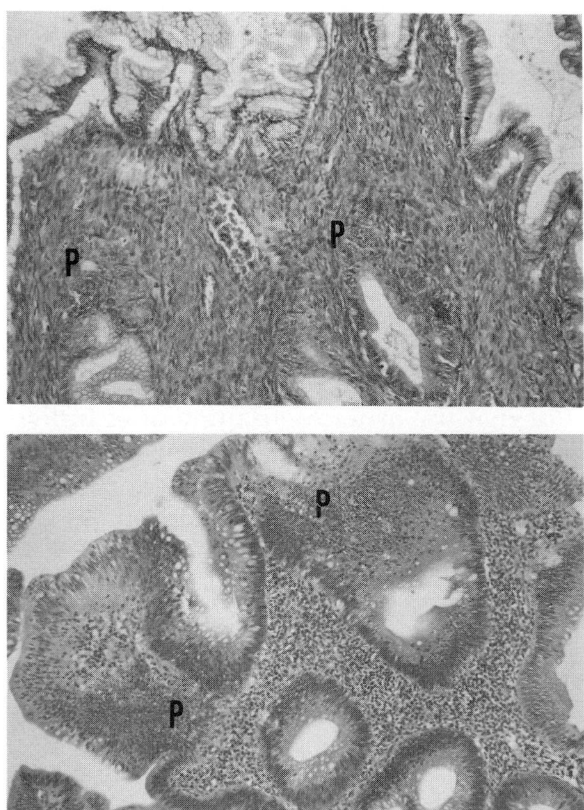

Fig. 6. Hypoxic milieu as a key factor in clonal selection in carcinogenesis. A. Emergence of foci of abnormal cells in an ovarian cyst. These adenoma cells have lost cellular polarity, and pile up one upon another along with nuclear alterations and mitosis (P). Vascular engorgement from pressure due to cystic expansion could have provided a hypoxic milieu. B. Emergence of cancerous foci in a rectal polyp. Numerous hypercellular adenomatous alveoli showing transition to malignant foci are observable, with loss of polarity and piling. These foci are located exactly distal and perpendicular to the direction of blood supply. (Hematoxylineosin stain. ×40.)

1980), invertebrates, vertebrates, and even mammals such as dolphins. In most studies, cancer metabolism is compared with that of the brain and muscles. Such comparisons must be viewed with caution, however. Although cancer cells do not rest, the comparisons have been made with resting brain and muscles rather than with those fully engaged in work. Secondly, most experimental animals are small and short-lived. Therefore, their metabolic rate and the metabolism of their neoplastic cells may be much higher than those of larger animals: one day in the life of a mouse approximates one month in a human (Makinodan 1977). Cancer cells may be compatible with anoxic and hypoglycemic milieux (Table 1).

Cancer Cell Reliance on the Primitive Fermentation Portion of Glycolysis, an ATP-independent Mechanism

Horowitz has stated that the evolution of the basic syntheses proceeded in a stepwise manner, involving one mutation at a time, but that the order of attainment of individual steps has been in the reverse direction from that in which synthesis proceeds in the chain, with the ultimate synthesis the first to be acquired in the course of evolution, the penultimate

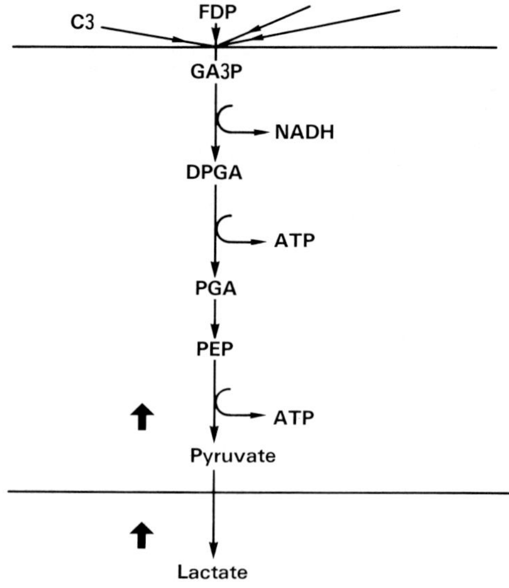

Fig. 7. The principle of primitive fermentation. When tricarbons are processed to yield pyruvate, there is no need for investment for ATP. This portion of glycolysis has been designated primitive fermentation (Nakamura 1982). These tricarbons could have been abundant in the primitive seas. Thus, the availability of ATP and absence of the need for ATP preinvestment seem to support the hypothesis of primitive fermentation.

step next, and so on (1945). Thus, the part of glycolysis in which tricarbons are transformed to lactate and the generation of ATP proceeds without any investment of ATP could have been one of the most primitive glycolytic processes, primitive fermentation (Fig. 7) (Nakamura 1982).

As shown in Fig. 8, a review of the biochemical pathways of fermentation among the prokaryotes, however, shows that all four pathways of glycolysis—Embden-Meyerhof, Entner-Doudoroff, pentose phosphate, and phosphoketolase—lead to the production of glyceroaldehyde-3-phosphate (GA3P) before pyruvate, which can then be fermented to lactate, ethanol, and so on (Metzler 1977). All of the hexoses require ATP or NAD$^+$ or NADP$^+$ as they enter the glycolytic pathways. Therefore, the portions of glycolysis prior to the production of GA3P could be evolutionarily more recent than

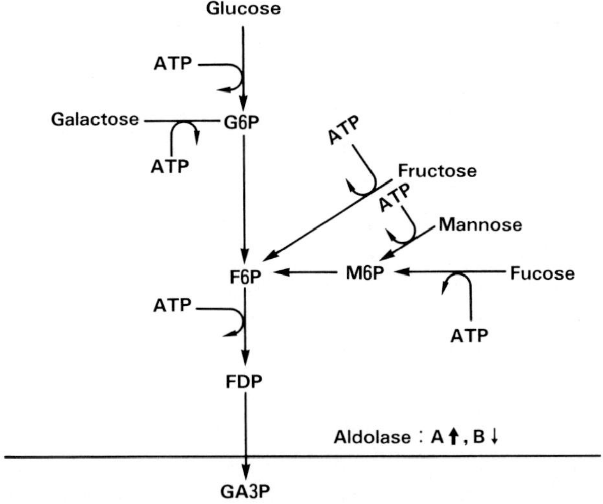

Fig. 8. Principle of low pK, low specificity. The glycolytic processes of hexoses other than glucose are of low pK and low specificity. They invariably demand pre-investment of ATP. As the tricarbons became less available, other materials including hexoses must have been used until the advent of photosynthesis supplied an enormous quantity of glucose. These necessitate an investment of 1 mol of ATP per mol hexose. Increased aldolase activation (Sugimura *et al.* 1972) may be purposefully related to the activation of primitive fermentation.

those thereafter. Because a variety of carbohydrates can be produced abiotically (Margulis 1981), extensive use of any of the hexoses could have been prevalent until the predominant to selective dependence of animal life on glucose eventually evolved. Cancer cells then might have retreated from the liberal and specific use of glucose to abundant consumption of nonspecific hexoses by increasing hexokinases (Shatton *et al*. 1969).

These enzymatic alterations give rise to a further evolutionary concept: isozyme evolution. Embryomuscular isozymes are prevalent among the undifferentiated cancers (Tsuiki 1973): pyruvate kinase (Sato *et al*. 1978), fructose-1-diphosphatase (Sato and Tsuiki 1968), aldolase (Sugimura *et al*. 1972), and hexokinase (Sato *et al*. 1978). The specific and efficient glycolytic enzyme, glucokinase, has been shown to decrease with increasing grades of malignancy. Enzymes of gluoconeogenesis such as fructose-1, 6-diphosphatase are remarkably reduced (Tsuiki 1973).

It seems appropriate to emphasize that these alterations may not simply represent embryonic reversion, but may bear important evolutionary significance. Cancer cells may be retreating from the swift and highly specific use of glucose. The severing of primitive from recent glycolysis seems to occur at the level of fructose-1, 6-diphosphatase (Tsuiki 1973; Weber 1977). Cancer cells may be struggling to run the prototype machinery of ATP and NADH production, but at slower rates and possibly at lower pH. An extensive review of the matter may be mandatory.

Reversion of the Krebs Cycle and Electron Transport System in Cancer

Similar alterations of evolutionary significance may take place in the Krebs cycle and mitochondrial electron transport system. The number of mitochondria may be reduced (Allard *et al*. 1953), their structure hypoplastic, and their activity deterioriated (Pedersen *et al*. 1970; Mehard *et al*. 1971; Stocco *et al*. 1980). Glutamine and glutamate are the major respiratory substrates in tumor cells, and the mitochondrial matrix enzymes involved in glutamate metabolism may be associated in a multi-enzyme cluster, resulting in various abnormalities.

In normal cells, malate coming into the mitochondria from the cytoplasm is oxidized to aspartate, to constitute the malate-aspartate shuttle (Fig. 9). However, in tumor cells, the incoming malate is oxidized primarily by mitochondrial malic enzyme to pyruvate, which is extruded, or it can be converted into citrate, which is also extruded (Moreadith and Lehninger 1984). Figure 10 illustrates the sequence of events, showing how the TCA or Krebs cycle is reverted and contracted. More ample use of glutamate in place of malate is probable, a phenomenon that can be taken advantage of in tumor imaging (Reiman *et al.* 1984). This may occur because in tumor mitochondria the matrix volume is small and the protein concentration high (Srere 1980). Because the cytoplasm dissolves enormous amounts of elements and compounds, its osmotic pressure inevitably increases. The cells can adjust the osmotic pressure by removing definite amounts of solutes by shedding, diluting, or, with the help of evolutionary modifi-cations, encasing the solutes in appropriate organelles such as the mitochondria. However, the water content of can-

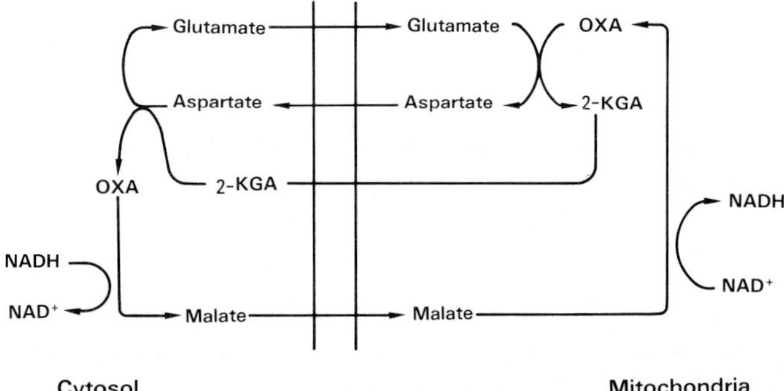

Fig. 9. The malate-aspartate shuttle as the connector of the TCA cycle to the mitochondrial electron transport system (1). The difficulty arises because the mitochondria are impermeable to NADH. All cells that generate NADH in the cytosol during aerobic glycolysis have a requirement that hydrogen shuttles connect to the electron transport system. In mammalian tissues, the major one is the malate-aspartate shuttle, which operates at no significant energy cost (Hochachka 1980).

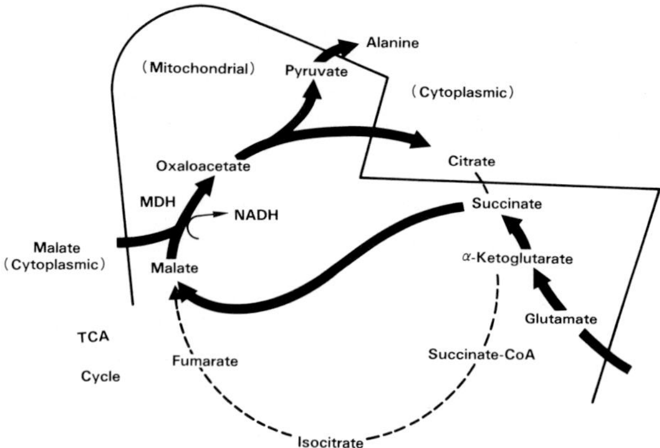

Fig. 10. The malate-aspartate shuttle as the connector of the TCA cycle to the mitochondrial electron transport system (2): Possible deviation in cancer cells. In Ehrlich ascites tumor cells, the formation of aspartate from glutamate is disorganized in such a way that alanine and citrate are produced and subsequently extruded from the mitochondria. Then the entire TCA cycle contracts to one analogous to that of green algae, and the transfer of the hydrogen to the mitochondrion is derailed (Nakamura 1982; Moreadith and Lehninger 1984).

cer cells is greater than that of normal cells (Craig and Waterhouse 1957), and there are definite differences in the concentrations of elements between the cytoplasm and nucleus (Smith *et al.* 1978). These data again add up to an evolutionary concept of cancer at the mitochondrial level because the described metabolic pathway resembles that of the green algae that flourished more than two billion years ago. The crucial importance of this type of observation cannot be overemphasized, especially in the construction of strategies for anticancer therapy and diagnosis.

Principle of Low pK, Low Specificity for Carbohydrate Metabolism in Cancer

Primitive aquatic animals lived on primitive sugars such as galactose, fructose, and mannose, on primitive proteins such as glycine, alanine, and glutamine, and on D-amino acids. Low pK or slow chemical reactions could have been well tolerated in the absence of abundant molecular oxygen: abundant use of tricarbons for effective production of ATP and NADH from elevated pyruvate kinase, the most primitive principal fermentation. Utilization of hexoses at the cost of one molecule of ATP per molecule of hexose, but with a low pK, could also have been well tolerated. In other words, the liberal use of glucose could have been the result of photosynthetic evolution, and therefore a reduction in gluconeogenesis would be a natural phenomenon in cancers (Tsuiki 1973), with the probable exception of terminal metastatic cachexia (Holrodye *et al.* 1979).

Low Specificity Principle in the Protein Metabolism of Cancer

Although protein metabolism has long been thought to be highly activated in cancer cells (Weber 1977), it is best to adhere to the assumption that human tumor cells proliferate more slowly than those in normal cell renewal systems. Still, the magnitude of the host's metabolism has to be increased if the bodily burden of the tumor exceeds certain limits. The turnover rate per se may not always be accelerated. The tumor uptake of D-amino acids in the Ehrlich tumor is greater than in the liver, pancreas, and other organs (Tamemasa *et al.* 1978). Among the amino acids studied, alanine and leucine are easily synthesized from simple inorganic materials, and both L- and D-types of amino acids could have been abundant in the primitive seas (Margulis 1981). These experimental results indicate a probable loss of specificity as compared with normal control organs.

A Tendency towards Pre-eukaryotic Metabolism: Methionine-dependence of Animal Tumors

The uptake of methionine in cancer has long been regarded as one of the major signs of hypermetabolism. Even when ^{11}C-labeled methionine is used, the assumption seems unshakeable (Kubota *et al.* 1988). Goseki *et al.* have consistently reported that experimental cancer cells are sensitive to methionine depletion, to the point of cancer cure (1984; 1987).

The rationale behind these observations could be as follows: (1) methionine is essential for the production of creatine phosphate (CP); (2) CP produces ATP (Baldwin 1957); (3) these reactions would enable cancer cells to survive without glucose, a phenomenon of muscle-like dependence of cancer on CP for ATP production; (4) conversely, in the absence of glucose, cancer cells may be dependent upon methionine for the generation of energy via CP; (5) therapeutic effects can be achieved by methionine depletion, resulting in cellular degeneration and ultimate cell loss (Goseki *et al*. 1984); and (6) although CP is limited to the vertebrates, the same principle may be applicable to tumors of the invertebrate animals: the arginine phosphate of such animals may be methylated by methionine, too.

The proposed clinical usefulness of the principle awaits further studies, because of the discrepancy between humans and the small animals.

Natural History of Tumor Growth

A tumor may proceed to cancer phanerosis as it emerges through processes of immortalization and transformation. When the size of a tumor or the number of tumor cells is taken into account, the entire course of a tumor can be represented by a curve something like that shown in Fig. 11. This may, in a sense, represent the natural history of tumor growth. While we do not think it possible yet to diagnose a cancer during its preclinical period, it may be possible to do so as soon as it advances to the clinical stage. During the clinical period, we presume that the tumor grows according to the following growth function:

$$Y = \frac{a}{1 + be^{-kt}}$$

Our clinical experience suggests that the point of inflection occurring at $a/2$ is the turning point for the development of overt cachexia. The precachectic portion of the curve is exponential, with a doubling time of $1/k$. The curve has a horizontal asymptote (Steel 1977). The value of a is about 10^{12} cancer cells, and $a/1+b$ is 10^5. Thus, b is about 10^7.

This logistic model implies that the growth rates of a tumor may change from time to time. The transplantation passages used with experimental tumors, cause tumors to grow more rapidly than primary tumors (Steel *et al*. 1971). The acute exacerbation of chronic myelogenous leukemia is another case. Undoubtedly, this is true with solid tumors as well. One possible explanation is that a primary tumor may consist of heterogeneous populations, and that the transplantation passage would permit clonal selection, such that rapid growers would prevail in subsequent transplantations (Hauschka 1961). The modern molecular biology of cancer, however, appears to suggest differently. Once established, the activated onocogenes increase the rate or velocity of proliferation of cancer cells. One candidate phenomenon may be gene amplification, in which DNA fragments containing oncogenes are abnormally increased. The changes are morphologically observable as the homogeneously staining regions or double minutes. These changes have been observed among human cancer cells obtained from terminal cachectic patients (Rowley 1984; Stark and Wohl 1984). Therefore, our original assumption that cancer cells proliferate slowly in their hypoxic milieu has to be changed by adding the following: "until they arrive at the cachectic inflection point where they begin to grow rapidly." This is obviously a compromised view, one that demands further confirmation. How can this switch to rapid growth be metabolically sustained, and what are the evolutionary implications?

Cancer as a Metabolic Host: Metabolic Strategies of Cancer against Host Patients

Our clinical experience suggests that the evolutionary implications of cancer metabolism should be discussed in two discrete categories: precachectic and cachectic. It should be emphasized, however, that the evolution of cancer advances from the precachectic to the cachectic.

The Precachectic Stage: Slow Tumor Growth under Hypoxia and Hypo-nourishment

Estimates of tumor doubling times and tumor cell cycle times (Steel 1977) have generally been carried out without regard to the natural history of the tumor, which indicates that tumor growth rates may change from time to time, even in single tumors (Fig. 11). Nonetheless, the intermitotic times of acute leukemias seem to be as long as 37 to 82 hours

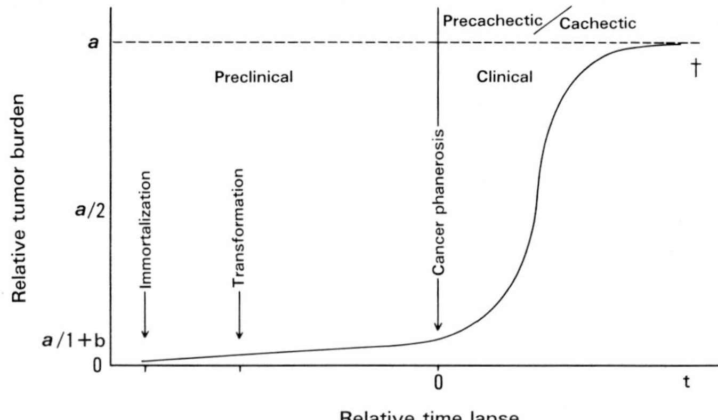

Fig. 11. Natural history of cancer in terms of cell number or burden and induction of cachexia. The curve can be simulated by a
logistic growth function: $Y=\dfrac{a}{1+be^{-kt}}$. The primary implication
of this type of simulation is that the rate of tumor growth may
change with time. This notion is in good agreement with our clinical impression of terminal patients. The experimental demonstration shown here suggests a possible underlying mechanism. While
it indicates that a cancer patient dies from an excessive tumor burden, he or she may die as a result of cachexia resulting from a multitude of humoral factors elaborated by the cancer, e.g., inhibitors
of energy metabolism.

    a=ultimate tumor size or burden
    b=clinically diagnosable tumor size
    k=rate constant

(Steel 1977). With solid tumors, the intermitotic times vary
widely, from 23 to 113 hours (Steel 1977), or 49.9 hours on
average (Sasaki *et al.* 1981). Therefore, the expansion of malignancy is not a problem of the speed at which tumor cells propagate, but a matter of delayed extinction or, conversely, prolonged persistence of the tumor cells that are born. Needless
to say, normal cell renewal systems are characterized by the
elimination of senescent cells and the introduction of a host
of newly born cells. The intermitotic times for such normal
cell renewal systems are less than 24 hours, as discussed earlier. When the number of cancer cells is within certain limits,
there may be no appreciable exploitation of the host patient
by the tumor, although cachectic effects are thought to occur
even when the tumor is very small (Steel 1977). Thus, the

tumor may propagate under a hypoxic, hyponutritious, but secured environment. This is in keeping with our anti-evolutionary view of malignancy.

The Cachectic Stage: Cancer as a Metabolic Host

Does cancer emerge with some kind of mission, or is it simply a random aberration? Even though cancer is a fitter variant that evolves from and is supported by the host (Cairns 1975; 1981), it may arise, in one way or another, as a result of modification of genetic materials that have been conveyed through generations beyond the barriers of species and probably of phylum as well. Therefore, it is possible that the metabolic changes that take place in cancer phanerosis might resemble those of evolutionary history. As discussed earlier, evolutionary changes may be manifested in the metabolic processes of cancer phanerosis.

Most of the physiological metabolic processes in humans are regulated by humoral factors that accompany various physical activities; so it is with cancer metabolism. At least, cancer metabolism can be influenced by probable "cancer factors." These factors may affect the cancer cells themselves or the host patient. Thus, the categorization of metabolic inter-

Table 2. Cancer as a metabolic host

Tumor to Tumor	Tumor to Host
A. Growth-promoting: Feeder-layer effect Tumor-adhesive glycoprotein	A. Short-ranging: TAF (tumor angiogenesis factor; currently, angiogenin) Leukemia-associated inhibitors Tumor invasion (laminin)
B. Growth-inhibiting: Prostaglandin D_2 to reduce metastasis Protein-synthesis inhibitor	B. Long-ranging: Distant metastasis Paraneoplastic syndromes Tumor-specific antigens Toxohormone, including asthenic factors and SOD inhibitors Activation of the Cori cycle Activation of protein kinase Granulocytosis-producing factor Immunosuppressive acidic protein CEA

play as tumor-to-tumor, tumor-to-host, and host-to-tumor shown in Table 2 is reasonable (Okuyama and Mishina 1985 a), although it does not necessarily list all the known factors and enzymes.

The "feeder effect" is a term originally used in tissue culture (Stoker and Sussman 1965), but its use can be expanded to *in vivo* situations if we consider a tumor cord in which necrotic cells lie next to the viable cell layer. Prostaglandin D_2 may reduce cancer metastasis through modification of the negative charges on the cellular membrane (Fitzpatrick and Stringfellow 1979; Stringfellow and Fitzpatrick 1979; Kondo *et al.* 1981). Tumor adhesive glycoprotein secreted by cancer cells induces their anatomical juxtaposition (Ishimaru *et al.* 1980). An inhibitor of protein synthesis has also been reported (Werner *et al.* 1973).

Among the factors in the tumor-to-host category, tumor angiogenesis factor (TAF), now called angiogenin, is relatively short-ranging, as discussed earlier. Tumor invasion seems to proceed through the production of substances that may break up the surrounding barriers of collagen (Liotta 1986).

A host of tumor products target the host and affect it in one way or another. If individual cancer cells are capable of producing factors, whether short- or long-ranging, distant metastasis itself may serve as a long-ranging effector. The so-called paraneoplastic syndrome is characterized by versatile, clinically active substances resembling hormones (Table 3) (Minna and Bunn 1982). Tumor-specific antigens are also being clarified. However, should any immunosuppresive factors be elaborated by the tumor (Tamura *et al.* 1981), the establishment of anticancer immunity can be endangered. Toxohormone (Nakahara and Fukuoka 1961) is now known to possess several biological and therefore cachectic activities; e.g. it induces anemia (Fujii and Okuda 1979), causes asthenia (Theologides 1982), and inhibits SOD (Leutehauser *et al.* 1984). Although not necessarily categorized as short- or long-ranging, leukemia-associated inhibitory factor (LAI) influences the proliferation of normal marrow cells (Chiyoda *et al.* 1978; Olofsson and Olsson 1980). This is intriguing since the phenomenon may affect normal cells and interfere with re-

Table 3. *Endocrine paraneoplastic syndromes*

Syndrome	Hormone	Tumor	Incidence (percent)
Cushing's syndrome	ACTH	Lung cancer—all types	0~2.0
		Small cell lung cancer	2.8~22
Inappropriate antidiuresis	AVP	Lung cancer—all types	0.9~2.0
		Small cell lung cancer	8~53
Nonmetastatic hypercalcemia	PTH	Lung cancer—all types	1.0~7.5
		Squamous cell lung cancer	15
		Other tumors	14
Gynecomastia		Lung cancer—all types	0.5~0.9
		Small cell lung cancer	2.0
Hyperthyroidism		Lung cancer	0~1.4
Calcitonin		Medullary carcinoma of the thyroid	
		Small cell lung cancer	
		Other lung cancer types	
		Breast cancer	0~70

(Reproduced from Minna and Bunn 1982)

covery from chemotherapeutic damage to the nucleus (Himori *et al*. 1983). Activation of the Cori cycle seems to be a rather late effect of malignancy (Holrodye *et al*. 1979). Many of the oncogenes are known to possess tyrosine kinase activity, and it is not surprising to see increased tyrosine levels in cancer patients (Bennegard *et al*. 1982).

There are several kinds of host-to-tumor interactions. Whether related to the tumor-specific antigens or not, many anticancer immune systems operate within the body, as described in textbooks of immunology (Alexander and Good 1977; Bellanti 1976). Because of the molecular diversity that would evolve as these immune mechanisms advanced along the line of evolution, the more highly differentiated an animal or organ, the greater its antigenic spectrum might be. Although this theorem has not been entirely substantiated, it seems probable because evolution itself has advanced through genetic increments that would likely be accompanied by antigenic increment.

Superoxide radicals, and probably other active oxygen moieties that arise endogenously within the body, are seen in the classical examples of spontaneous tumor regression following acute infections, especially streptococcal infection (Nauts *et al.* 1953). Corticosteroids may also be important in terms of anticancer effects if the phenomenon of apoptosis (Kerr and Searle 1980) is taken into account. The primary function of these steroids is to enable the host to adapt to acute emergencies that require the supply of energy at the expense of host cells like lymphocytes as well as glycolysis (Kobayashi 1983): the target cells are destroyed and phagocytosed. Such may be the evolutionary significance of this phenomenon.

Although it has yet to be proven, prostaglandin D_2 seems to contribute in one way or another to this phenomenon in that brain tumors, even if they are highly malignant, seldom metastasize extracranially, but relentlessly destroy the brain tissue (Robbins and Cotran 1976). This phenomenon is presumably dependent upon the abundant distribution of prostaglandin D_2 in the brain (Shimizu *et al.* 1979).

A special category, parasite-to-tumor, appears to be necessary when the antitumor effects of various microbial products are considered. Many of the bacterial and mycotic parasites that harbor within host humans may elaborate antineoplastic substances. From the clinical point of view, host-mediated anticancer agents like OK-432 (NBC-B116209) and lentinan are interesting in that they are capable of activating immune systems, leading to major therapeutic effects in selected cases (Okamoto *et al.* 1972; Okuyama and Mishina 1986a; Hamuro and Chihara 1984; Okuyama and Mishina 1987b).

At least two more factors deserve mention: (1) those directed to cell membranes and (2) those directed to proto-oncogenes. The first group includes Bestatin, from *Streptomyces olivoreticuli* (Umezawa 1978). It is cytostatic in the sense that it may inhibit cancer metastasis (Svanberg and Elisson 1983; Pimm 1986), and it is capable of inducing redifferentiation of cancer cells in human patients as well as in cultured cells (Okuyama and Mishina 1984a, c; Okuyama *et al.* 1983d; 1985b). Herbimycin inhibits intracellular *src* kinase (Uehara *et al.* 1985) and induces redifferentiation of transformed cells *in vitro*. These agents may constitute a special category of anticancer agents.

It is necessary to return to the problem of oxygenation in tumor tissues and proliferation of cancer cells. It is true that tumor tissues can be well oxygenated. A detailed oximetric study of an experimental murine mammary adenocarcinoma *in vivo* demonstrated areas of hyperoxidation as well as hypoxic regions in the same tumor samples (Cole *et al.* 1983). The oxygen distribution in a tumor cord seems to represent a similar phenomenon in terms of multplication of cancer cells (Tannock 1968): hyperoxic in the vicinity of the vascular endothelium, and hypoxic to anoxic in the peripheral necrotic areas. The main difference, however, lies in the total dependence of the latter upon oxygen tension in the blood passing through the cord vessel. Positron emission tomography (PET) is well known for its accurate *in vivo* quantitation of metabolic changes. Comparison of oxygen uptake has shown that human tumors take up identical quantities of oxygen as normal brain and muscles (Harada 1973; Kubota *et al.* 1983). In interpreting these data, it is necessary to take into account the fact that the latter tissues are at rest during investigation while tumors do not rest and are being measured at maximum activity, unless hampered by G_0 cells.

Before proceeding further, a biological time comparison between rodents and humans would be useful. A rough estimate is that one day in the life of a mouse corresponds to one month in a human (Makinodan 1977). Even in the mouse, most primary spontaneous tumors possess relatively long cell cycle times and grow rather slowly (Steel 1977).

The question then arises of how cancer cells increase so enormously if not through rapid proliferation. One possible explanation may be that cancer cells, once generated, do not mature or die off through senescence (Steel 1977; Cooper *et al.* 1972). As the number of myeloblasts increases, a reciprocal decrease in the labeling index (with tritiated thymidine) occurs in the marrow of patients with CML (Steel 1977). Thus, exploitation of the host patient by an increasing number of cancer cells is highly probable, yet is not necessarily the result of rapid cancer cell proliferation. The above discussion of evolutionary significance thus seems to be valid, even in the advent of the cachectic period: slow growth under hypoxia and hyponutrition.

In addition to exploitating energy materials, cancer may affect the host patient through several cachexia-producing mechanisms. As discussed in the section on tumor-to-host interrelationships, the role of toxohormone may be of prime importance. It leads to an intractable anemia through the depletion of transferrin, and decreases the plasma levels of catalase. These properties of toxohormone support our theory that cancer represents a devolution towards the pre-eukaryotic state. Toxohormone would convert the muscles to hypoxic metabolizers, and their enzymes would become M enzymes, which function best under hypoxia (Ibrahin *et al.* 1981).

Cachexia as Sequelae of Submission to Cancer, the Metabolic Host

Cachexia denotes the morbidity of somatic cells of a cancer-bearing host. What is cancer cachexia? How does it ensue? Does it have any evolutionary implications? Subjectively, cachexia is the feeling of asthenia; objectively, it is the loss of body mass. Patients first appear almost normal, but in selected cases may present signs of increased metabolism. This increase has long been thought to result from exploitation caused by the rapid proliferation of cancer cells. But as we have seen, cancer cells do not necessarily proliferate rapidly. They are slow growers under hypoxia and hyponutrition. How then can they appear hypermetabolic? First, terminal cachectic patients with a huge primary tumor or numerous metastases would have an enormous cancer cell burden even if the cells proliferated slowly. The *energy expenditure* of cancer patients is greater than that of non-cancer controls (Lundholm *et al.* 1979; Lindmark *et al.* 1984). The energy-producing mechanisms of such patients are naturally inefficient. As discussed earlier, the energy mechanisms of cancer cells may involve (1) primitive fermentation, (2) a primitve TCA cycle, and (3) deficient mitochondrial workup. This combination is far from efficient, and the host has to pay for the increased molecules of ATP by increasing the Cori cycling of lactate to glucose (Holroyde *et al.* 1979). This cycle requires 6 M of ATP to produce 1 M of glucose, and is therefore highly inefficient. The primitive TCA cycle can be run with the new isozyme of maleate dehydrogenase (Grisham *et al.* 1983), making full use of glutamate (Reitzer *et al.* 1979;

Zielke *et al.* 1976). The maleate-aspartate shuttle can be blocked, causing the electron transport system to malfunction (Moreadith and Lehninger 1984). Thus, the evolutionarily well-developed factory for ATP production is incapacitated by reverting towards the pre-eukaryotic state. A sense of asthenia would occur, even in the absence of obvious signs of muscular depletion, as a result of defective ATP production. Cancer itself could thus have directed the patient toward pre-eukaryotism.

Asthenia: Cancer's Prevailing Metabolic Displacement

Cancer has been defined as a population of cells that may propagate endlessly, ultimately leading to the death of the host. It is characterized by overhydration, low SOD levels, and reduced capacity for excision repair of DNA damage. Cancer has to secure an environment in which oxygen toxicity is negligible. It then has to endure undernutrition, controlling cellular growth as well. It has to live principally on primitive fermentation. All of these changes are known to characterize oncofetalism, and we have just seen that they can be regarded as an evolutionary and phylogenetic reversion. In the preceding sections, our focus has been mainly on the metabolism of tumor cells and cachexia rather than the problem of asthenia.

Asthenia in cancer may be a remote manifestation of the disease which is induced by substances released from the tumor that can alter the metabolism and function of tumor-free host tissues (Theologides 1982): when blood from a fatigued subject is injected into a rested subject, manifestations of fatigue are produced. In selected cancer patients, carcinomatous neuropathy or a myasthenic state may be responsible for muscular weakness, independent of cancer cachexia. In patients with small cell carcinomas of the lung, the Eaton-Lumbert syndrome, it may be seen as a result of the production and liberation of substances that are capable of inducing a neuromuscular transmission defect (Minna and Bunn 1982). The changes in remote white muscles are astonishing in that the weakness is due not only to their atrophy but also to their metabolic shift from aerobic to highly anaerobic glycolysis because of increased (anaerobic) M-type LDH isozyme. The transplanted tumors are thought to induce the appropriate gene of the muscle fiber to produce isozyme, resulting in metabolic changes toward the glycolytic pathway (Theologides 1982). These changes do not appear to be limited to the skeletal muscles. On close examination, arterioles in the vicinity of a large hepatoma have been found to lose normal medial muscular structures and become asthenic (Fig. 5) (Suzuki *et al.* 1987). TAF, or angiogenin, secreted from a tumor induces hypoxic neovascularization in its vicinity. The same or different agent(s) or inhibitors of SOD or toxohormone from the tumor may also be trying to secure a hypoxic milieu by affecting the greater vasculature. Thus, the cachectic period in the history of a cancer is multifarious, and the weakness of cancer patients can be seen to have evolutionary significance as well.

When the arterial concentrations of various substances in cancer patients were compared with those from appropriate controls, levels of free fatty acids and tyrosine were elevated

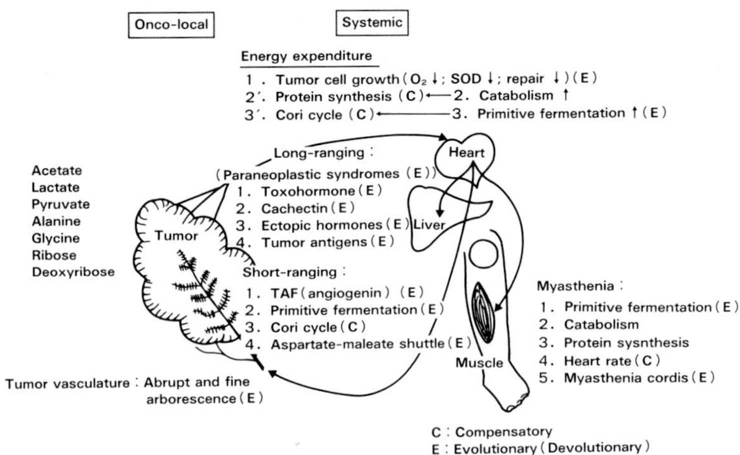

Fig. 12. Cancer cachexia as forced pre-eukaryotic life: a schematized view. A major distinction was made between the onco-local and systemic types. Onco-local: An abrupt and fine aroborescence of tumor vessels in the presence of TAF, dependence on primitive fermentation and on the use of archaic substrates such as lactate, pyruvate, and glycine as listed. Systemic effects may be devolutionary, too.

while that of alanine was reduced (Bennegard *et al.* 1982). The increment of free fatty acids may represent compensation for reduced glycolysis. The mosaicism of protein metabolism demands an explanation: (1) cancer hyponutrition requires secondary sugar sources, and protein catabolism would supply a large quantity of energy; (2) protein synthesis, in contrast, requires tyrosine more urgently than alanine, because of the phenol base. From the chemical evolutionary point of view, tyrosine is more recent than alanine (Margulis 1981). In this regard, tyrosine metabolism resembles Cori cycle activation in metastatic cachexia (Fig. 12).

Possible Therapeutic Strategies against Cancer Cachexia

The best therapy for cancer cachexia is undoubtedly the elimination of cancer cells from the patient's body. Clinical improvement is common following "successful" treatment by surgery, chemotherapy, and/or radiotherapy.

In clinical oncology, we are confronted by patients with advanced cachexia. It has been suggested that an appropriate antimetabolite that would successfully and harmlessly block the Cori cycle is needed along with adequate parenteral alimentation (Gold 1968; Gruffs *et al.* 1979).

Although the level fluctuates, hypozincemia seems to be a constant finding in cancer patients. Chemotherapeutics such as vincristine may aggravate it through leakage (Fletcher *et al.* 1975). We routinely use zinc supplementation, especially in cases of radiation and chemotherapy (Okuyama *et al.* 1983a). This supplementation is expected to counteract the Cu, ZnSOD depletion and protein degradation caused by toxohormone (Lundholm *et al.* 1981; Leuthauser *et al.* 1984).

Cancer Cachexia and the Oncogene Theory of Cancer

Cancer cachexia is the end stage of cancer phanerosis. As discussed above, it consists of several apparently conflicting clinical and metabolic abnormalities. Our assumption, however, is that everything converges in an evolutionary archaic model of pre-eurkaryotism, whether functional or morphological, or both. Some tumor marker genes are reported to cluster near the cellular oncogenes (Siegfried *et al.* 1986). We may go one step further: during the immortalization stage of carcinogenesis, the gene for MnSOD is destroyed (Oberley and Oberley 1984). Transformed cells have actually been shown to be devoid of MnSOD activity (Loven *et al.* 1984). The experiments of Loven *et al.* on transformation, however, all involved superoxide radical types (paraquat and X-rays). Because the resultant cancer cells have to survive, present carcinogenesis must be a way of finding a new refuge where cancer cells are secure even without MnSOD, i.e., pre-eukaryotic life. Nonetheless, how can this degree of selection be possible when the distribution of these free radicals along DNA molecules is not necessarily selective? Radiation damage to DNA is repairable in principle. There may be sites of *locus minoris resistaentiae* in terms of repairability. The formation of 8-hydroxy-guanine in the murine liver *in vivo* was much less than that formed from *in vitro* irradiation (Kasai *et al.* 1986). This observation may indicate lesser DNA damage and possibly greater repairability, presumably except for selected sites of *locus minoris*. Are the candidate sites closely related to proto-oncogenes? Further investigation will be needed to solve these problems.

Summary

Leukemias resulting from unrepaired DNA or disintegrative type—the most archaic; an additional transformational events are needed in solid tumors. The retroviral infection-neoploastic conversion may be the most novel——
——S. Okuyama and H. Mishina,
Radiology, *1988*

Cancer as an Evolutionary and Devolutionary Phenomenon

Several evolutionary principles seem to be involved in cancer and the process of carcinogenesis. Our understanding of cancer, which is derived from our experience in treating malignancies by radiotherapy and chemotherapy, is that it may represent a devolution of normal cells to an environment similar to that of primitive aquatic life, or slow proliferation under a hypoxic, hyponutritious milieu, with no urgent need for DNA repair. The evolutionary aspects of carcinogenesis are reflected in (1) the nonepithelial-epithelial tumor shift, (2) the evolutionary nature of atomic bomb radiation carcinogenesis, and (3) reiteration of the nonepithelial-epithelial tumor shift in Fanconi's anemia, one of the cancer-prone diseases. Carcinogenesis may proceed by immortalization, transformation, and phanerosis, all of which may be backed up by appropriate oncogenesis. Because of devolution, cancer may exert its effects on the host through a metabolic process: slow growth sustained by primitive fermentation and TCA cycle, and a defective maleate-aspartate shuttle. Carcinogenesis itself seems to be evolving, and may be classified into the disintegrative leukemias, the oldest; disintegrative carcinomas, the next oldest; compensatory lymphomas, the third oldest; and neoplasms resulting from viruses, the most recent.

II. EVOLUTIONARY CONCEPTS AS THE BASES OF ANTICANCER STRATEGIES

Chapter 7

Tetracycline Targeting of the Pre-eukaryotic *locus minoris*

> *Two concepts new to biology: (1) The most fundamental division in the living world is between the pre-eukaryotic and the eukaryotic organisms; (2) the evolution of symbioses.*
> ——*Lynn Margulis*, Biology, *1981*

Because radiotherapy and surgery may induce intractable radiation dermatitis and eventual radiation ulcers, these techniques should be avoided in treating tumor regrowths or metastases in fields of previous irradiation. The law of probabilistic cell killing requires that large doses of radiation be given, even in radiotherapy for small tumorous nodules. Therefore, novel techniques that facilitate local tumor control without untoward hazard to the host are needed.

Tetracyclines have been employed in the treatment of malignant pleurisy, where they induce serosal fibrosis (Rubinson and Bolooki 1972). Because these prokaryocytic antibiotics have been shown to be cytocidal *in vitro* (Okuyama and Mishina 1982b; Okuyama *et al.* 1984c), we thought it worthwhile to investigate the probable therapeutic effects of intratumoral injection of tetracyclines into skin metastases of human malignancies. The favorable results (Okuyama *et al.* 1987a) were thought to support our assumption that cancer cells have pre-eukaryotic properties (Setala 1984; Okuyama and Mishina 1984b; Kroon and van den Bogert 1985; van den Bogert *et al.* 1986). Such studies may well support the hypothesis of endosymbiotic evolution of the eukaryotic cells (Margulis 1981).

Table 1. Treatment of skin metastases of malignancies by intra/peri-tumoral administration of doxycycline: Excellent local control

Patient	Primary	Skin metastases	Responses	Local control	Remarks
1. I. M. F 34y	Odontosarcoma	1.5×5 mm 2.21×16 mm	Disappeared Reduced	21 months Removed*	Alive and active
2. W. S. F 51y	Breast cancer	5×5 mm	Disappeared	5 months	Died from perforation of the intestinum
3. K. Y. F 71y	Breast cancer	5×4 mm	Disappeared	13 months	Alive and active
4. K. K. F 37y	Breast cancer	3×3 mm	Disappeared	9 months	Died from liver metastasis
5. A. K. M 37y	Neck tumor (Squam. c.c.)	50×30 mm	Ineffective	—	Switched to radiochemotherapy
6. S. S. F 53y	Lip cancer (Squam. c.c.)	3×5 mm	Disappeared	1 month	Prior radiochemotherapy, ineffective
7. T. S. F 52y	Thyroid cancer	3×5 mm	Disappeared	19 months	Alive and active

* Extirpated en bloc. Histopathological examination revealed tumor cell loss from the sites of tumor cords (Fig. 1).

Experimental Use of Doxycycline

Cultured murine FM3A mammary adenocarcinoma cells were exposed to varying doses of doxycycline and incubated in a standard CO_2 incubator for 48 hr. Cells were counted with a standard hemocytometer.

Thirty 6-month-old male Wistar rats were fasted overnight and intraperitoneally injected with aliquots of normal saline or doses of doxycycline (50, 100, or 200 mg per rat). The blood concentrations of Cu and Zn were determined by atomic absorptiometry. The high-density lipoprotein (HDL) concentration was estimated by the method of Noma *et al.* (1978).

Doxycycline was injected into skin metastases from a variety of tumors (Table 1). Seven patients in the Department of Radiology, Tohoku Rosai Hospital, Sendai, were treated with intratumoral injections of 0.3 to 0.6 ml or 6 to 12 mg of undiluted doxycycline. The patients had already undergone surgery on their primary tumors. The injections were carried out daily, two or three times a week, or once every two weeks at the convenience of the outpatient. Therapeutic effectiveness was evaluated by regression or disappearance of the nodules and the length of time free from local regrowth.

Evaluation of Results

Figure 1 is a dose-response curve for FM3A cells exposed to doxycycline. The higher the dose, the more cells were killed. Doxycycline at 50-100 mg per rat has been shown capable of mobilizing Zn and HDL-cholesterol, inducing hypocuprozincemia and hypo-HDL-cholesterolemia, and even prompting death at 200 mg (Table 2).

Tumor regression was observed in six of the seven patients (Table 1). Local recurrence was not seen for one to 21 months, although two out of the seven died because of progression of their primary disease. Large tumors appeared not to respond to treatment. Histological examination of the tumor tissues revealed that the so-called tumor cords seemed emptied of tumor cells (Fig. 2). Thus, intra- and peritumoral injections of doxycycline seemed useful.

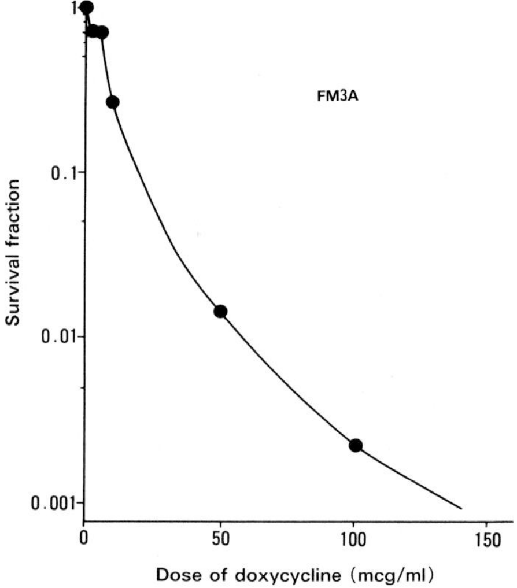

Fig. 1. Dose-response curve for doxycycline in FM3A murine mammary adenocarcinoma cells *in vitro*. Total cell killing rather than marginal killing was observed at higher doses.

Table 2. Doxycycline induces hypocuprozincemia and hypo-HDL-cholesterolemia in the rat

Time	Injectate (dose/rat)	Number of rats	Zn (μg/ml)	Cu (μg/ml)	HDL-chol (mg/ml)
1 hr	Saline	5	168.2± 7.4	139.2±18.1	44.8± 3.6
	200 mg DOX	6	206.0±19.4	125.7± 6.5	79.2±31.1
24 hr	Saline	6	157.7±16.8	153.1± 5.5	32.0± 6.3
	50 mg DOX	6	125.0±13.9	127.2± 9.5	25.4± 4.8
	100 mg DOX	3	105.7±15.3	111.0±11.3	20.7± 2.1

Values are means±S.D.

With or without their mobilization, doxycycline (DOX) induced reduction of the plasma concentrations of Zn, Cu and HDL-cholesterol.

Because of their biological uniqueness, the protein synthesis of eukaryotic cells may not be affected by doxycycline (Alberts *et al.* 1983). However, recent advances in the biochemical analysis of mitochondrial protein synthesis and oxidative phosphorylation suggest that protein synthesis can be blocked to produce selective cytostatic effects on cancer cells both *in vivo* and *in vitro* (Kroon and van den Bogert 1985; van den Bogert *et al.* 1986). Therefore, the observed anticancer effects may arise initially from cell killing through the chelation of

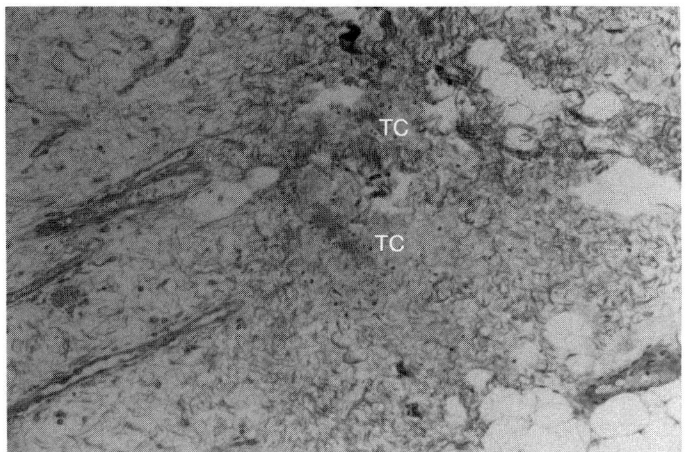

Fig. 2. Effects of intratumoral administration of doxycycline on human malignant cells. Areas of acellularity are thought to represent empty tumor cords (TC), as leaked doxycycline could have killed the tumor cells.

heavy metals and the resultant inactivation of relevant vital enzymes like superoxide dismutase (Okuyama and Mishina 1981a), causing instability of the mitochondrial membranes (Chapvil *et al.* 1972), DNA polymerase (Slater *et al.* 1971), and enzymes involved in mitochondrial protein synthesis, causing inhibition of oxidative phosphorylation (Kroon and van den Bogert 1985; van den Bogert *et al.* 1986), as well as through depletion of HDL-cholesterol from the cell membranes, presumably causing the disintegration of cancer cells (Bierman and Glomset 1981). It should also be noted that neoplastic cells tend to revert along the line of evolution to "pre-eukaryotic status" (Okuyama and Mishina 1984b; 1985c, d; 1986b; Setala 1984).

Thus, tetracyclines provide a novel mode of cancer cell elimination, whose usefulness cannot be overexaggerated. This is a topical treatment aimed at the probable *loci minores resistentiae* of evolutionary, and therefore endosymbiotic, origin (Margulis 1981).

Taking skin thickness into account, palpable tumors 6 mm in diameter may approximate nodules 2 mm in diameter consisting of 10^6 cells (Steel 1977). The *in vitro* potency of doxycy-cline at 100-150 μg/ml for 48 hr is a cell kill of 10^3 (Okuyama and Mishina 1982b; Okuyama *et al.* 1984c). The concentration of undiluted doxcycline is one-thousand times greater. A repetitive course of this agent would certainly enable cancer cell to be eradicated if the cell cycle times were sufficiently long.

The technique can be expanded to the eradication of viable tumor cells remaining after radiotherapy and chemotherapy. Because the injection of doxycycline is painful, patients need be informed and appropriate analgesics need to be readied. In view of the pain accompanying doxycyclcine, teramycin for intramuscular injections is advisable, as it contains xylocaine for pain control. Larger tumor masses can be treated by repetitive injection. Although transient fibrotic sequelae may be indistinguishable from residual cancer nodules, tenderness would persist if the nodules contained tumorous tissues of appreciable size.

Chapter 8

The Radiosensitivity of Cancer

Je le pensé, et Dieu le guérit.
——*Ambroise Paré (1517-1590)*, Surgery

Radiotherapy as an Anticancer Treatment

Although the statement "Kampf dem Krebs. Krebs ist heilbar" is attributed to Roentgen, we have not yet scrutinized how he came to use X-rays for the treatment of cancer. According to Casarett (1968), the biological effects of radiation were first detected by Daniel of Vanderbilt University, in April 1896, within four months of Roentgen's initial report: irradiation of the skull resulted in the loss of hair. In 1899, two Swedish physicians, Stenbeck and Sjogren, claimed the first radiation cure in the removal of a skin tumor from the tip of a patient's nose. A reduction in the size of the spleen of a leukemic patient was reported in 1903 by Senn of Chicago. The path leading to modern cancer radiotherapy has been long and difficult for both patients and radiotherapists. The era of Bragg's radiotherapy is just ending, and radiotherapists are still dependent on conventional, low-LET irradiation.

Radiotherapy as Local Chemotherapy
Selectivity

Radiotherapy seems to have "selective" effectiveness. Irradiation of a deep tumor mass, for example, may well eradicate the mass without causing any serious reactions in the overlying normal tissues of skin, muscles, or heart (Fig. 1).

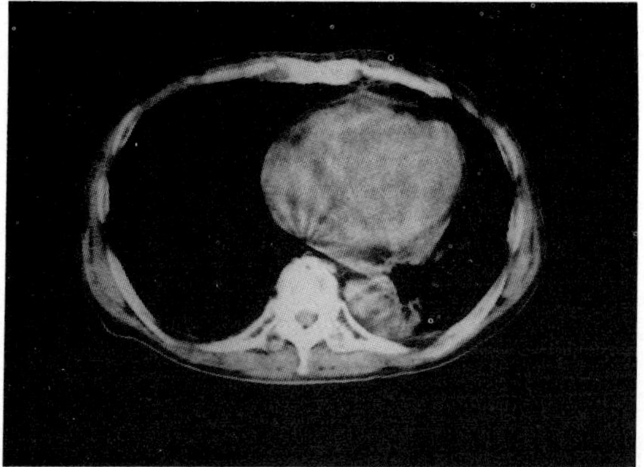

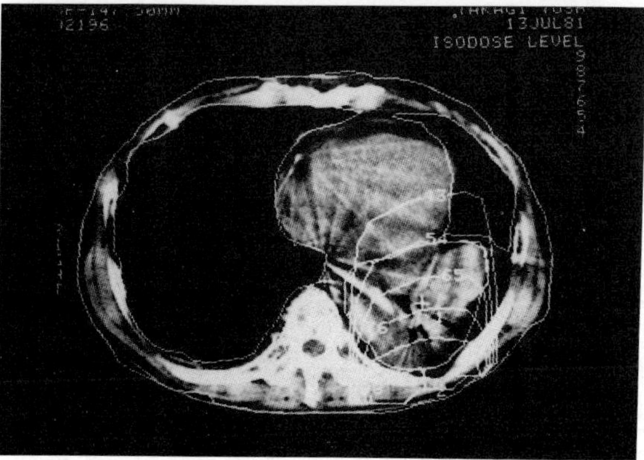

Fig. 1. Origin of the selectivity of radiotherapy of cancer (1). Although the dose to the skin is double that to the tumor, the tumor dissolves with time, while the overlying skin does not. Radiotherapy is a local chemotherapy that proceeds according to a different therapeutic process.

This selectivity proved so fascinating that we wanted to explore its origin. In addition, whenever we attempted to develop techniques to improve radiotherapeutic efficiency, we found ourselves confronting the origin of this selectivity. We eventually arrived at the conclusion that radiotherapy is a local chemotherapy of relatively high specificity (Okuyama and Mishina 1982a, c). This conclusion may sound fantastic unless viewed quantitatively and in terms of a few substances. Superoxide is one such substance (Fig. 2).

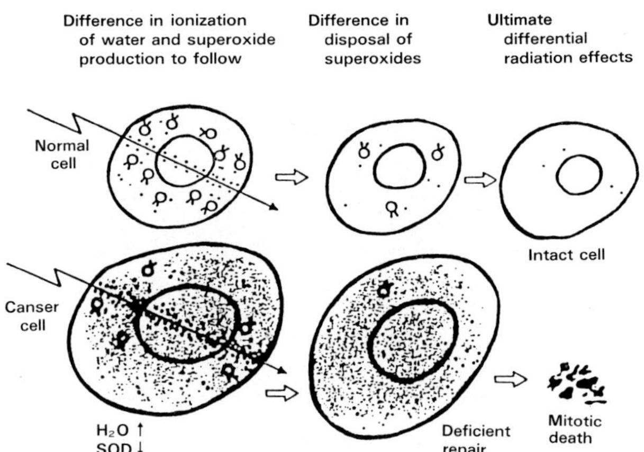

Fig. 2. Origin of the selectivity of radiotherapy of cancer (2): increased water density in cancer cells, decreased superoxide dismutase, and reduced capacity for excision repair of DNA damage. These changes support the evolutionary concept of cancer (Okuyama and Mishina 1984).

Production of Superoxide Radicals

Radiotherapeutic irradiation is essentially a heavy bombardment of high energy photons, causing water molecules in the tumor tissue to release electrons (the Compton effect). The ejected electrons are soon taken up by oxygen molecules to produce superoxide radicals ($\cdot O_2^-$). The radiotherapeutic selectivity of cancer tissues implies that their water density is greater than that in normal tissues, and this is indeed the case (Craig and Waterhouse 1957; Damadian 1971; Okuyama *et al.* 1979a). Magnetic resonance imaging of cancers rests on this same phenomenon (Fig. 3). The greater the water density, the greater the number of ionizations. To answer why cancers have a higher water density, we assumed a probable reversion to the time when life existed deep in the sea. The hydrostatic pressure in the deep sea could be counteracted by increasing intracellular solutes in the cytoplasm, a finding that has been confirmed (Smith *et al.* 1978). The reciprocal principle for normal cells, with their greater degree of differentiation, would be the enclosure of the cytoplasmic solutes in appropriate microorganelles, such as the mitochondrial enclosure of the electron transport system. Thus, cancer cells would have to be

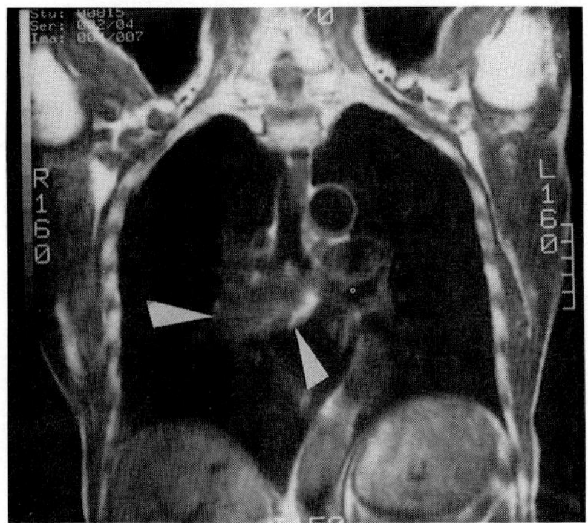

Fig. 3. Origin of the selectivity of radiotherapy of cancer (3). The increased water content of this lung cancer expanding to the mediastinum is clearly delineated by MRI, although silicotic changes are also seen scattered throughout the lung fields.

"wet" as a result of devolution. However, according to the observations and hypothesis of Setala (1984), they are "dry."

Devolution to Primitive Hypoxic Life as the Second Mechanism of Selectivity

The primary evidence for hypoxic devolution comes from the angiographic observation of abrupt, fine arborization of tumor nutrient vessels, in contrast to the gradual, incremental arborization of those nourishing normal tissues (Fig. 4). Although the number of fine vessels is increased, the actual blood and oxygen supply to the tumor is reduced. This type of vascular structure seems to resemble Hunter's vascular circle (Brookes 1971; Okuyama 1987). The structure helps to reduce the blood pressure entering the target bone structures, buffering the possible wide-ranging fluctuations in systemic blood pressure, and to secure even blood and oxygen supply to the target. The function of this structure could not be offset even by prostaglandin E_1, a vasodilator (Tomiie *et al.* 1982).

The hypothesis of cancer's preference for a hypoxic milieu seems to be substantiated by observations of reduced superoxide dismutase (SOD) in a host of experimental tumors (Pes-

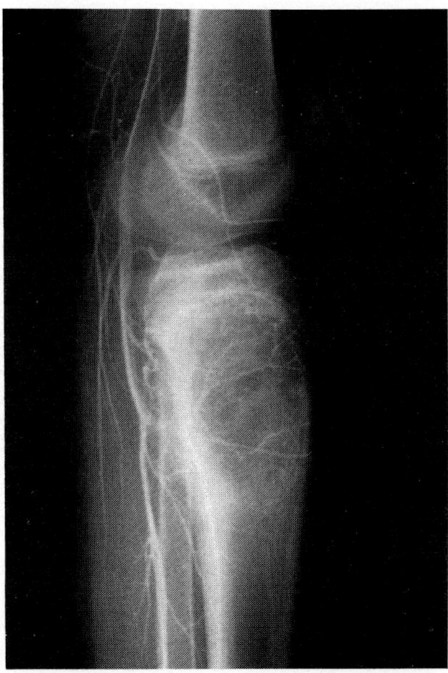

Fig. 4.   Tumor angiogram showing abrupt, fine arborization in a case of osteosarcoma. This type of vasculature may help to secure a hypoxic milieu. Normal vessels, in contrast, would show gradual tapering.

kin *et al.* 1977; Oberley and Buettner 1979). Two types of SOD are known to occur in mammalian cells: Cu, ZnSOD and MnSOD. Malignant cells are thought to lack MnSOD (Oberley and Buettner 1979). Thus, a selective superoxide toxicity to cancer cells would be expected if Cu, ZnSOD could be sufficiently copper- and probably zinc-chelated. This idea was tested *in vitro* and *in vivo* with D-penicillamine (Okuyama and Mishina 1981a). A sublethal dose of the agent induced hyperlipoperoxidemia and hypocupremia in aged rats. Treatment of cancer cells *in vitro* and *in vivo* with D-penicillamine resulted in appreciable suppression of cell multiplication and inhibition of tumor growth. Erythropoiesis did not seem to be affected. Thus, cancer cells may be "hypoxic growers."

Cancer cells would be expected to be more vulnerable to superoxide toxicity because they may lack the ability to efficiently dispose of such radicals (Fig. 2). In spite of reports of its absence from (experimental) tumor cells (Oberley and

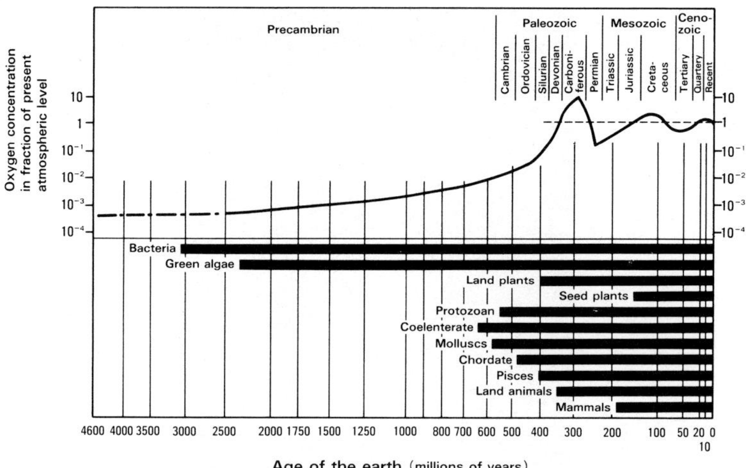

Fig. 5.   Changes in atmospheric oxygen concentration with the aging of the earth. The acquisition of Cu, ZnSOD could have taken place around the Carboniferous Period, 420 million years ago (Asada 1976), when the atmospheric oxygen levels rose steeply (Berkner and Marshall 1965). The increase may explain the high level of SOD activity in lung cancer, and the slight decline in cancers of the mammalian symbol organs (Sykes *et al.* 1978). (Two figures from Berkner and Marshall 1965 and Patterson 1978 were combined)

Buettner 1979; Loven *et al.* 1984), measurable MnSOD has been reported in human lung cancer cells (Iizuka *et al.* 1984). Total SOD activity may vary greatly depending on the organ of origin (Sykes *et al.* 1978). Nonetheless, changes in SOD molecules are central events in carcinogenesis and therefore in radiotherapeutic efficacy (Loven *et al.* 1984; Okuyama and Mishina 1985h). This phenomenon can tentatively be assumed to represent the devolution of such cells to an era before the Carboniferous Period, when the atmospheric oxygen concentrations rose steeply (Fig. 5).

Defective DNA Repair as the Third Evolutionary Mechanism of Cancer Radiosensitivity

The third assumed evolutionary mechanism behind the radiosensitivity of cancer cells is their probable defective excision repair, as suggested elsewhere (Yatani *et al.* 1983). There are three major mechanisms to repair DNA damage, regardless of etiology: (1) photoreactivation, (2) excision repair, and (3) recombinational repair, and their acquisition is thought to have taken place in that order (Kondo 1972). Their evolution is closely related to the atmospheric oxygen concentration and therefore, conversely, to the intensity of the actinic ultraviolet rays reaching the earth: oxygen molecules are disintegrated by ultraviolet radiation in the air to yield ozone. Ozone forms a layer that absorbs ultraviolet rays, thereby reducing the intensity of ultraviolet rays reaching the ground.

Photoreactivation is dedicated to the treatment of ultraviolet-induced thymine dimers, a type of repair that has already been lost in mammalians (Kondo 1972). Excision repair was also originally intended to treat ultraviolet-induced dimers and nicks in DNA, but it is capable of repairing damage from ionizing radiation, that from chemotherapy with mitomycin C, and so on (Kondo 1972). Any deficiency in this property in cancer cells would probably increase the therapeutic efficiency of radiotherapy and chemotherapy. Cancer cells are primarily defective (Yatani *et al.* 1983). However, this principle is potentially expandable. They can be rendered so by agents that interfere with the activity of DNA polymerase I: bleomycin and neocarzinostatin (Terasima *et al.* 1970; Matsuzawa *et al.* 1976; Okuyama and Matsuzawa 1979; Mueller *et al.* 1979; Okuyama and Mishina 1980). This principle can be termed "perpetuation" (Okuyama and Matsuzawa 1979; Okuyama and Mishina 1980). Inhibitors of this type are more common (Nakatsugawa and Sugawara 1982).

Thus, cancer cells may be selectively radiosensitive because of their devolutionary complexity. Radiotherapy is a *local* chemotherapy because its ionizing influence does not extend beyond the limits of the photon path. It is a local *chemotherapy* because its actual effects are substantiated initially by the chemically active superoxide radicals. We are currently investigating a possible fourth evolutionary category of cancer cell death: endosymbiotic disintegration.

Evolutionary Origin of the Varying Radiosensitivities of Cancers from Different Primary Organ Systems

Cancers originating in different organs have differing sensitivity to irradiation. Most breast cancers are likely to be cured with 40 Gy, while those of the lung may not be cured with as much as 50-60 Gy. Radiotherapists have not been able to give scientific precision to their studies because they have not succeeded in substantiating their radiation dose data with any known toxic or protective materials. Table 1 is a descriptive classification of organs and their neoplasms according to their radiotherapeutic responsiveness. Radiotherapeutic cell death is mitotic. Irradiated cells die because they cannot go through the stages of mitosis as chromosomal abnormalities become apparent. Therefore, irradiated organs or tissues that contain greater numbers of mitotable cells have greater radiosensitivity. According to the first law of Bergonié-Tribondeau, the radiosensitivity of an organ can be predicted by its mitotic prospect (Rubin and Casarett 1968).

Table 1. Origin of the radiosensitivity of cancer of different primary organ systems (1). A conventional classification of various tissues in decreasing order of relative radiosensitivity.

Tissues	Relative radio-sensitivity	Neoplasms
Lymphoid, hemopoietic (marrow), spermatogenic epithelium, ovarian follicular epithelium, intestinal epithelium	High	Lymphoma, leukemia, seminoma, dygerminoma
Oropharyngeal stratified epithelium, epidermal epithelium, urinary bladder epithelium, esophageal epithelium, gastric gland epithelium	Fairly high	Squamous cell carcinoma (oropharynx, skin, esophagus, cervix uteri)
Interstitial connective tissue, vessels, growing cartilage and bone	Medium	Astrocytoma
Mature cartilage and bone, mucous or serous gland epithelium, renal epithelium, hepatic epithelium, thyroid epithelium	Fair low	Adenocarcinoma (breast, liver, kidney), osteosarcoma, chondrosarcoma
Neuronal tissue, muscular tissue	Low	Ganglioneurofibroma, leiomyosarcoma, rhabomyosarcoma

While this law predicts probable radiation damage to intervening normal organs and tissues, it does not provide any information concerning the radiosensitivity of neoplasms arising in these organs.

Evolutionary Implication of SOD Content of Tumors: A Measure of Radiosensitivity?

There have been no comprehensive or systematic studies on the SOD content of major human organ systems. Therefore, data on surgical materials provide a beginning (Table 2) (Sykes *et al.* 1978). The original data of Sykes *et al.* have been rearranged according to the evolutionary age of the individual organs: prevertebral (full development prior to the appearance of vertebral structure such as muscle), poikilothermic, homeothermic, and mammalian. The gonads are separately categorized as "evolutionarily secured" because of their genetic implications. Any errors in the genetic material of the

Table 2. Origin of the radiosensitivity of cancers of different primary organ systems (2). The organ systems are classified according to their apparent evolutionary history, with their SOD activity, as reported by Sykes *et al.* (1978), listed alongside (Okuyama and Mishina 1985a).

	Evolutionary age	Organ system	Tumor	SOD content*
I	Evolutionarily secured	Testis Ovary	—— Carcinomas	 $6.1\pm8.9(6)$** $(1/6)$***
II	A Mammalian evolution	Breast Uterus Prostate	Cancers Cervical ca. ——	$7.7\pm13.9(10)$ $(2/10)$ $5.1(1)$
	B Homeothermic evolution	Lung Thyroid	Cancers ——	$45.1\pm228.1(3)$ (3.3)
	C Poikilothermic evolution	Stomach Colon Brain Bone	Cancer Cancers Astrocytoma Melanoma	$0.4(1)$ $29.3\pm44.1(18)$ $(10/18)$ $1.6(1)$ $0.25(1)$
	D Prevertebral	Soft tissue	Leiomyosarcoma	$1.3(1)$

* units/g tumor
**Number of tumor studied
***Number of tumors exceeding 10 units of SOD per g tumor

gonads can be crucial to the species (*horror autotoxicus*), and have to be eliminated (Okuyama and Mishina 1985h). The data are compared with variations in the radiosensitivity of the principal tumor or a representative tumor of each organ system (Fig. 6) (Okuyama and Mishina 1985h). The data help

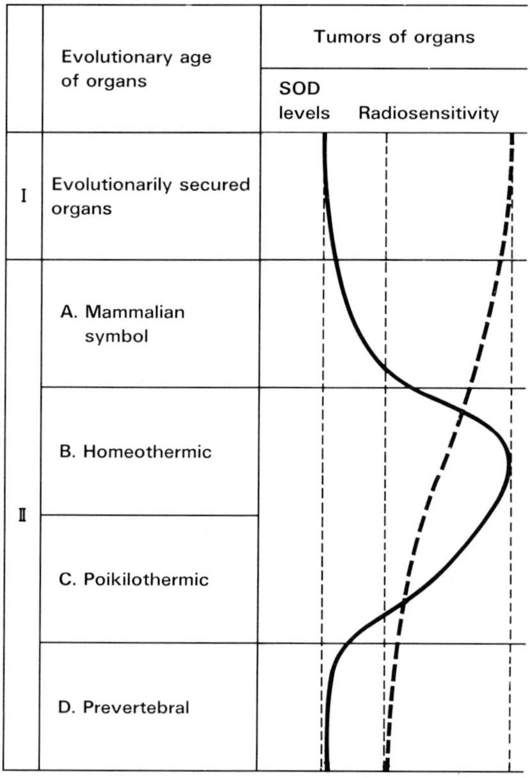

Fig. 6. Origin of the radiosensitivity of cancers of different primary organ systems (3). Radiosensitivity was expressed in terms of curative doses in rad (not shown here) based on Fletcher's (1973) data for most cancers and Asakawa's (1982) data for stomach cancers. The SOD content explains the radiosensitivity of tumors of the evolutionarily secured (gonadal) and mammalian symbol organs, and the radioresistance of lung cancers. The radioresistance of nonepithelial tumors and that of prevertebral tumors must be explained differently.

to elucidate the probable role of SOD in the varying radiosensitivity of neoplasms of different organ systems. The figure shows the greatest radiosensitivity coupled with a low SOD content in the gonadal tumor, as expected. A second feature is that the radioresistance of lung cancer parallels the elevated SOD activity. This could have been closely related to the evolution of homeothermic life as atmospheric oxygen concentration increased during the Carboniferous Period.

A clear exception is found in the prevertebral tissues, where the strong radioresistance is not accompanied by any increase in SOD activity. This contradiction deserves special comment. As represented by fibroblasts, the prevertebral organ cells are more proliferative under a hypoxic rather than a hyperoxic milieu (Bradley *et al.* 1978; Kan and Yamane 1983). Melanocytes are transitional, and melanomas, too, are hypoxic growers (Joyce and Vincent 1983). These cells would naturally not require as much SOD activity as those of the respiratory system. In other words, hypoxia may preserve the tumor cells because of less efficient production of superoxide radicals. Thus, the SOD content of a tumor can be a measure of its radiosensitivity so long as it arises in one of the vertebral organ systems or the gonads.

The radiosensitivity of a tumor may be expressed by formulating various contributory factors as follows:

$$S = f(W \cdot O \cdot D \cdot T \cdot d \cdot R \cdot E \cdot M \cdot B)$$

where S stands for the radiosensitivity of the tumor; W, water content (proton density); O, partial oxygen pressure *in loco*; D, content of superoxide dismutase; T, temperature; d, DNA density; R, reciprocal of the capacity for repair; E, biological effectiveness; M, mitotic prospects; and B, biological amplification. In cancer cells, W is greater than in normal cells, while O and R are both lower, as discussed earlier. Changes in W, O, and D are largely dependent upon temperature because they represent "chemical reactions." Because irradiated cells die as a result of mitotic difficulty, tumors of higher mitotic frequency (M) would probably exhibit greater radiosensitivity. E is unity for X-rays and gamma-rays. It is 10 for alpha particle rays and neutron beams.

Origin of Different Radiosensitivities of Different Histological Diagnoses

Different therapeutic plans are usually employed for different histological types of tumors of the same primary source. In lung cancer, for instance, we give a course of 1.5 Gy per day and 45 Gy in total for squamous cell carcinomas. For adenocarcinomas of the lung, we may give a course of 2.5 Gy per day and 70 Gy in total.

One way to determine why the dose schedule has to be changed from one carcinoma to another is to measure the SOD activity of different histological types of one category of cancer. This was done with lung cancers (Table 3) (Iizuka *et al.* 1984). Measurable amounts of MnSOD are reportedly present in specimens of human lung cancers, a finding that contradicts the reports of Oberley's group on experimental animal cells (Loven *et al.* 1981). Secondly, there are definite differences in MnSOD activity between different histological types of cancers; activity was the greatest in adenocarcinoma. These differences probably account to a large extent for the differences in radiosensitivity between different histopathologic types of tumors.

Apoptosis as the Fourth Evolutionary Mechanism for the Elimination of Radiation-damaged Cancer Cells

Apoptosis is the death of a single cell in a tissue (Lennox and Lennox 1986). Cell death may take place in any tissue, at any time, for any reason, pathological or normal, as in the case of digit formation during histogenesis (Kerr and Searle

Table 3. MnSOD content in human lung cancers and normal lung

Carcinoma type	Carcinoma, μg enzyme/mg protein	Uninvolved, μg enzyme/mg protein	P-value
Adenocarcinoma	41.0 ± 3.88 (26)	17.3 ± 2.17 (20)	$<.001$
Squamous cell carcinoma	33.9 ± 3.87 (11)	21.1 ± 5.19 (7)	$<.10$
Large cell carcinoma	29.6 ± 6.13 (3)	26.0 ± 8.29 (2)	NS

Values are means $\pm$ SE. Numbers in parentheses are numbers of patients. Statistical analysis was performed by Student's *t*-test.

NS = not significant.

MnSOD content may be different among different histological types of cancers of the same organ system (Iizuka *et al.* 1984)

1980). From the standpoint of evolution, cells in the testis that have committed DNA error(s), regardless of etiology, have to be eliminated. Apoptosis would help to overcome life-threatening emergencies by supplying energy through corticosteroid secretion followed by cytolysis, as in the case of stress lympholysis (Kobayashi 1980). Cell loss also occurs after radiotherapy and chemotherapy. However, cell loss after radiotherapy does not include cell death at high radiation doses, i.e., kilorads, but is thought to represent cancer cell death from routine fractionated doses of 100 to 300 rad. Cell killing at higher doses can be a demonstration of the *potential* of doing so. There is no 100% guarantee that cell loss occurs at lower doses, especially those of routine daily fractionation. In this regard, apoptosis may be an appropriate explanation, one that has evolutionary implications.

Exfoliation as a Mode of Cancer Cell Loss Contributing to the Different Radiosensitivities of Different Histological Types
Other important factors contribute to these differences in

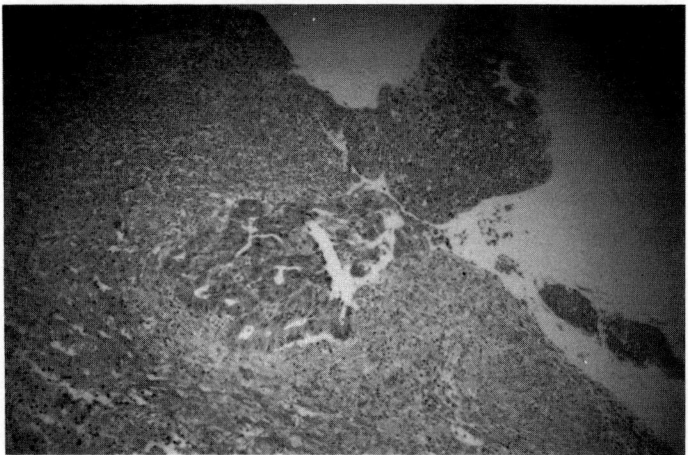

Fig. 7. Effects of radiochemotherapy with low-dose irradiation on rectal carcinoma (1). The low-dose radiotherapy may promote exfoliation of cohorts of cancer cells into the rectal lumen. This regression may be the reverse arborization seen in the spread of the cancer cells (Okuyama and Mishina 1984; Iwama and Takahashi 1983).

radiosensitivity. The ability to effect DNA repair can be important. However, certain biological mechanisms seem to be essential for the disposal of radiation-damaged but viable cancer cells. Exfoliation is one such mechanism, as shown for

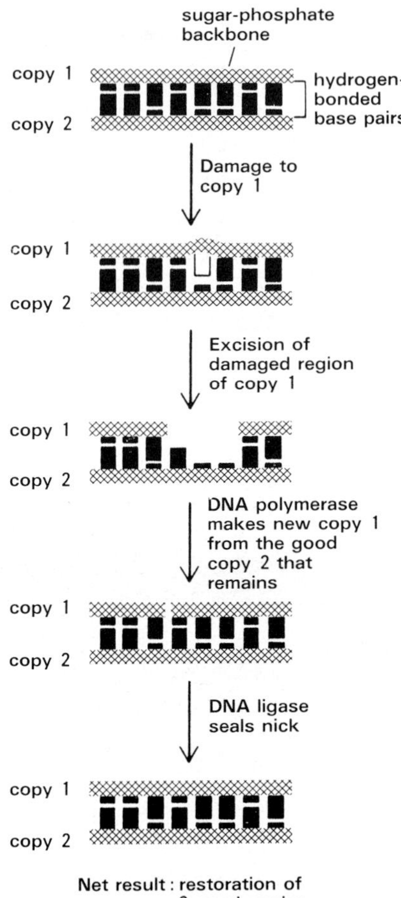

Fig. 8. Excision repair of DNA: Illustration of excision and restoration, two reactions fundamental to DNA repair. Restoration involves two steps: (1) DNA polymerase fills the gap created by the excision and (2) DNA ligase seals the nick left in the repaired strand. Nick sealing consists of the reformation of a broken phosphodiester bond (Alberts *et al.* 1983). This type of repair could have been acquired billions of years ago when ultraviolet rays were still intense because of the low oxygen concentration in air (Kondo 1972)

irradiated rectal cancer (Fig. 7) (Okuyama *et al.* 1984b). Rectal cancer cells grow and spread through the submucosa in an arborescent way (Iwama and Takahashi 1983). When treated, the normal tissue architecture is well preserved, but the rectal cancer cells can regress from the submucosa and eventually exfoliate into the rectal lumen. This tendency may be common rather then occasional. When a series of irradiated and extirpated specimens were re-examined and compared with those treated by chemotherapy followed by surgery, definite improvement was seen. The general tendency was toward reduction in contiguous and lymphatic spread at the time of surgery and increased confinement of the disease

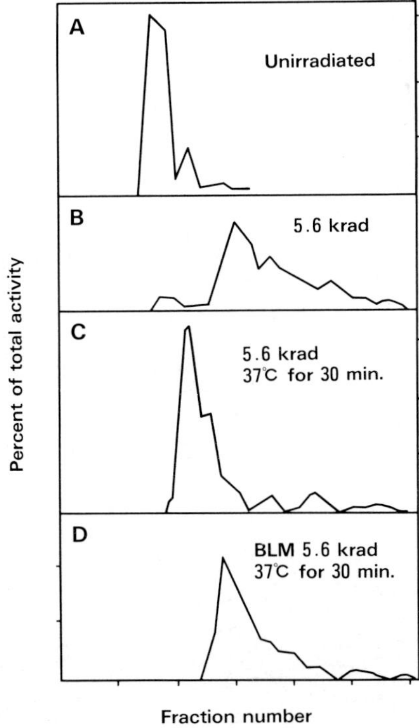

Fig. 9. Perpetuation of repairable radiation damage in DNA: An ultracentrifugal study on DNA from murine L cells. The radiation-induced DNA breaks, which are eventually repaired by rejoining, were "perpetuated" by consecutive bleomycin (Terasima *et al.* 1970). Here, bleomycin interferes with DNA polymerase beta (Mueller *et al.* 1979).

within the rectal wall. The same mechanism may operate in other combinations of cancerous and normal tissue.

Evolutionary Background of Excision Repair

Excision repair itself could have been acquired relatively early in evolution, perhaps 2.5-2.8 billion years ago (Kondo 1972). Its primary function is to get rid of defective portions of DNA. Restoration of the lost information can be achieved by copying the corresponding portions of the remaining DNA (Fig. 8). The homologous genes for this kind of repair are found in yeast as well as in human beings (van Duin *et al.* 1986). It would be useful to know whether there are quantitative or qualitative differences in gene expression between tumors of different organ systems and different histopathologic types, and whether these differences are sufficient to produce differences in radiosensitivity.

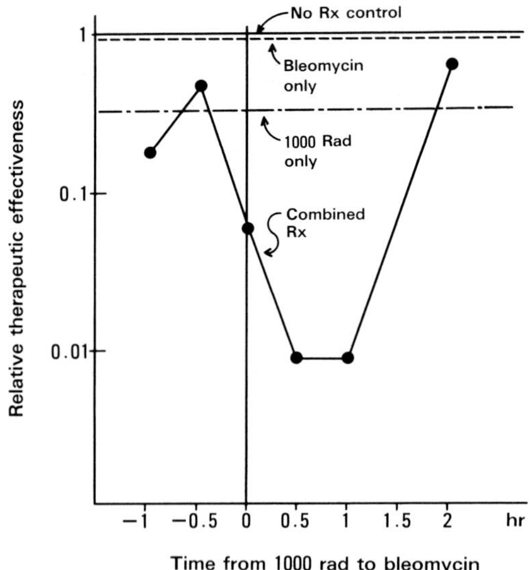

Fig. 10. Synergistic effect of consecutive bleomycin and radiotherapy. Consecutive bleomycin at 0.5 to 1 hr postirradiation increased the therapeutic effect of radiation (Okuyama and Matsuzawa 1979; Okuyama and Mishina 1980).

Clinical Implications of Excision Repair: Perpetuation Principle of Radiotherapy

It is possible to take advantage of evolutionary excision repair by *perpetuating* radiation-induced, repairable DNA damage, if that kind of repair is defective to any appreciable degree, as suggested by Yatani *et al.* (1982). This principle was clearly demonstrated *in vitro* with bleomycin by Terasima *et al.* (1970) (Fig. 9). In our *in vivo* studies in the rabbit, the time at which the perpetuating agents were administered appeared critical (Fig. 10) (Okuyama and Matsuzawa 1979). In head and neck tumors, the principle was applied to appreciably reduce radiation doses (Mishina *et al.* 1986). Other perpetuators are also available: neocarzinostatin (Okuyama and Mishina 1980; Mueller *et al.* 1979) and cordycepin, an inhibitor of adenosine deaminase (Nakatsugawa and Sugawara 1980). The perpetuation principle can probably be expanded to the domain of chemotherapy as well.

Chapter 9

The Chemosensitivity of Cancer

> *Bleomycin is one of the least toxic drugs to plants. Plants have constantly been exposed to sunlight since their appearance on earth, and are accordingly potent enough to repair nicked DNA.*
> ——*Hamao   Umezawa   (1914-1986),*
> Pharmacology

Evolutionary Implications of Current Anticancer Chemotherapeutics

The contemporary classifications of chemotherapeutic agents are not always self-explanatory to the clinician. To facilitate a better understanding of chemotherapeutic mechanisms and to assist in planning their administration, a new classification is presented in Table 1. It is designed to cover the proliferative structures and functions of cancer cells, i.e., DNA, mitochondria, or mitosis, and will aid in understanding the evolutionary concept of cancer cell chemosensitivity.

DNA type   These agents in this category interfere in one way or another with the DNA synthesis. They include metabolic inhibitors of DNA synthesis per se, like 5-fluorouracil and methotrexate, and agents that interfere with the mechanical aspects of synthesis—for example, nicking by bleomycin and mitomycin C, intercalation by actinomycin D, and cross-linking by alkylating agents (Goodman and Gilman 1975). The latter two therapeutic categories probably have in common the excision repair of DNA damage (Alberts *et al.* 1983). Their chemotherapeutic efficacy can be diminished by repair of previously induced, repairable DNA damage. For example, the damage incurred by mitomycin C is repaired within 24 hr of treatment. This type of DNA repair was reportedly

Table 1. Classification of cancer chemotherapeutics

Target type	Drug types	Drug	Remarks
DNA type	DNA synthesis inhibitors	5–Fluorouracil	
	DNA damage	Mitomycin C	
		Cyclophospha-mide	
		Cisplatin	
		Bleomycin	
RNA type		L–asparaginase	
		Actinomycin D	
		Adriamycin	
Mitotic	Metaphase arrest	Vincristine	
		Vinblastine	
Mitochondrial	Tetracyclines	Vibramycin	Okuyama *et al.* 1987
		Teramycin	(Kroon *et al.* 1985)
Receptor	Corticosteroids		
	Sex hormones		
Tumor antigen	Monoclonal antibodies		
Anti-oncogene/ oncogene products		Herbimycin	(Uehara *et al.* 1986)

N.B., Names in parentheses denote reporters of experimental studies.

acquired nearly 3 billion years ago (Kondo 1972). It requires DNA polymerase β whose action can be blocked by certain agents. Our experiments suggest that bleomycin at small doses blocks DNA polymerase to interfere with repair of DNA damage created by cisplatin (Fig. 1), while neocarzino-statin acts against that created by bleomycin at large doses (Okuyama and Mishina 1980). The net effects can be designated the "perpetuation principle" of chemotherapy (Okuyama and Mishina 1981b; 1982a, c; 1983a).

RNA type   Agents in this category interfere with the metabolism of transcription of the template gene(s) in DNA to RNA. L-asparaginase, actinomycin D, and adriamycin belong to this group.

Mitotic type   Vincristine and vinblastine induce metaphase arrest, leading to the death of cancer cells. Mitosis may be one of the major *loci minores resistentiae,* for the process of mitosis consists of several endosymbiotic structures (Mar-

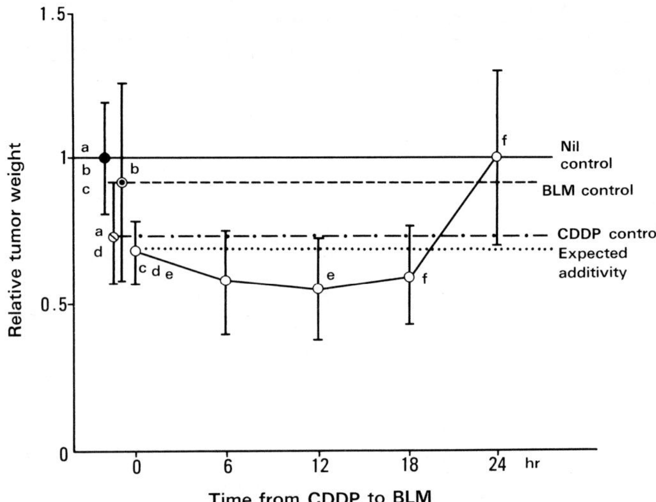

Fig. 1. Synergistic effect of consecutive bleomycin on alkylating chemotherapy. The therapeutic effect of cisplatin (CDDP) was augmented for 6-18 hours post-CDDP by the consecutive administration of bleomycin (Okuyama and Mishina 1980). Although the DNA damage incurred by alkylation is repairable, bleomycin could have interfered with repair by inhibiting the DNA polymerase. Similar perpetuating activity can be expected for neocarzinostatin (Okuyama and Mishina 1980; Mueller *et al.* 1979).

gulis 1981), and is therefore vulnerable to such agents. Thus, this type can also be seen in evolutionary terms.

Mitochondrial type   Mitochondria are also endosymbiotic structures (Margulis 1980). However, little attention had been paid to them in terms of anticancer potential until direct anticancer effects started being observed with tetracyclines, which are antibacterial agents (Okuyama *et al.* 1984c; 1987a). We found that cancer may express prokaryotic or pre-eukaryotic properties that can be targeted to cancer cell death. Kroon and his associates independently observed that mitochondrial protein synthesis can be the target of tetracyclines (Kroon and van den Bogert 1985; van den Bogert *et al.* 1986). However, our data indicate that cellular membranes are also critical structures, because the dosage of intratumoral injections for human cancers is high, and in the experimental rat model, the prompt changes in serum HDL-cholesterol are sufficiently drastic (Okuyama *et al.* 1987a).

Receptor type   The corticosteroids are lympholytic. Sex hormones are capable of destroying cancer cells that possess compatible receptors in sufficient amounts: estrogens for prostatic cancers, and androgens for breast cancers. The concept can be expanded beyond the evolutionary background. Cases of lung cancer can be treated with synthetic progesterone (Fig. 2) (Okuyama and Mishina 1989), as suggested earlier (Chaudhuri *et al.* 1982; Mattern *et al.* 1985). The evolutionary implication of corticosteroids may be apoptosis, or individual cell death in tissues (Kerr and Searle 1980), possibly designed to energize the host at the cost of tissue cells in situations like escaping danger or chasing game (Kobayashi 1980).

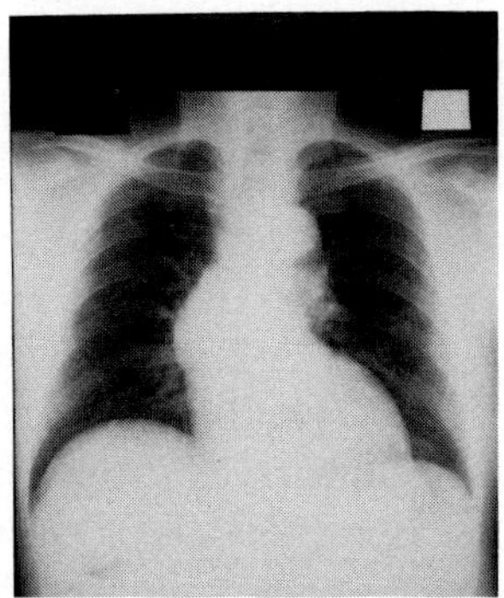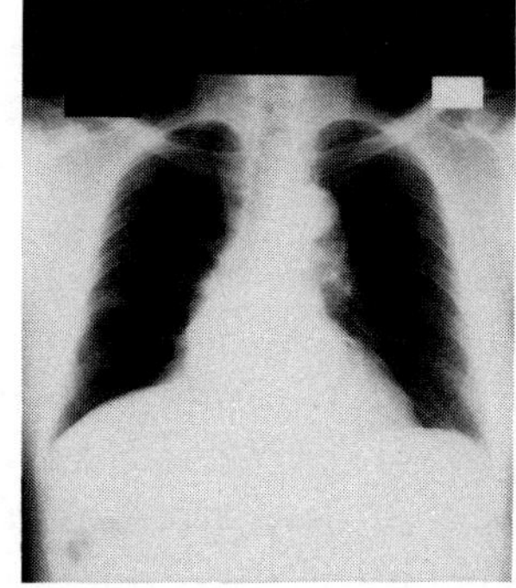

Fig. 2.   Effects of medroxyprogesterone acetate on male lung cancer. The patient, a male 76 years of age, was referred to us for possible radiotherapy of bilateral hilar lung cancer. He was known to have had an episode of myocardial infarction followed by anginal spells. He was not thought to be a candidate for radiotherapy, and was placed on synthetic progesterone (400 mg t.i.d.) along with a low dose of carmofur. A pronounced therapeutic effect was observed (Okuyama and Mishina 1988b). Thus, the receptor type of anticancer therapy can be expanded beyond the mammalian breast and uterine cancers. The underlying mechanism may be one of receptor expressions of devolution followed by evolutionary apoptosis.

A second group of the receptor type of anticancer agents seems likely. Bestatin, a specific leucine aminopeptidase inhibitor, is capble of immunostimulation (Umezawa 1977). However, its direct binding to cancer cells appears to induce their redifferentiation, however primitive the signs may be, and to entice cancer cell death (Okuyama and Mishina 1984a, c; Okuyama *et al*. 1985b).

Cancer antigen type   The concept of anticancer immunity may have been originated by Ehrlich (Bellanti 1971). Recent advances in monoclonal antibody preparation are expected to provide specific, potent anticancer antibodies. Recent progress with mediators of immune reactions also appears promising. Anti-cancer immunity is not a recent evolutionary development (Kumagai 1985). As is discussed elsewhere (Okuyama and Mishina 1987a), the T immunity could have emerged 500 million years ago with the appearance of vertebrates. B immunity seems to have developed about 350 million years ago, when land animals appeared. The mammalians appeared nearly 200 million years ago. The evolutionary steps in the development of immunity may be indicative of a similar step-by-step development of antigenicity, or, in other words, the elaboration of new tissues and organs. The mammalian symbol organs, for instance, may have unique antigens that would not have been observed in early evolution. Newer species have novel self-markers. Being out of the water, the land animals needed humoral immunity to establish their "self" against constant viral and bacterial invaders. T immunity may have characterized the aquatic semi-vertebrates, permitting T-cells to patrol the body to counteract invaders. NK cells could have emerged prior to T-cells. These cells are highly sensitive to radiation, and therefore to superoxide anions. This particular property of NK cell indicates that they could have emerged when the atmospheric oxygen concentrations were still low. Thus, immune systems could have been evolutionarily stratified, as could anticancer immunity itself. Immunotherapy for myelophthisis carcinomatosa from cancers of the mammalian symbol organs such as the breast and prostate with OK-432, a viable streptococcal preparation, is frequently effective.

A second aspect of cancer anitigenicity may be related to the devolution of cancer. Recent advances in the assay of tumor markers indicate (1) that there are gross antigens such as TPA that may be common to a wide range of tumors, (2) that a second group of tumor markers may represent the untoward expression of cryptic antigens that have been masked by dint of normal differentiation of the relevant organ system, e.g., CEA and AFP, and by logic, (3) that apparent ectopic antigenic expression may also take place, as in the case of CEA positivity in small cell carcinoma of the lung and malignant lymphoma. It seems noteworthy that similar diversification may take place with the elaboration of hormones, as in lung cancers of Eaton-Lambert syndrome, and the expression of receptors, as in the above-mentioned case of lung cancer for progesterone. Because protein synthesis is controlled by genes, these antigenic peculiarities, by analogy, have to be oncogene-controlled. Nonetheless, the most potent anti-cancer immune modes appear to be the quasispecific rather than the specific ones, as will be discussed more fully in the next chapter.

Anti-oncogene/oncogene products   This category of medicine is expected to include prevention against the development of cancers, in addition to the treatment of established neoplasms. Herbimycin is known to act on the *ras*-gene products of cancer cells and to cause such cells to redifferentiate (Uehara *et al.* 1985). This could be developed to form a new principle of treatment. The search for emerogenes (anti-oncogenes or tumor suppressor genes) should also be encouraged (Klein 1987).

Evolutionary and Strategic Reinforcement of Chemotherapy: Selective Concentration and the Principle of Perpetuation

Because clinicians are strongly interested in any appreciable improvement in cancer treatment, it is important to determine what the evolutionary perspective of chemotherapy offers in this regard.

Selective Concentration of Drugs in the Tumor

The effects of chemotherapy depend upon the drug concentration at the target site and patient tolerance. Selective concentration can be achieved in various ways (Table 2): (1) concentration by specific affinity, (2) selective spatial concentration, and (3) selective temporal concentration (Okuyama and Mishina 1982a, c). Among these, the technique of induced hypertension chemotherapy (IHC) appears the most evolutionary (Suzuki *et al.* 1981; Sato *et al.* 1981; Sato 1987).

Tumor vasculature provides a hypoxic milieu (Algire and Chalkley 1945; Cole *et al.* 1983) that can hinder drug delivery to cancer cells. This situation can be overcome by the use of angiotensin II (Suzuki *et al.* 1981; Burton *et al.* 1985). When systemic blood pressure is elevated by an intravenous administration of angiotensin II, the local, tumoral blood pressure also rises. This rise can be maintained as long as the agent is infused, and chemotherapeutic efficacy is enhanced. Signifi cant clinical effectiveness has been observed (Sato *et al.* 1981; Sato 1987). Nonetheless, it remains to be determined whether IHC helps to solve the practical problem of the nonhomo-

Table 2.   Principle of selective concentration in cancer therapy

Mechanism	Relevant examples
1. Concentration by specific affinity	Antigenicity-oriented immunotherapy like ^{131}I–CEA.
	Hormonal receptor therapy of breast and prostate cancer, lympholysis.
2. Selective spatial concentration	Direct impregnation.
	Selective arterial infusion/embolization.
	Vascular maceration with proteases.
	Topical concentration by inflammation, inhibition of drug metabolism, enzyme induction or activation within cancer tissues.
	Heat application.
	Low-dose irradiation.
	Cellular membrane modulation.
3. Selective temporal concentration	Cell cycle phase-specific chemotherapy.
	Continuous low-dose infusion of cell cycle phase-specific chemotherapeutics.

geneous structure and function of larger human tumors, thus preventing local regrowth in the long run.

Principle of Perpetuation of Repairable Chemotherapeutic DNA Damage

The DNA damage incurred by radiotherapy is repairable, and can be perpetuated with bleomycin (Terasima *et al.* 1970; Okuyama and Matsuzawa 1979). Because alkylating chemotherapeutics are "radiomimetics," we wonder if their DNA damage could be similarly perpetuated with bleomycin. This question was the point of departure for our studies (Okuyama and Mishina 1980; 1983a). As with radiotherapy, the effects of chemotherapy can also be probabilistic. In a volume of irradiated tumor, there are three categories of cells: (1) lethally damaged, (2) damaged but repairable, and (3) intact (Fig. 3). If portions of the repairable damage can be kept unrepaired, the resultant therapeutic size can be increased that much more. One drug acts as an inducer of repairable DNA damage, while a second, consecutive, agent inhibits the repair. This second agent is thus a perpetuator. This is the fundamental idea of the perpetuation principle, which may have a biochemical background as well (Mueller *et al.* 1979).

Figure 1 shows an experimental result achieved with cisplatin, an inducer, and bleomycin, a perpetuator (Okuyama and

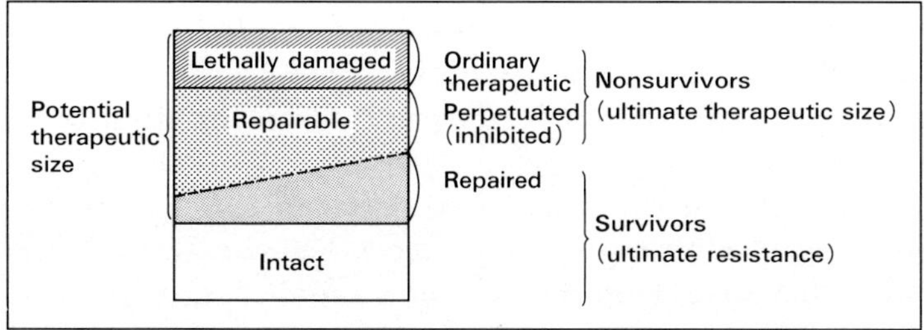

Fig. 3. Perpetuation principle of radiotherapy and chemotherapy indicating three functional categories ranging from damaged to intact. The principle aims to enhance the ultimate potential therapeutic size, which would otherwise be reduced through repair over time (Okuyama and Mishina 1982a, c).

Table 3. Probable relation of DNA lesions to perpetuation schedules. With single strand lesions, the optimal perpetuator timings were shorter than with double strand lesions.

	Inducer	DNA lesion	Perpetuator	Consecutive schedule
I.	Mainly single strand lesions:			
	Radiation	Single strand scission[a]	Bleomycin*	0.5 to 1 hr** Min to 6 hr
	Bleomycin*	Nicking and single strand scission	Actinomycin D[b] Neocarzino-statin	1 hr***
II.	Mainly double strand lesions:			
	Cyclophosphamide	Cross-linking[c]	Bleomycin	18 to 24 hr period***
	Cis-Diammine-dichloroplatinum (II)	Cross-linking[d]	Bleomycin	Up to 18 to 24 hr***

a. Any textbook of radiology or radiobiology.
b. Smith and Wilson (1970).
c. Any textbook of cancer chemotherapy or pharmacology.
d. Van deu Berg *et al.* 1977
* Large doses as an inducer, but much smaller doses as a perpetuator or repair inhibitor.
** Rabbit V2 epidermoid carcinoma, lung colony assay.
*** Rat AH109A adenocarcinoma, footpat tumor assay.

Mishina 1980). Unlike the combination of radiotherapy and bleomycin, in which the effective duration of perpetuation was 0.5 to 2 hr postirradiation, the duration with the cisplatin-bleomycin combination was 6 to 18 hr. Different perpetuation times can be expected with other combinations (Table 3). The length of effective perpetuation seems to be closely related to whether the DNA lesions are single or double strand lesions.

However subtle the difference between cancer and normal tissue, chemotherapeutic perpetuation can be an evolutionary principle, because defective excision repair is one of the devolutionary characteristics of cancer (Yatani *et al.* 1983; Gibson *et al.* 1985; David *et al.* 1985). Thus, evolutionary considerations are likely to facilitate further development of anticancer chemotherapy.

Chapter 10

The Principles of Tumor Imaging

> *Knowing that the metabolic activity of malignant tumors is higher than that of normal tissues, attempts have been made to diagnose tumors; they were not very successful.*
> ——*Yasuhiko Ito (1932–1983)*, Nuclear Medicine

Our first attempt to discuss cancer as an anti-evolutionary phenomenon, or devolution, began with our consideration of the origin of the radiosensitivity of cancer cells (Okuyama and Mishina 1984b). When we prepared a paper for PET 85, Sendai, we again found ouselves holding an evolutionary concept in attempting to understand the complex mechanisms of tumor imaging with radionuclides. As has already been described and discussed elsewhere, this led us to a better understanding of cancer cachexia as well. We had long been perplexed by the bizarre configurations of redifferentiation presented by cancer cells exposed to bestatin (Okuyama and Mishina 1984c; Okuyama *et al.* 1985b), and a satisfactory answer to that question again seemed to come from the concept of devolution.

Tumor imaging is a dynamic process: the radiopharmaceutical approaches the tumor, enters it, and is excreted (Fig. 1) (Okuyama 1973; Okuyama *et al.* 1977; Ito and Muranaka 1982). An image is obtained when the radiopharmaceutical inflow and/or deposition is increased in the tumor or when its retention in the tumor is prolonged.

Biological Discrimination of Cancer

It has been stated that the greatest difficulty in cancer chemotherapy stems from insufficient biological discrimination

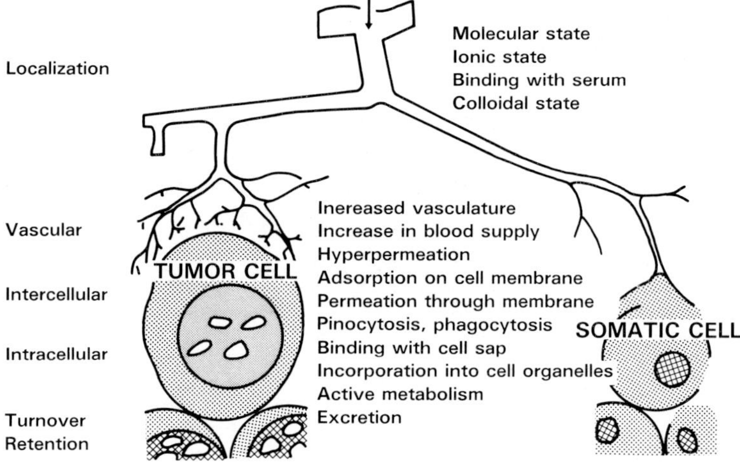

Fig. 1. Deposition of "tumor affinitive" radiopharmaceuticals. Any radiopharmaceutical administered intravenously approaches the tumor via vessels, extravasates, is adsorbed on the cell membrane, enters the cell and/or binds to cytoplasm or organelles. Radiopharmaceuticals may reside in any of these compartments, singly or in combination (Okuyama 1973; Okuyama *et al.* 1977; Ito and Muranaka 1982). The endosymbiotic hypothesis of Margulis (1981) can be used to look for abnormalities.

between cancer cells and normal host cells (Tanaka 1972). The purpose of tumor imaging is to make this discrimination and demonstrate it in radionuclide scintigraphy. Current discrimination is mostly based on empirical, relative concepts rather than being logical and absolute. We hope to develop logical ways of approaching discrimination.

Cancer Biology Leading to Legible Tumor Imaging: Principles of Tumor Imaging

The following evolutionary principles of tumor imaging may be useful in furthering the understanding of tumor imaging and the principles that underlie it.

The Principle of Hypoxia/Hypoperfusion

Cancer may represent an unusual population of cells that

proliferate slowly under a hypoxic milieu. The angiographic demonstration of tumor vessels in capillary phase may depend on the delayed passage of contrast media. Tumor vessels are characterized by fine arborescence that has an abrupt onset (Yamaura 1971). Because abrupt, fine aborization would permit an abrupt drop in blood pressure (Suwa *et al.* 1963), and because oxygen and nutrients are distributed among an enormous number of cancer cells, a definite decrease in blood pressure would be expected. This is the principle of hypoxia/hypoperfusion in cancer. When we inject aliquots of ^{99m}Tc pertechnetium or ^{67}Ga, a faint, transient accumulation of radionuclides can be visualized during the early period of injection. This change is not necessarily a guarantee of the long-supposed hypervascularity of a tumor.

The second feature of the hypoxia/hypoperfusion principle is hyponutrition due to inappropriate metabolic uptake and disposal of certain categories of substances. This can be taken advantage of with fluorohexoses (Table 1) (Ido 1986), D-amino acids (Tamemasa *et al.* 1978), or synthetic amino acids (Kubota *et al.* 1984; Ishiwata *et al.* 1988). Slower incorporation into proteins or slower oxidation or metabolic blockade can all be responsible for radionuclide retention in cancer cells. The D-amino acids may have definite evolutionary significance as they differ from the normal or physiological L-types.

The third aspect of this principle is related to the probable increased use of methionine in the process of ATP production, a result of devolution: cancer cells depend on creatine

Table 1. Tumor deposition of labelled fluorohexoses in the rat (Ido 1986)

Labelled fluorohexose	Tumor	Time (min)	Tumor uptake (% dose/g)	Tumor-to-organ Blood	Muscle
^{11}C–glucose	AH109A	10	1.2±0.2	1.00	3.57
^{11}C–fructose	AH109A	10	0.7±0.1	1.31	2.62
^{18}F–deoxy-fluoroglucose	AH109A	60	2.7±0.6	22.1	6.46
^{18}F–D–fluoromannose	AH109A	60	2.7±0.8	29.4	5.41
^{18}F–D–fluorogalactose	AH109A	60	1.4±0.2	5.27	13.7
^{18}F–L–2-deoxy-fluoro-glucose	AH109A	60	0.30±0.03	1.11	3.33

phosphate for energy rather than glucose (Baldwin 1957; Goseki *et al.* 1984; 1987). Viable cancer cell delineation with ^{11}C-labeled methionine (Kubota *et al.* 1988) would thus rest on an evolutionary basis of cancer.

The Principle of Primitive Fermentation

The biochemical characterization of cancers has been difficult because of two extremely different views: one hypothesizing rapid growth under hypervascularity and hypernutrition and the other, slow growth under hypoxia and hyponutrition. We have taken a third view, a composite or mosaic theorem: (1) Intratumoral oxygen distribution can be nonhomogeneous (Cole *et al.* 1983). This situation is graphically demonstrated by the cross-sectional anatomy of a tumor cord (Steel 1977). (2) The SOD content of different kinds of human tumors varies widely (Sykes *et al.* 1978). (3) Average cell cycle times for human cancers are as long as 50 hours (Sasaki *et al.* 1981), while the normal range is 24–30 hours (Lipkin *et al.* 1959; Westerveld *et al.* 1971; Zosimovska and Ljapunova 1966). (4) According to Horowitz's law of biochemical evolution (1945), the lowest tricarbon portions of glycolysis are evolutionarily the most primitive (Nakamura 1982). These reactions can proceed without any pre-investment of ATP, while reactions involving "fueling" with glucose and other hexoses demand preheating with ATP. As cancer cells prefer slow proliferation under a hypoxic milieu, the formation of lactate from pyruvate is increased. This can be taken advantage of in tumor imaging with ^{11}C-labelled pyruvate (Fig. 2) (Suzuki *et al.* 1985). The label is retained in the cancer cells for some time.

A second approach to the problem is to take advantage of the probable selective preference of tumors for a specific metabolism(s), the result of devolution. Although no new cancer-specific metabolisms have yet been established, galactose utilization by the embryonic and infantile liver can be regained as a result of hepatomagenesis (Fukuda et al. 1986), and hepatomas can be selectively visualized by ^{18}F-labeled D-galactose (Yamaguchi *et al.* 1986; 1988).

Thus, tumor imaging per se can take on an evolutionary meaning in selected cases.

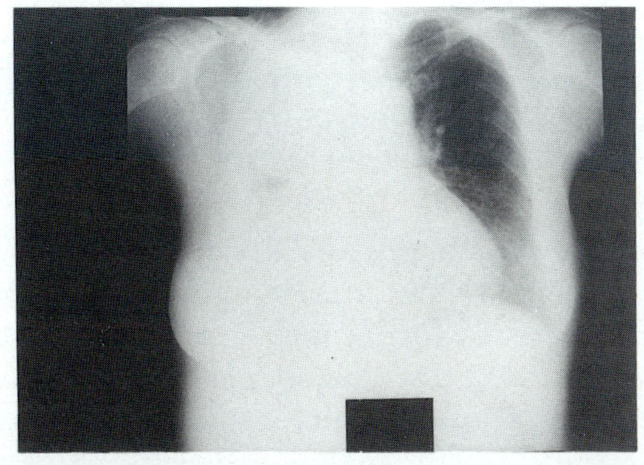

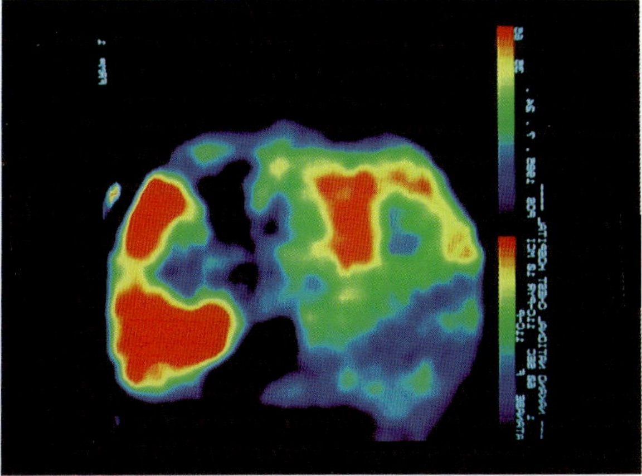

Fig. 2. The principle of primitive fermentation. Tumor imaging with ^{11}C-pyruvate (Suzuki *et al*. 1985). Metastatic tumors in the right lung are delineated positively. The sternal marrow also shows uptake of the radiopharmaceutical. This tumor imaging technique may have an evolutionary background.

The Principle of Low pK, Low Specificity

In the primitive seas, where the biodistribution of hexoses could have been rather homogeneous, hexokinases were indispensable. However, as the green algae acquired the capacity to produce abundant glucose through photosynthesis, animals must have adapted themselves by acquiring glucokinase of high pK and high specificity. If cancers represent a return to the primitive marine environment, they would have to depend upon hexoses other than glucose. The reported tumor imaging with labelled galactose and mannose (Fukuda *et al.* 1982) as well as that with FDG (^{18}F-labelled deoxyglucose) may thus have evolutionary significance.

Mitochondrial Principle

Mitochondria, which possess a type of DNA that is different from nuclear DNA, are thought to be endosymbionts and to contribute to the formation of eukaryotic cells (Margulis 1981). Because of their devolution, cancer cells may undergo a variety of changes, some of which can be used for tumor imaging. One example is the malate-aspartate shuttle, which is essential to ensure the use of NADH in the electron transport system, because mitochondrial membranes are impermeable to NADH. The hydrogen atom in NADH is transferred onto malate, which then enters the mitochondrion. Electronic balance is achieved by the extrusion of aspartate. In cancer cells, however, extrinsic malate is immediately oxidized by malic enzyme and eventually extruded as alanine after being aminated from glutamate. Concomitantly, citrate is formed and extruded (Moreadith and Lehninger 1984). Thus, the amine is misused, and the shuttle reverts to the age of green algae (Fig. 10, chapter 6). Glutamate incorporation would thus be increased in cancer cells, where it would contribute to tumor imaging with ^{13}N glutamate (Reiman *et al.* 1982).

The Lysosomal Principle

Lysosomes may also be the descendants of endosymbionts (Margulis 1981), and would devolve as a result of carcinogenesis, appearing coarser and more fragile than normal (Fig. 3) (Takeda *et al.* 1978). In addition to their morphological dysdifferentiation, their phagocytic function can also become abnormal (Takeda and Takusagawa 1978). Labelling of viable cancer cells is thus possible (Ito *et al.* 1971). Tumor labeling with ^{67}Ga (Edwards and Hayes 1969) seems not only to involve active uptake by the cancer cells (Kobayashi 1986; Higashi *et al.* 1988) but retention of the label within the cell (Fig. 4) (Muranaka *et al.* 1980), specifically in the diseased lysosomes (Takeda *et al.* 1978). A similar situation holds true for tumor imaging with ^{111}In chloride (Uchida *et al.* 1976). Thus,

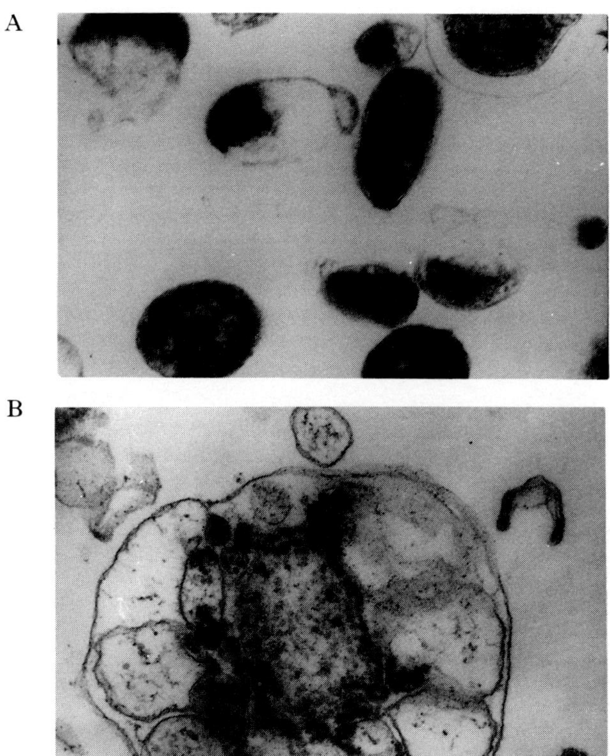

Fig. 3. The lysosomal principle of tumor imaging. Electron microscopic view of the lysosomes. A. Normal liver lysosomes. B. Abnormal lysosomes of a Morris hepatoma (Takeda and Takusagawa 1978). The swollen, adherent lysosomes may not be functioning properly: there are electron-dense microbodies in the center of this lysosomal conglomerate. This may indicate retention of slowly phagocytosed materials that have failed to be digested and expelled.

tumor imaging with ^{67}Ga and ^{111}In reflects the evolutionary concept of cancer.

The Receptor Principle of Tumor Imaging

The so-called receptor type of imaging has been extensively investigated, particularly in the field of brain neurology, where ^{11}C-labelled pharmaceuticals are used, among others. Although no reports of this type of imaging seem to have been published, it is likely that tumor imaging agents of this

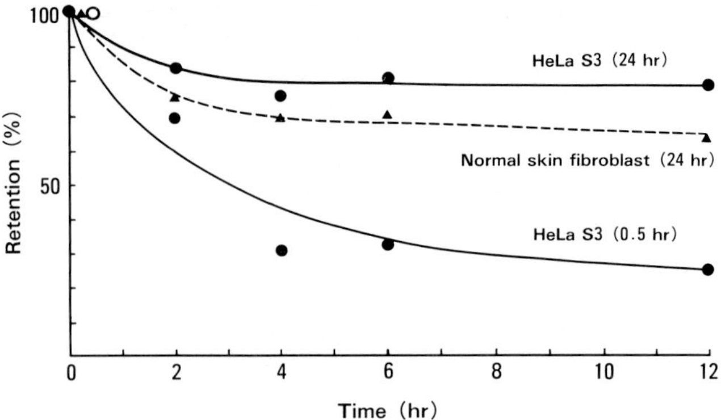

Fig. 4. The lysosomal principle of tumor imaging (2). Retention of radiogallium by cancer cells is clearly demonstrated in this experimental model (Muranaka *et al.* 1980). It took approximately 15 years for us to arrive at a plausible scientific explanation for the radiogallium imaging of cancer (Ito *et al.* 1971).

type will be developed in line with the evolutionary concept of cancer.

The Principle of Tumor Antigenicity

Given the recent remarkable advances in monoclonal antibody techniques, definite progress in the area of tumor antigenicity seems probable. The major problem will be in the development of tumor antigens with high labelling specificity. Antigens of symbiotic etiology need to be investigated as well.

The Principle of Oncogene/Oncogene Products

It is unclear whether specific oncogenes can be labelled. It may, however, be possible to neutralize oncogene products. In an *in vitro* system, the microinjection of a specific monoclonal antibody against oncogene products, e.g., cellular *ras* proteins, was seen to neutralize the activity of *ras* protein within the injected cells (Stacey *et al.* 1986). This same design can be propagated to label larger numbers of cancer cells. The cancer margins can also be labelled as soon as gene products relative to cancer invasion and metastasis are identified and harvested in amounts sufficient to permit preparation for clinical use. The techniques of gene manipulation would be of benefit in helping to define strategies.

The Tumor Structure Principle

The tumor structure pirnciple includes tumor vasculature, which has already been included in the principle of hypoxia/hypoperfusion and is of definite evolutionary significance. As the tumor continues to grow, vessels become tortuous and rupture here and there. Foci of hemorrhage and thrombosis also emerge. These tortuous, hemorrhagic/thrombotic vessels can be labelled with ^{131}I-MAA (Arimizu *et al.* 1972). The thrombosis can also be marked with ^{131}I-fibrinogen (Hisada *et al.* 1968). A technique for imaging small cancer foci by labelling TAF, or, more specifically, angiogenin, should also be developed.

The tumor imaging agents so far developed appear to have been empirical or incidental, as in the case of ^{67}Ga, or of limited specificity, as in the case of ^{131}I-fibrinogen. What is urgently needed now is a strategic plan for the development of tumor imaging agents that takes advantage of the definite biological distinction between what is normal and what is cancerous, and the ability to distribute these agents throughout the tumor or body. We believe that the evolutionary concept of cancer will aid in the designing of such agents.

Chapter 11

Strategic Cancer Therapy

> *The virtue of ECIB (extracorporeal irra-
> diation of blood) in treating CLL is sim-
> ply that there are no general toxic effects
> as encountered with chemotherapy and
> general radiation therapy (^{32}P or whole
> body radiation) or no local damage as
> seen after extensive splenic irradiation.*
> ——Eugene P. Cronkite, Hematology,
> *1967*

Introduction

One of the prerequisites of clinical medicine is a sound
diagnostic/therapeutic philosophy. When treating a patient, a
clinician needs to be aware of the patient's disease history as
well as the natural history of that disease. The initial therapeutic targets and the immediate consequences of treatment need
to be assessed. The means of achieving therapeutic benefits
must be available, as must those of alleviating therapeutic
hazards such as radiation dermatitis. It should also be possible
to plan a sequence of therapeutic events. Such a plan, while
clearly important, is not always easy to put into practice. The
need for practical ways to improve therapeutic planning led us,
about 10 years ago, to search for simple yet adequate ways of
planning and prescribing anticancer therapy. Our interim solution was to categorize anticancer therapy along the lines of ini-
tiation/perpetuation/biological aftermath, based on the recognition that any one of the current anticancer therapies was inadequate by itself and that synergistic cooperation among the
various modalities of treatment was clearly needed. The results were an attempt at logical integration (Okuyama and
Mishina 1981b; 1982c; 1985a, e). The origin of this concept
was the selective radiotherapy of leukemia cells by extracorporeal irradiation of the blood (Cronkite 1967). We came to
realize that such integration may have an evolutionary back-

ground, because carcinogenesis itself may be "devolutionary" (Okuyama and Mishina 1984b; Setala 1984). The evolutionary concepts of cancer may thus lead to the practical integration of various anticancer modalities.

Merits of Anticancer Therapy and Limitations Demanding Positive Strategic Measures

A variety of anticancer therapies exist: radiotherapy, chemotherapy, immunotherapy, and surgery. Each treatment modality is associated with a particular anticancer philosophy built upon its therapeutic effectiveness in a particular type of cancer. Table 1 summarizes the probable advantages and disadvantages of each modality of treatment. In brief, there seems to be a need for the strategic incorporation of different modalities of treatment with appropriate timeliness. An awareness of the probable advantages and disadvantages of each form of therapy would certainly orient the attending physicians to the entire scope of treatment available to the patients.

Table 1. Advantages and disadvantages of radiotherapy, chemotherapy, and surgery, and positive strategic anticancer measures

	Advantages	Disadvantages	Strategic tactics
Radio-therapy	Collimation DNA damage	Localness Log killing (probabilistic) Tissue tolerance Repairability	B = Biological amplifications (immunotherapy, rescue) PR = Perpetuation T = Particle RT
Chemo-therapy	Systemic effect Wide-range of subcellular targets	Log killing Tolerance Repair Tumor concentration	B (immunotherapy, rescue) PC = Perpetuation S = Spatial/temporal concentration
Surgery	Possible local completeness (no log kill)	Spilling	Presurgical RT* Postsurgical RT*

* RT = radiotherapy

Because we are radiologists, our plan centered around radiotherapy: the efficacy of radiotherapy and chemotherapy as it relates to the evolutionary history of cancer. The vulnerability of cancer to irradiation and chemotherapy was viewed in evolutionary terms. Surgery is not evolutionary; it is revolutionary. It has the potential in selected cases to effect complete removal of cancer cells. Nonetheless, surgery may have to adapt itself to other modalities of cancer treatment because of the possible spilling and scattering of cancer cells into the field of surgery or the movement of such cells into the circulation (Maki *et al.* 1963b). The many inoperable cases should also be noted here.

In order to facilitate interdisciplinary cooperation, a plan incorporating the different principles of treatment is proposed. It is hoped that this concept will aid the attending physician in developing an integrated scientific overview of the particular cancer to be treated.

Rationale for the Strategic Incorporation of Different Modalities of Treatment

Prospects and Limitations of Radiotherapy, a Local Chemotherapy

Radiotherapy is a local chemotherapy. The therapeutic effects of radiotherapy start with the ionization or ejection of electrons from water molecules and the production of superoxide radicals that are capable of inducing a host of chemical reactions, including damaging DNA. This knowledge is important because it facilitates the enhancement of therapeutic effects and the development of protective measures.

The definite advantage of radiotherapy lies in its collimation. In addition to its therapeutic effects, it also helps to confine side effects within the field of irradiation. Its therapeutic target is nuclear DNA, damage to which leads to (1) mitotic death and/or (2) apoptosis (intermitotic death).

Several limitations curtail the usefulnes of radiotherapy: (1) localized treatment, as in the case of surgery; (2) log kill or probabilistic limitation (Fig. 1) (Withers 1980); (3) repair of previously incurred DNA damage; and (4) damage to the surrounding normal tissue. These limitations have to be over-

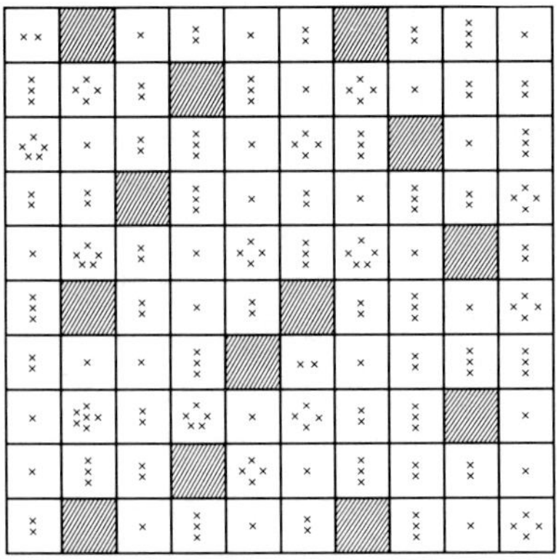

$$\lambda = 2$$

Fig. 1. Log kill limitation of radiotherapy. Radiation photons hit sensitive targets in a probabilistic manner, as demonstrated here (Withers 1981). The same principle would apply to chemotherapy where drug molecules are to represent the photons for radiotherapy.

come in one way or another, and the suggested techniques are listed in Table 2.

T stands for the effective *transfer* of radiation energy, such as in good collimation or selective irradiation, as in the case of ECIB (Cronkite 1967), and neutron capture therapy (Farr *et al.* 1954) or high energy transfer (LET) radiotherapy, including particle radiotherapy (Archambeau *et al.* 1974). The use of hypoxic sensitizers or D-penicillamine as an SOD inhibitor (Okuyama *et al.* 1981a) is also relevant here. The design of lymphocytosis induction by means of administration of lymphocytosis producing factors of biological or synthetic origin may deserve evaluation in the treatment of chronic lymphocytic leukemia and immunosuppression through ECIB (Okuyama *et al.* 1970).

The *repairable* DNA damage can be *perpetuated* (*PR*) by interfering with the repair processes in one way or another (Terasima *et al.* 1970; Matsuzawa *et al.* 1972; Okuyama and Mishina 1980). The effect is additive (Mueller *et al.* 1979). Cordycepin can also be employed in the same way (Nakatsugawa and Sugawara 1982). Thus, the perpetuation principle seems to operate both *in vitro* and *in vivo* at the experimental level. In cancer patients, tumor regression is expedited,

Table 2. Consecutive and strategic integration of principles of radiotherapy: *T-PR-B*

Symbol	Principle	Mechanism	Practical techniques	Remarks
T	Energy transfer	Selective transfer	Collimation	
			ECIB (extracorporeal irradiation of blood)	Cronkite 1971 (Okuyama 1970)
		Increased interactions	Increased water density in cancer	(Damadian 1971
			Neutron capture therapy	Farr 1954
			Heavy particle radiotherapy	Archambeau 1974
		Increased capture/ decreased disposal	Hypoxic cell sensitizers	(Okuyama 1980; 1981)
			Inhibition of superoxide dismutase	Okuyama 1982a; b
PR	Perpetuation of DNA damage	Inhibition and perpetuation of DNA damage	Bleomycin as perpetuator	(Terasima 1970) (Nakatsugawa 1982)
			Cordycepin, perpetuator	
			Aclacinomycin, perpetuator	(Miyamoto 1983)
		Immunity (Quasi specific)	GVH reaction	(Truitt 1976) Weiden 1981
B	Biological amplifications		BCG	(Old 1959) Mathe 1969
			Streptococcus (OK–432)	(Okamoto 1959)
			Basidiomyces (PSK, lentinan, and sizofilan)	(Chihara 1969) Furue 1987
			Sendai virus	(Matsuya 1979)
		Emperipolesis (specific)		Okuyama 1979
			Streptococcus (OK–432)	(Sasaki 1980)
		Apoptosis "Exfoliation"		Kerr 1980
			Exfoliation	Okuyama 1984 Mishina 1988
			Redifferentiation (Bestatin, PGD$_2$)	Okuyama 1985
			Surgery	
		Rescue	Cytochrome *c* effect (cytochrome *c*)	Okuyama 1982c 1983b
			(*ubiquinone*)	Mishina 1977
			(*hyperbaric oxygen*)	
			Lysozyme	Okuyama 1988

Names in parentheses under Remarks denote experimental researchers.

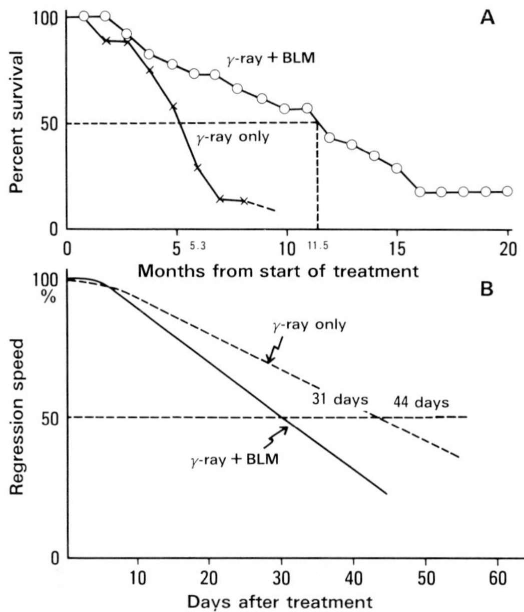

Fig. 2. Perpetuation of repairable radiation damage to DNA (1): A clinical study on lung cancer. Bleomycin was intravenously administered 0.5 to 1 hr post-irradiation. A. Regression of the tumor during consecutive radiation-bleomycin therapy; B. Survival curve of patients (Okuyama *et al*. 1975; Okuyama and Matsuzawa 1979). To prevent untoward development of hemoptysis from tumor necrosis (Okuyama *et al*. 1978), bleomycin in oil emulsion appears preferable (Mishina *et al*. 1985).

and prolongation of survival can be expected (Fig. 2). This type of perpetuating radiochemotherapy of head and neck tumors can further be reinforced with additional cisplatin (CDDP). A dose of 160 mg of CDDP was found capable of saving on average 20 Gy and 90 mg of bleomycin when the therapeutic effects were strictly evaluated by repetitive bi-optic negative conversion (Fig. 3) (Mishina *et al*. 1986). The 5-year survival rate for maxillary cancer was as high as 75% (Saijo *et al*. 1986). When histopathological examinations were carried out on a separate series, peculiar nuclear changes, presumably leading to cell loss through apoptosis rather than mitotic death, were to be seen (Fig. 4) (Okuyama *et al*. 1989a). The same principle has successfully been expanded to cases of esophageal cancer (Mishina and Okuyama 1983). Thus,

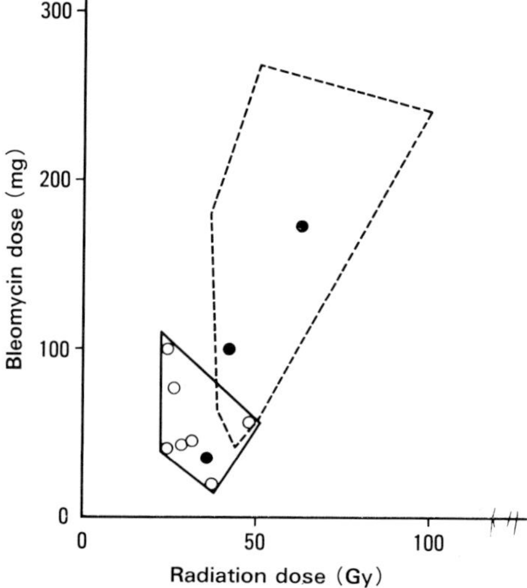

Fig. 3. Perpetuation of repairable radiation damage to DNA (2): Dose reduction with cisplatin. The combined effects of radiation, bleomycin, and tegafur on head and neck tumors were evaluated by repetitive biopsy. The dose-effect of radiation and bleomycin for negative conversion was confined to the upper region (dotted line). With the addition of cisplatin, radiation (1500 rad) and bleomycin (100 mg) doses are reduced.

the perpetuation principle of radiotherapy may simulate and strengthen the evolutionary phenomenon of apoptosis (Kerr and Searle 1980).

It is symbolically represented as *PR*, or the perpetuation of repairable radiotherapeutic damage, in Table 2.

B stands for *biological amplifications* of any type that serve to benefit the patient. They can be supplementary to chemotherapy and/or radiotherapy. Biological amplification includes two distinct categories of treatment: (1) biological measures that increase therapeutic efficacy by overcoming the log kill limitation, and (2) measures that protect surrounding normal tissues from radiation damage and rescue already incurred radiation damage, to increase tissue tolerance. An appreciable degree of protection and rescue can be achieved by simply administering cytochrome *c* or topically applying ubiquinone ointment (Okuyama and Mishina 1982d; 1983b).

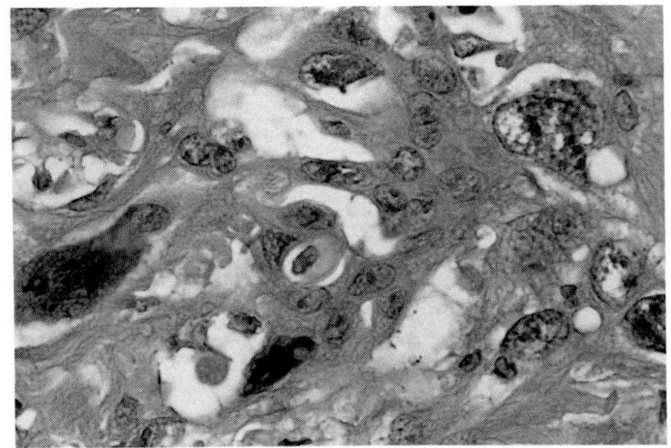

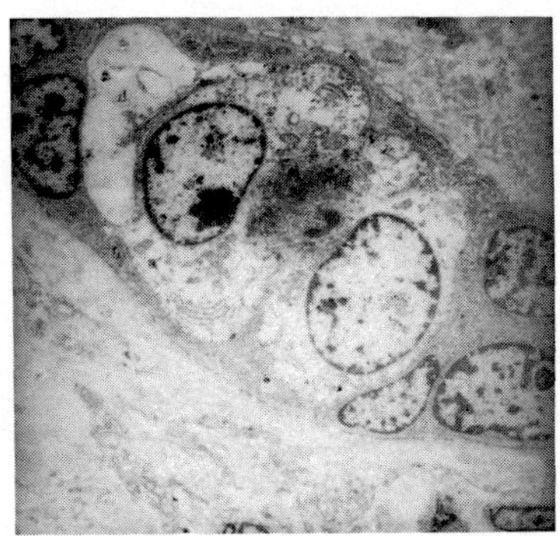

Fig. 4. Perpetuation of repairable radiation damage to DNA (3): Nuclear changes following radiochemotherapy with bleomycin. A case of maxillary cancer in a 45-year-old man. An autopsy was performed following a course of radiochemotherapy to 2250 rad, 100 mg of bleomycin, and 280 mg of cisplatin. Trails of cancer cells showing bizarre nuclear configurations are seen. The sequence of events in the nuclei can be presumed to represent apoptosis: chromatin condensation, margination, and fragmentation, ending in cytolysis. A. Photomicrograph; B. Electron micrograph (Okuyama *et al.* 1988a; Krishan 1973; Kerr and Searle 1980). Thus, the perpetuation principle may be taking advantage of the evolutionary nature of cancer cells or evolutionary discrimination of the increased vulnerability of cancer cells to radiochemotherapy.

The scope of anticancer immunotherapy is extremely limited, and no specific regimens are currently available. Our suggestion here is naturally a compromise: (1) quasispecific immunotherapy in terms of cross-immunity, mostly by employing viable BCG or a streptococcal preparation (OK-432) and (2) immunostimulation through the activation of T-cell subsets and/or NK cells (PSK, Lentinan and Sizofilan, and Bestatin). However, several problems need to be confronted: (1) tumor antigenicity, (2) T-cell imbalances in cancer patients, and (3) cancer exposure. At present, there appear to be no universal tumor antigens, just tumor-associated antigens (TAA) (Sulitzeanu 1985). TAA are not always selective enough for specific tumor systems. For example, the monoclonal antibodies against melanoma exhibit cross-reactivity even after absorption for irrelevant tissues (Sulitzeanu 1985). Cross-reacting organ/tumor tissues are largely confined to those of the central nervous system or those of mesenchymal origin among vertebrates (Table 3). Melanocytes are derived from the central nervous system, and the latter evolved with the advent of the vertebrates. Thus, they may respond to tissue antigens that are evolutionarily more primitive, e.g.,

Table 3. Cross-reactivity of monoclonal antibodies to melanoma tumor-associated antigens: Probable absence of consistent tumor specificity (modified from D. Sulitzeanu 1985). Of 35 monoclonal antibodies to melanoma TAA, only four were solely reactive to melanomas, while the remainder cross-reacted to other neoplasms of different primary tumors or normal tissues or amniofetal cells. When their relative distribution was examined, the majority of cross-reactions were found to be confined to TAAs of those organ categories representing early vertebral life, but not to those from organs of recent evolution or to the gonadal (evolutionarily secured presumably through immune tolerance or horror autotoxicus). See Figure 5.

Organ category	Cross-reactions	Overall incidence
Evolutionarily secured	0	0%
Mammalian symbol	1	
Homeothermic	1	
Poikilothermic	1	
"Epithelial"	14	32%
Neuroepithelial	18	
Renal	4	
Sarcomas	3	
Prevertebral (hematopoietic)	2	51%
Amniofetal antigens	9	17%

those for the kidney, as well those for elements of the central nervous system. Conversely, they may not embrace antigens that specify the newer organs that symbolize mammalian evolution, e.g., the breast and prostate. Accordingly, if evolution adds new antigens as new tissues and organs appear, TAAs may be stratified with regard to advancing evolution, with cancers of the mammalian symbol organs exhibiting the greatest cross-reactivity with other organs and tumors (Fig. 5). If this were true, it would enable us to evaluate specific anticancer immunity for the purposes of diagnosis and treatment. The cross-reactivity of BCG and OK-432 is well documented (Sawamura 1986; Sasaki and Kunimatsu 1980).

The second feature of cancer immunity seems to be

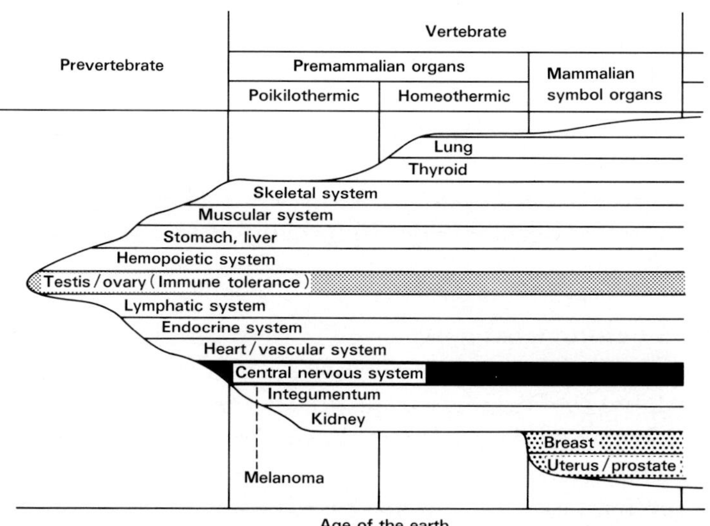

Fig. 5. Evolution of tumor antigens along the line of organ evolution: Hypothetical model. Tumor antigens could have evolved along with the evolution of different organ systems: monoclonal antibodies to melanomas show cross-reactivity that is limited to those that can be specified by their own evolutionary history. Melanocytes are of neural origin (Bloom and Fawcett 1975), while the neuroepithelium would be an organ of prehomeothermic vertebral life. Thus, it is logical that melanoma antigens would not react with those of the homeothermic or mammalian symbol organs as well as the gonads, the evolutionarily secured organs, through the immune tolerance.

immunosuppression, possibly owing to T-cell imbalance (Dillman and Koziol 1983; Kumano *et al.* 1985). This is characterized by a relative increase in suppressor cells. Suppressor cells are primarily cytotoxic effector cells, while helper cells enable B-cells to function properly. Both helper and suppressor cells emerge and differentiate in the thymus (Reinherz and Schlossman 1980). Suppressor cells appear to be more archaic than helper cells. The latter are connected with B-cells or specific immunity, as indicated by the radiosensitivity and the putative recent origin of specific humoral immunity (Kumagai 1985). Experiments on the induction of suppressor cells from the helper cell population are intriguing in this regard (Thomas *et al.* 1981; 1982). Suppression could be a modified cytotoxic function, while the helper function could be a discrete branching along the line of evolution. The full development of the B-cell system could have taken place in homeothermic life, probably in birds, in which the bursa of Fabricius is the central lymphoid organ for the B-cell system (Good 1971). These organ systems that originated or developed fully during the homeothermic period are relatively radioresistant because of the high atmospheric oxygen concentration (Berkner and Marshall 1965; Patterson 1978). The helper and B cells, which could have appeared with the advent of homeothermic life, may be radioresistant, while NK and cytotoxic/suppressor cells may be radiosensitive. In carcinogenesis, the suppression of specific immunity may be required by the tumor to eliminate probable aggression at tumor antigen sites by host immunity. Interestingly, however, the NK cell population, which is not necessarily decreased in cancer patients, can be increased after a course of peroral Bestatin (Kumano *et al.* 1985).

The third problem with cancer immunotherapy is its potency and/or penetrability. Single tumors are known to be heterogeneous in terms of morphology and sensitivity to radiotherapy and chemotherapy. The same rule may apply to immunotherapy as well. Nonetheless, there seem to be several ways to increase the vulnerability of cancer cells to immune attack (Schlager *et al.* 1978a, b). According to Schlager *et al.*, experimental tumor cells can be rendered more sensitive to humoral immune attacks by irradiating them or exposing them to chemotherapeutics like actinomycin-D and adriamycin. It is not clear whether or not such treatments would induce similar changes against attacks by cellular immunity.

The effectiveness of GVH reactions from transplanted allogeneic marrow cells in the treatment of leukemias (Masaoka and Inoue 1986) is interesting in that the principle may take advantage of the self-recognition function of the T cell system (Truitt and Pollard 1976; Weiden *et al.* 1981). In the case of choriocarcinomas, their definite therapeutic effectiveness becomes apparent only when radiotherapy and/or chemotherapy is effective, or when the numbers of remaining choriocarcinoma cells fall below certain threshold levels. This is a typical *T-B* or *S-B* scheme in which the biological amplifications (*B*) consist of GVH reactions between the fetal quasi-antigens and the immune system of the host mother (Alexander and Good 1977). The antigenic expression of experimental tumor cells is thought to change as a result of irradiation or exposure to chemotherapeutics (Tachibana 1974). Tachibana's review indicated that the histocompatibility genes would increase as cell cycle times were prolonged by such treatment, but not without exceptions.

The principal anticancer effect of mycotic preparations such as PSK, Lentinan, and Sizofilan may be their priming of lymphocytes to attack cancer cells. Figure 6 is intended to illustrate how lymphocytes infiltrate cancer tissues, approach cells, and destroy them when the cancer-bearing host is treated with such agents (Hamuro *et al.* 1980). The underlying mechanisms are known to involve activation of macrophages, induction of interleukins 1, 2, and 3, and activation of NK and T cells along with the specific antibody-dependent cell-mediated cytotoxicity (Fig. 7), as discussed elsewhere (Aoki 1984; Furue 1987). Their therapeutic prospects appear good as long as they are coupled with adequate chemotherapy (Hamuro and Chihara 1984).

OK-432 as a Nonspecific to Quasispecific Anticancer Immunogen

Table 4 shows the therapeutic results from OK-432 inhalation immunotherapy (Mishina and Okuyama 1987). The preparation was suspended in 3 to 5 ml of saline at doses of 0.2

Table 4. Cancer therapy by inhalation of OK-432

Primary cancer	Radiotherapy/ patients	Radiation dose (Gy)	OK-432*			Survival (months)	Therapeutic response (CR)	Surgery
			IV	IH	Tumor			
Breast	(+)/12	29.9±4.3		12/12		14.5±9.3	11	1
	(−)/4		1/4	4/4	1/4		4	0
Uterine	(−)/1		1/1	1/1		30	1	0
Prostatic	(+)/1	20		1/1		48	1	0
Head and neck	(+)/15	31.2±7.7	3/15	15/15		11.6±9.1	15	0
	(−)/1			1/1			1	1
Lung	(+)/1	40		1/1		12	1	0
	(−)/2		2/2	2/2		6, 24	2	0
Stomach	(+)/1	5	1/1	1/1		10	1	0
Rectum	(+)/1	20	1/1	1/1		3	1	0
Liver	(+)/1	32	1/1	1/1		28	1	0
Parotid	(+)/1	40	1/1	1/1		9	1	0
Scalp	(+)/1	35	1/1	1/1		4	1	0

* IV: intravenous injection; IH: inhalation; Tumor: sprinkled over the cancerous ulcers.

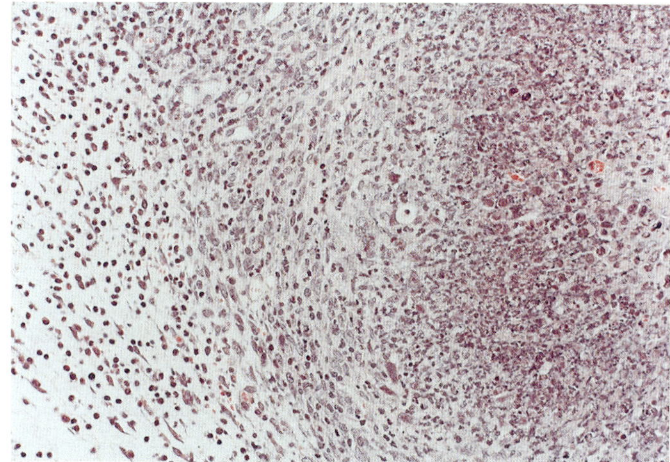

Fig. 6. Anticancer immune reaction enhanced by lentinan, an extract of *Lentinus edodes*; an experimental demonstration. Lymphocytes are seen infiltrating the tumor nests. The reaction itself can also be quasispecific. (Hematoxylin-esosin stain.) (Hamuro *et al*. 1980).

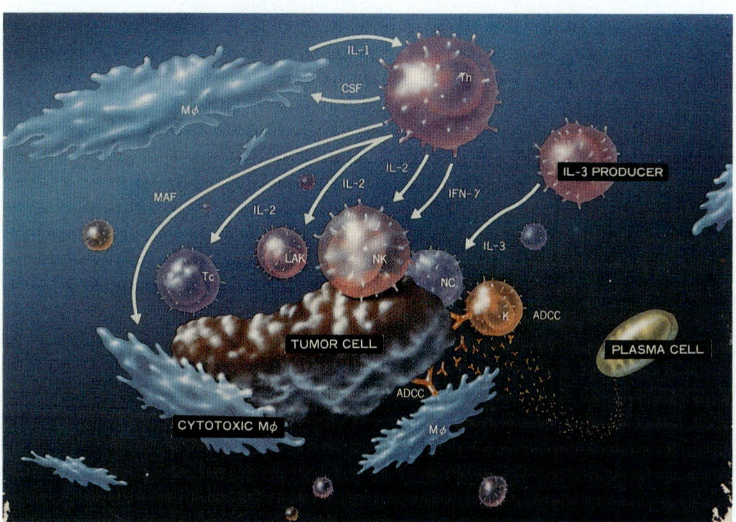

Fig. 7. The quasispecific immune reactions schematized. Most of the anticancer effects are primarily quasispecific, involving the macrophages, lymphokines, and NK cells. The schema indicates nature's endorsement of the devolutionary alteration of carcinogenesis.

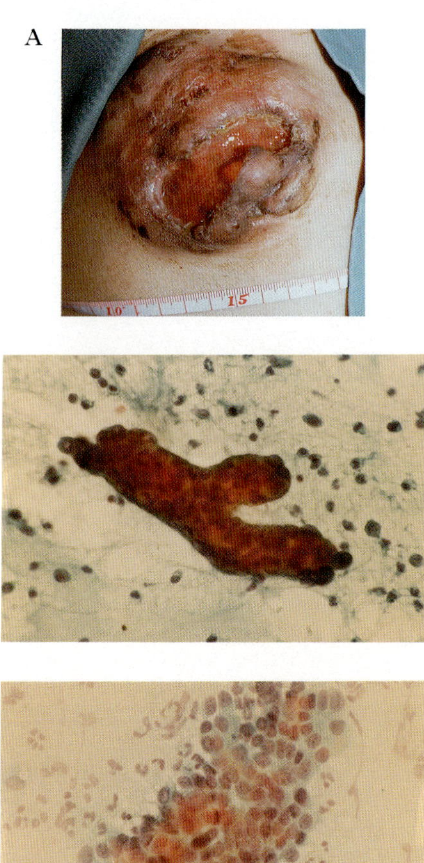

Fig. 11. Exfoliation as a mode of anticancer therapy: A case of breast cancer. A. A huge mass of inflammatory breast cancer. There were three large cancerous ulcers at the time of referral. Units of OK-432 powder were sprinkled over the ulcers as the entire right breast was irradiated to 200 rad five days a week. B and C. As the regression became obvious, a sequential cytological study of the healing breast cancer was undertaken by touch preparation. Cancer cells exfoliated en bloc and were tightly bound to each other. Some time after powdering with OK-432, the cells appeared loosened and became infiltrated by neutophils and lymphocytes. As their external portions became loose enough, the masses of cancer cells started falling off. The next layer of cancer cells would then be exposed to OK-432 the next day (Mishina *et al*. 1989).

to 5 units for nebulization. The results in a variety of cancer patients were excellent. The probable underlying mechanisms are (1) cross-antigen immunization between the streptococcus and tumor cells (Sasaki and Kunimatsu 1980), and (2) potent immunization through the respiratory system (Alexander and Good 1977), like that of antituberculosis immunity in pulmonary tuberculosis. The evolutionary impli-

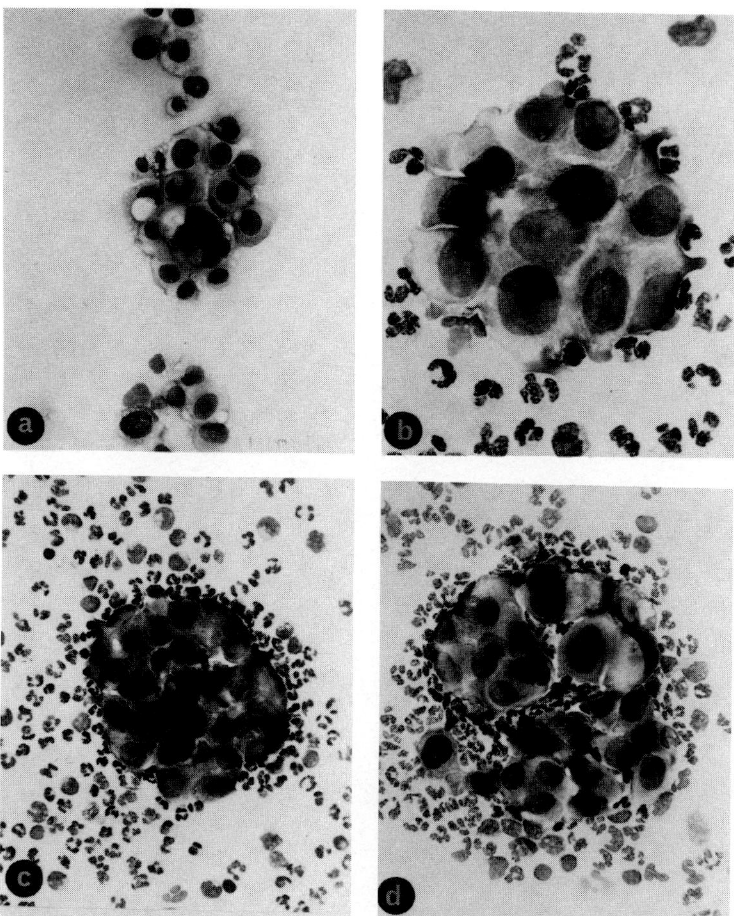

Fig. 8. Clinical evaluation of the nonspecific to quasispecific immunotherapy (1): Role of neutrophil leukocytes. OK-432 induces neutrophil leukocytes to attack cancer cells (Torisu *et al.* 1985).

cations of the cross-reactivity of tumors have already been discussed above.

An *in vivo*, cellular, anticancer event can be analyzed by using cancerous serositides such as ascites. When temporal changes in the number of cancer cells and neutrophils in ascites were followed up after an intraperitoneal introduction of OK-432, the cancer cells were found to disappear as the number of phagocytes surged (Fujimura *et al.* 1983). Figure 8 shows how such neutrophils attack cancer cells (Torisu *et al.* 1985). The fluidity of the ascites may expedite the phenomenon by several times at least (Torisu and Katano 1980). The same agent may also seduce macrophages into contact with cancer cells, leading to their eventual death (Fig. 9) (Toge *et al.* 1986). The probable activation of pulmonary alveolar macrophages through the inhalation of OK-432 is also relevant (Mishina and Okuyama 1987a). Direct, intratumoral impregnation of the agent would induce similar cellular reactions against cancer cells. We recently tried to expand the principle by introducing a saline suspension of OK-432 into the gut peranum or through the artificial stoma to alleviate cancerous peritonitis from, and eventually to combat,

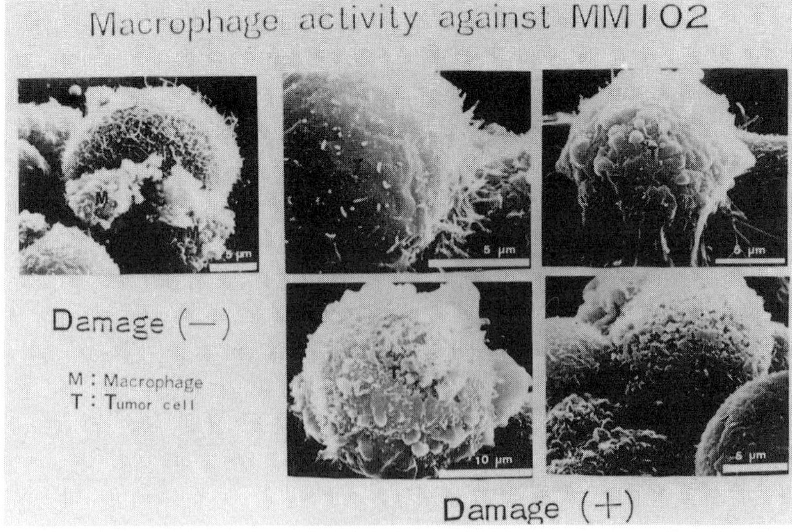

Fig. 9. Clinical evaluation of the nonspecific to quasispecific immunotherapy (2): Role of macrophages. OK-432 induces the macrophages to attack cancer cells (Toge *et al.* 1986).

retroperitoneal metastases from rectal cancer. The results seemed promising (Mishina and Okuyama 1989b). The substantial anticancer effect may be derived from the production of superoxide and other active oxygen molecules, which is common to both macrophages and neutrophils (Newburger *et al.* 1980; Weiss and LoBuglio 1980; Jong and Klebanoff 1980; Tomioka and Saito 1979). The secondary activation of T-cell immunity via the production of interferon (Saito *et al.* 1982) and interleukins (Ichimura *et al.* 1983) can also be important in the presence of factor(s) elaborated by the cancer cells themselves (Matsubara *et al.* 1980). Such a factor(s) is capable of inducing topical and systemic inflammations that might contribute to the redistribution of anticancer drugs (Okuyama *et al.* 1978a). Thus, the archaism of anticancer cellular events is in accordance with the devolutionary commitment of cancer cells. Coley's toxin could also involve the same or similar nonspecific to quasispecific immune reactions (Nauts *et al.* 1953).

PSK, Lentinan and Sizofilan as Quasispecific Immunogens
These agents are also closely related to macrophages, NK cells, and T- and B-cells in producing their anticancer activity. However, their effects seem to be in the domain of quasispecific immunity. They do not possess any of the effects of OK-432 in terms of hyperthermia and topical inflammations.
TNF and Schwartzman reaction as a quasispecific immunity
According to Fukushi (1983), the Schwartzmann reaction of hemorrhagic necrosis of experimental tumors was employed to titrate the biological potency of *Salmonella* endotoxicin in the 1960s. The phenomenon's therapeutic usefulness was expanded later as it was seen to be substantiated by serum factors (TNF) (Carswell *et al.* 1975; Ribi *et al.* 1975). Clinical application based on the phenomenon will be possible as soon as the active principles are understood (Fukushi *et al.* 1986). Should the phenomenon involve any specific antigenicity of the tumors to be treated, cross-antigenicity could be responsible.

It should be mentioned again that these immunological anticancer therapies are nonetheless nonspecific to quasispecific, and their principal mechanisms presumably predate the emergence of the chordates, when T-cell immunity could have started (Good *et al.* 1965). Bleomycin is known to selectively eliminate suppressor cells (Morikawa *et al.* 1985). Nonetheless, it remains to be seen whether it would enhance specific anticancer immunity in humans generally. The effectiveness of these therapies on cancer may conversely betray the devolutionary property of such cells in terms of antigenicity.

Additional biological amplifications are removal of cancer cells by surgery or by exfoliation, and induction of redifferentiation (Table 2).   Surgery carries the potential of overcoming the log kill limitation, especially following a course of adequate radiotherapy (tumor bed effect) (Withers 1980). Exfoliation can also be expedited (Okuyama *et al.* 1984b). The induction of redifferentiation can be seen as functional exfoliation, for the redifferentiated cells may die off or persist within the body but terminate their aggressive malignancy. Bestatin can be of importance in this regard (Okuyama *et al.* 1985b). If cancer cells are suspended in serosal effusions, they can be killed differently: (1) by OK-432-induced polymorphonuclear leukocytes probably through the secretion of "local humoral" factors such as superoxide radicals (Torisu 1981); (2) by lymphocytes through the emperipolesis (Fig. 10) (Okuyama *et al.* 1979b), a property which could be archaic, but which we are unable to reinforce; and (3) by the intrapleural introduction of tetracyclines (Rubinson and Bolooki 1972), whose antipleurisy effect can be produced by sclerosing activity (Thorsrud 1965) and cell kill (Okuyama *et al.* 1984c; 1987a).

Exfoliation implies separation and shedding of surface cells from the epithelium. The idea can be expanded to a mode of cancer cell loss from the body (Okuyama *et al.* 1984b). When we closely examined surgical specimens of rectal cancers preoperatively irradiated to 30 Gy and treated with tegafur and bleomycin, pronounced improvement was seen in terms of Dukes' staging. The nests of residual cancer cells appeared to have approached the luminal surfaces, and eventually to have fallen off (Fig. 7, chapter 8). This trend may represent a reversal of the arborescent growths of colonic cancers (Iwama and Takahashi 1983).

A second feature of exfoliation is that the exfoliation of in-

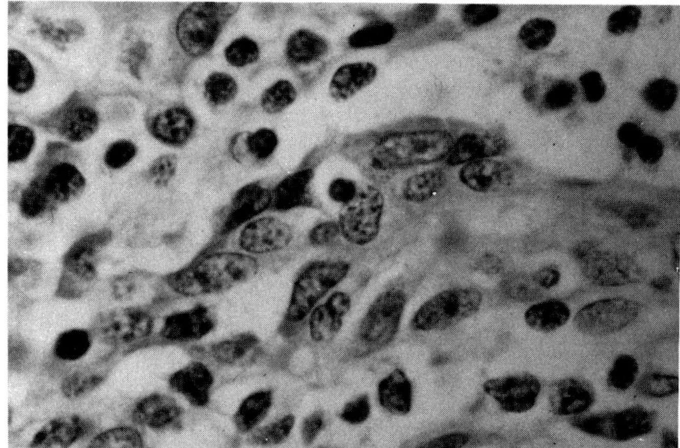

Fig. 10. Clinical evaluation of nonspecific to quasispecific immunotherapy (3): Role of lymphocytes in emperipolesis. A surgical specimen from gastric cancer reveals sites of emperipolesis, an invasion of cancer cells by lymphocytes. No specific conditions that would encourage this type of attack cancer are known (Okuyama *et al*. 1979).

dividual cancer cells can be expedited by the topical application of OK-432 (Mishina *et al*. 1988). During a course of radiotherapy for breast cancer in which cancerous infiltration had taken place in one breast to the point of inflammatory breast cancer, a powdered form of the streptococcal preparation was scattered over the ulcerative lesions (Fig. 11A). A sequential follow-up study by touch preparation revealed trails of the irradiated cells infiltrated and interspersed by lymphocytes and polymorphonuclears leukocytes (Fig. 11B) (Mishina *et al*. 1989a). The lymphocytic infiltrates themselves may also help to break cellular junctions and sequester cancer cells. A similar exfoliative mechanism may be involved in the improved therapeutic results among patients with head and neck tumors (Saijo *et al*. 1987). It is not, however, necessarily applicable to their metastatic lesions deep in the tissue, which are resistant to the same radiochemotherapy. Exfoliation would remove the viable and necrobiotic cancer cells along with the dead ones. In contrast, their failure to exfoliate entices regrowth. The intercellular tight junctions are vulnerable to irradiation, but such damage is repairable (Porvaznik 1979). The streptococci are lymphophilic, and induce blisters or interstitial edema (Ackerman 1978). The same effect on cancer cells is probable, as in our studies. The same or similar exfoliative mechanisms may also contribute to the extraordinary effectiveness of radiotherapy against head and neck tumors (Mishina *et al.* 1986; Saijo *et al.* 1987) as well as that of OK-432 inhalation therapy against lung cancer (Mishina and Okuyama 1987a), although such exfoliation, should it be retained beyond a certain length of time, would encourage re-transplantation (Maki *et al.* 1963a). The exfoliation itself can thus be seen as an evolutionary means of cancer surveillance and treatment.

Surgery, a form of manual "exfoliation," seems to provide a means of overcoming the log kill limitation, and its probability of doing so is increasing day by day.

The plethora of blood in polycythemia vera may require frequent exsanguination. Efficient exsanguination can be achieved by mobilizing into circulation fractions of the blood volume anchored in the spleen and incrasing the blood concentration. This can be done by administering adrenalin hypodermically (Okuyama *et al.* 1983b).

Redifferentiation is an induced exfoliation (Cooper 1972). Bestatin has been shown capable of inducing redifferentiation of cancer cells, as observed in cases of breast cancer (Okuyama *et al.* 1985b). Although still experimental, herbimycin may have similar potential, but through different pathways (Uehara *et al.* 1984).

The rescue of normal tissues in the radiation field from radiation damage has long been a problem, in spite of various efforts. The damage, especially in the form of ulcers, eventually leads to carcinogenesis if not properly treated. The main response has been to encourage ATP production by the damaged epithelial cells. The effect of cytochrome c, which was originally described for an *in vitro* system of recovering mitochondrial oxidative phosphorylation (van Bekkum 1956), is potent, according to our clinical and experimental results (Okuyama and Mishina 1982d; 1983b). Similar effects against radiation ulcers can be obtained with hyperbaric oxygen therapy (Mishina *et al.* 1977). In addition to the cytochrome c effect, hyperbaric oxygen therapy could help to generate active oxygen molecules that would eradicate the intractable infectious inhabitants of the radiation ulcers.

A second prospect in the treatment of intractable radiation ulcers is the ample use of lysozymal preparations (Okuyama *et al.* 1989b). Figure 12 demonstrates what happened to an intractable ulcer which had resulted from surgery for malignant endothelial sarcoma following 100 Gy to the skin. The ulcer started healing within two weeks of the application of a lysozymal ointment, steadily decreased in size, and eventually healed.

It appears that radiation dermatitis and ulcers, as well as damage to other normal tissues, are aided by materials that encourage *in loco* ATP production. These materials are originally "intrinsic" and have been acquired through the long history of evolution under stringent natural radiation. Thus, the treatment of radiation damage in humans also carries evolutionary implications.

Strategic Integration of Radiotherapeutic Principles: *T-PR-B*

The basic idea of integrating radiotherapeutic principles is to reinforce the initial DNA damage incurred by irradiation through the perpetuating procedure; therefore, *T-PR*. Cancer cells remaining because of the limitations imposed by log kill or probabilistic killing may be eliminated by biological amplifications or by increasing the tolerance of normal tissues by rescue or protective measures. The strategic integration of radiotherapy can thus be expressed by *T-PR-B* (Table 2). This order of integration is not fixed. The protective regimen may be dispensed during the course of radiotherapy. Biological amplification can be expanded to cancer cell elimination by surgery. We think it appropriate in most cases to perform surgery after radiotherapy in order to overcome the log kill limitation.

Strategic Integration for Chemotherapy: *S-PC-B*

The principle of strategic chemotherapy is not different from that of radiotherapy. In place of *T* and *PR*, we have *S*, for *selective* concentration of chemotherapeutics, and *PC*, for *perpetuation* of the repairable *chemotherapeutic* DNA damage (Table 5).

Agents with specific tumor affinity such as hormonal antagonists seem to possess an extraordinary potential for the future. The lympholytic potency of adrenocorticoids has long been noted (Fauci and Dale 1975). Although similar antineoplastic effects have been considered in connection with predni-

Table 5. Principles of cancer therapy: *S-PC-B*

Symbol	Principle	Mechanism	Practical techniques	Remarks
		Specific affinity	Antigenicity-oriented immunotherapy	
			Hormonal therapy	
S	Selective concentration	Spatial concentration	Direct impregnation	Okuyama 1987
				Ishii 1985
				Fukushi 1985
			Drug after removing effusates	Rubinson 1972
				Hayashi 1983
			Selection of routes	Mishina 1987b
			Induced hypertension	(Suzuki 1981)
				Sato 1981
			Concentration by inflammation, inhibition of drug metabolism, enzyme induction/activation, metallothionen, or fosfomycin	Okuyama 1978 (Hojo 1976) (Naganuma 1985) Tanaka 1983, 1985
			Embolization/chemical	Suzuki 1981
			Cellular membrane modulation	
		Temporal concentration	Cell cycle phase-specific	Tannock 1978
			Continuous, low-dose infusion	Shimoyama 1973
PC	Perpetuation of DNA damage	Inhibition and perpetuation of DNA damage	Cisplatin-bleomycin	(Okuyama 1980)
			Bleomycin-neocarzinostatin	Israel 1983
				Okuyama 1980
			Adriamycin-neocarzinostatin	Okuyama 1988
B	Biological amplification	Apoptosis	Corticosteroids	(Kerr 1980)
				(Saito 1971)
			Immunity (quasispecific; specific)	
			Exfoliation	

Names in parentheses denote experimental reporters.

Table 6. Effects of prednisolone on development of metastasis to the liver in gastric cancer patients. Larger doses of the agent were seen to significantly reduce the probability of developing cancer metastasis to the liver (Saito *et al.* 1973).

Degree of metastasis	Anticancer agents		No anticancer agents
	Ps* 500 mg	Ps* 500 or less	No Ps*
−	52.6% (20/38)	24.1% (7/29)	36.0% (9/25)
		29.6% (16/54)	
+	26.3% (10/38)	10.3% (3/29)	24.0% (6/25)
		16.7% (9/54)	
╫	13.2% (5/38)	24.1% (7/29)	12.0 (3/25)
		18.5% (10/54)	
╫╫	7.9% (3/38)	41.3% (12/29)	28.0 (7/25)
		35.2% (19/54)	

* Ps: Prednisolone.

solone, strong evidence to support this assumption appears to be lacking except that of Saito *et al.* (1967; 1973). When a large dose of prednisolone was administered, the chemotherapeutic effects were definitely increased in terms of survival after tumor transplantation and metastatic development, whereas the agent itself appeared to have no observable anticancer effects (Saito *et al.* 1967). A definite reduction in the development of metastases to the liver and lung was observed in patients with stomach cancer (Table 6) (Saito *et al.* 1973). Direct cancer cell toxicity caused by apoptosis is probable from large doses of corticosteroids, as suggested elsewhere (Kobayashi 1980; Kerr and Searle 1981): one of the primary functions of the metabolic endocrine systems is to supply energy in cases of emergency, such as chasing or being chased, at the expense of the host's own cells and tissues. This may also constitute an evolutionary aspect of cancer therapy.

Chemotherapeutic concentrations in tumor tissues may not necessarily be sufficient for effective chemotherapy, necessitating reinforcement along the spatial or temporal dimension. Our experience with OK-432 indicates that it increases the tumoral accretion of chemotherapeutics to an appreciable degree (Okuyama *et al.* 1978a), probably as a result of increased local tumor blood flow (Kudo *et al.* 1985). Spatial concentration can be attained by direct intratumoral or intracavitary administration. In general, the intratumoral injection of chemotherapeutics is hazardous because of local necrotic sequelae. However, tetracyclines can be safely administered for selective anticancer effects (Okuyama *et al.* 1987a). The pleural and vesical cavities are guarded by the mesothelium and transitional epithelium, respectively, and selected anticancer agents can be administered intrapleurally (aclacinomycin) (Hayashi and Konno 1983) and intravesically (mitomycin C and adriamycin) (Ogawa *et al.* 1983; Hellstein *et al.* 1983).

Although cell cycle-specific designs for chemotherapy can produce temporal concentration, their reliability in the treatment of humans has been criticized (Tannock 1978). As clinicians, we are more inclined to employ alkylating agents or radiomimetics whose anticancer DNA damage can be potentiated through the perpetuation principle (PC) (Okuyama and Mishina 1980). When this principle was strictly observed by administering a continuous low-dose infusion of bleomycin following a large dose of cisplatin, excellent theraputic results were reported (Israel *et al.* 1983). The combination of cisplatin and bleomycin may be simulated by cisplatin and neocarzinostatin or higher doses of bleomycin and neocarzinostatin (Okuyama and Mishina 1980). Other combinations may also be developed. In a study using lymphoid cells, cyclophosphamide alone seemed capable of perpetuating the DNA damage it had already caused (David *et al.* 1985).

DNA repair may have evolutionary significance, especially in light of the constant menace from ultraviolet rays and ionizing radiation on the one hand and a host of alkylating agents in the environmnet on the other (Singer 1985). The vulnerable molecular sites of DNA damage are "selected" (Gibson *et al.* 1985; Montesano *et al.* 1985). There are a number of repair-deficient syndromes that might be genetic, for example, Fanconi's anemia and xeroderma pigmentosum, as well as certain cases of rheumatoid arthritis (Harris and Lawley 1985). The genes that may be involved in these repair mechanisms are being identified (Naumovski and Friedberg 1983; van Duin *et al.* 1986). Proficient repair would decrease the cytotoxic effects of chemicals (Setlow 1985). Variations in

DNA repair among cancer cells would account for the different sensitivities to alkylating chemotherapy (Lawley and Brookes 1965; Gibson *et al.* 1985). Thus, cancer chemotherapy with radiomimetics also has evolutionary significance.

Evolutionary Implications of the Strategic Integration of *T-PR-B* and *S-PC-B*.

The probable evolutionary significance of these integrations can be deduced from discussions on the origin of radiosensitivity and chemosensitivity elsewhere in this book.

The preparation of an anticancer plan for each patient would probably facilitate the strategic integration of treatment, review, and informed revision. New therapeutic developments could easily be incorporated into ongoing therapeutic plans, an important consideration in today's climate of active research.

Thus, the usefulness of this type of strategic integration cannot be overemphasized.

Chapter 12

Redifferentiation of Cancer Cells: Bestatin, Estradiol, and Prostaglandin D_2

> *The differentiated cell does not divide for the remainder of its life-span——(and) will inevitably be lost.*
> ——*E. H. Cooper*, Pathology, *1972*

Introduction

The means to induce cancer cell redifferentiation, when it becomes available, will be invaluable in several clinical situations: (1) application to residual cancer cells left as a result of the log kill limitation of radiotherapy and/or chemotherapy; (2) application to cancer cells disseminated at the time of surgery; (3) application to widespread small metastases; and (4) probable maintenance of induced remissions. Past experimental and clinical research (Okuyama *et al.* 1978c; Awano and Matsuzawa 1977; Okuyama *et al.* 1983c) prompted us to carry out investigations on Bestatin (Okuyama *et al.* 1983d; Okuyama and Mishina 1984a; 1985b). We have become convinced that cancer cell redifferentiation can be induced clinically with Bestatin and appropriate hormones.

Bestatin is a small molecular weight product of *Streptomyces olivoreticuli* (Umezawa 1979) (Fig. 1). Through binding to hydrolytic enzymes on the cell surface, it may induce

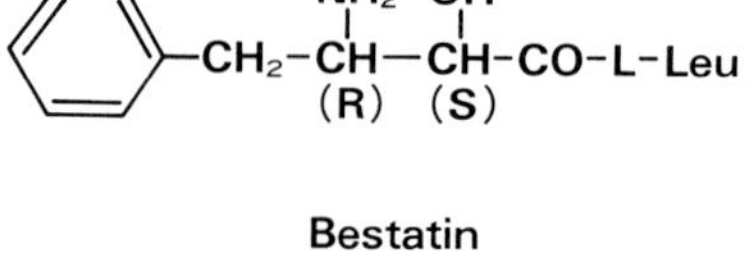

$$\text{C}_6\text{H}_5\text{—CH}_2\text{—}\underset{\underset{(R)}{|}}{\overset{\overset{NH_2}{|}}{\text{CH}}}\text{—}\underset{\underset{(S)}{|}}{\overset{\overset{OH}{|}}{\text{CH}}}\text{-CO-L-Leu}$$

Bestatin

Fig. 1. Chemical structure of Bestatin (Umezawa 1979).

Bestatin binds to hydrolytic enzymes on cell surface

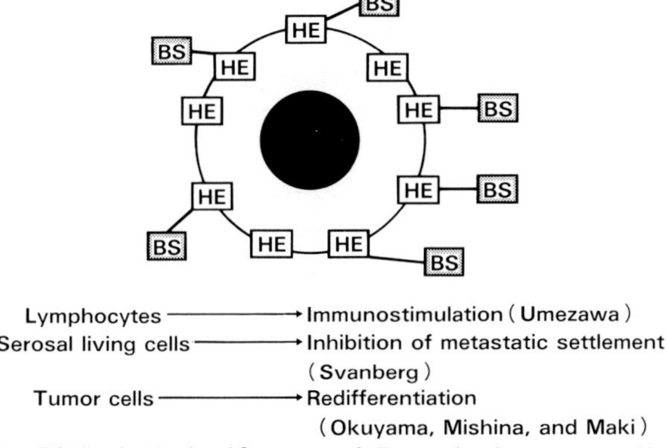

Lymphocytes ──────────→ Immunostimulation (Umezawa)
Serosal living cells ──────→ Inhibition of metastatic settlement
(Svanberg)
Tumor cells ───────────→ Redifferentiation
(Okuyama, Mishina, and Maki)

Fig. 2. Biological significance of Bestatin in mammalian cells. BS=Bestatin; HE=hydrolytic enzyme (Okuyama *et al.* 1985).

immunostimulation when it binds to lymphocytes (Fig. 2). It may also prevent metastatic cancer cells from settling in normal tissues (Svanberg and Elisson 1983) by inhibiting hydrolytic enzymes that can be activated as soon as cancer cells approach (Birbeck and Wheatley 1965; Baba 1966). The question of what happens to cancer cells when they are sufficiently coated with Bestatin molecules served as the motivation for our investigation into the probable induction of cancer redifferentiation (Okuyama *et al.* 1985b).

Both the inducibility of redifferentiation of leukemia and cancer cells and the aptitude for spontaneous regression of neoplasms appear to have evolutionary implications.

Experimental Materials and Methods

Culture of FM3A undifferentiated murine mammary adenocarcinoma cells   FM3A cells originated in a C_3H mouse (Nakano 1966). Experimental redifferentiation of these cells with gallium element has already been reported (Awano and Matsuzawa 1977). In this experiment, cells were cultured at 1.5×10 cells per dish in Eagle's MEM ($-Ca^{+2}$) supplemented with 10% calf serum under an atmosphere of 5% CO_2. Bestatin (Fig. 1), supplied by Nippon Kayaku, Tokyo, was dissolved in distilled water at a concentration of 30 mg/ml. The solution was diluted with physiological saline as needed. Estradiol benzoate suspended in saline was employed, and testosterone propionate was used. Prostaglandin D_2 supplied by Ono Pharmaceutical, Osaka, was dissolved in saline just prior to use. The viable cell count was determined by a hemocytometer, using 0.25% trypan blue solution.

General experimental plan   The experimental plan was as follows: Bestatin was added to the cell culture on day 0; estradiol or testosterone was added on day 3; and microscopic examination of the dishes for "redifferentiated" cells was carried out on days 3 to 6.

Culture of M1 murine leukemia cells   M1 cells derived from spontaneous myeloid leukemia in SL mice can be induced to redifferentiate into normal macrophages and granulocytes (Ichikawa 1969). The cells were cultured in RPMI 1640 medium supplemented with 5% FCS (fetal calf serum). Streptomycin and penicillin were added to the culture medium at concentrations of 100 μg per ml and 100 U per ml, respectively.

Phenotypic redifferentiation   Phenotypic redifferentiation was defined as the assumption by cells of any bizarre con-

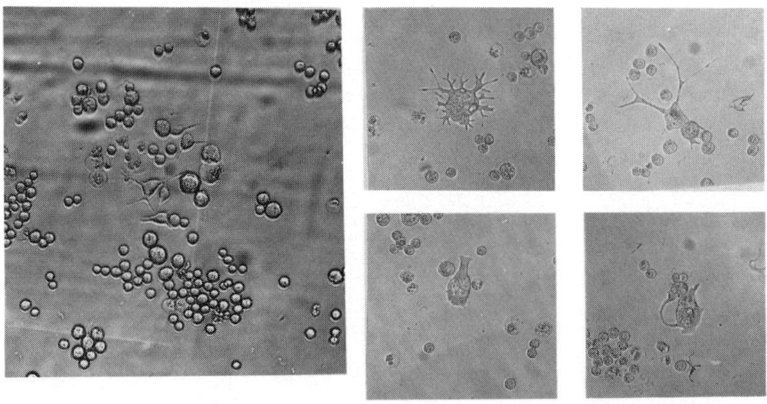

Fig. 3.   Redifferentiating effect of Bestatin on FM3A undifferentiated murine mammary adenocarcinoma cells *in vitro*. Induction of morphological differentiation by bizarre configurations is characteristic: neuron-like, goblet cell-like, etc.

figurations different from the round shape seen in the control culture (Fig. 3). Bizarre, pleomorphic alterations of the Bestatin-treated cancer cells were observed. Goblet cell-like, neuron-like, and macrophage-like configurations were seen, in addition to others. The number of redifferentiated cells in each dish was counted, a viable count made, and redifferentiation index (R.I.) computed (the number of redifferentiated cells per million viable cells).

In the M1 cells, phenotypic redifferentiation was measured in terms of the expression of Fc receptors (FcR) on leukemia cells as well as development of phagocytosis. The FcR was determined by microscopic observation of antibody-coated sheep erythrocytes. Phagocytosis was measured by injestion of 1.1 μm latex particles (Dow Chemical).

Measurement of the cell volume, flow cytometry, tritium TdR uptake studies, cell electrophoresis, and scanning electron microscopic studies were also carried out.

Experimental Results

Marginal cell kill with Bestatin   Marginal cell kill was observed in dose studies with Bestatin.

Reduction of saturation density and cell loss with Bestatin singly and in combination with estradiol   When temporal follow-up studies were carried out, a reduction in the saturation density was observed (Fig. 4) (Okuyama and Mishina 1984a). An increased fall in viable cell count was seen when estradiol was added to the Bestatin-containing culture at the beginning of the plateau (Fig. 5) (Okuyama and Mishina 1984c).

Redifferentiation potential of Bestatin   Occasional cells with bizarre configurations were observed even among the untreated cells. However, the R.I. rose nearly five-fold in response to 300 μg per ml or more of Bestatin as determined on day 3 of the incubation (Fig. 6). Enlargement of the individual round cells was also a conspicuous feature.

Effects on redifferentiation of estradiol singly or in combination with Bestatin   Estradiol was only marginally effective in killing FM3A cells until it became cytotoxic at the high dose of 750 U per ml. Appreciable cell kill was observed at lower doses when the hormone was administered following three-

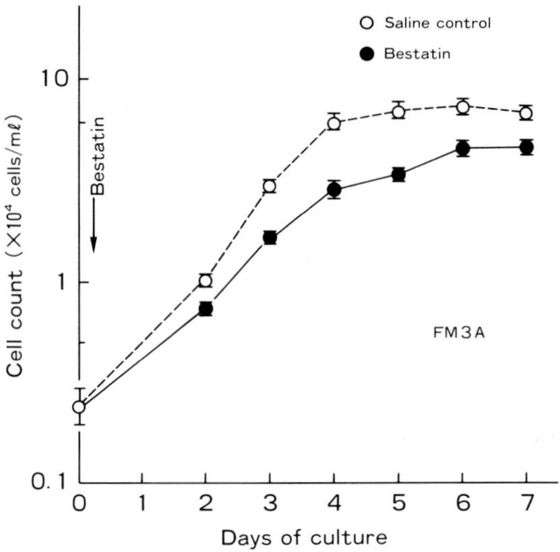

Fig. 4. Temporal response to Bestatin of FM3A cells *in vitro*. Reduction in the saturation density was observed. This finding was thought to indicate the induction of cancer redifferentiation (Okuyama *et al*. 1985).

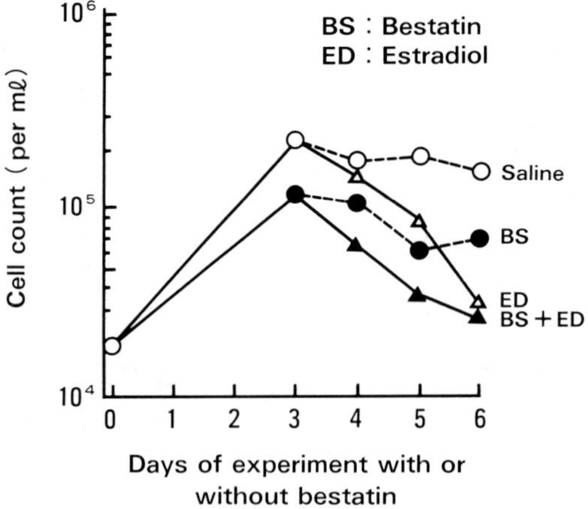

Fig. 5. Cancer cell loss induced in FM3A cells *in vitro* by the consecutive Bestatin-hormone regimen. Bestatin was added to the culture medium on day 0, and estradiol on day 3. (Okuyama *et al*. 1983a,b; 1985).

day exposure to Bestatin (Fig. 5). Under the microscope, the Bestatin-estradiol treated cells appeared larger than those of the saline control (Fig. 7). An additional conspicuous feature was the assupmtion of sessile configurations. Both estradiol

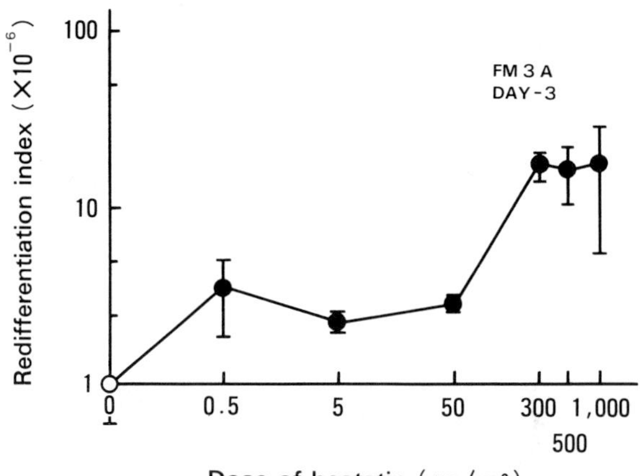

Fig. 6. Redifferentiation potential of Bestatin (1). Effect of Bestatin alone on FM3A cells *in vitro*. The effect appeared to be limited to the higher doses (Okuyama and Mishina 1985a).

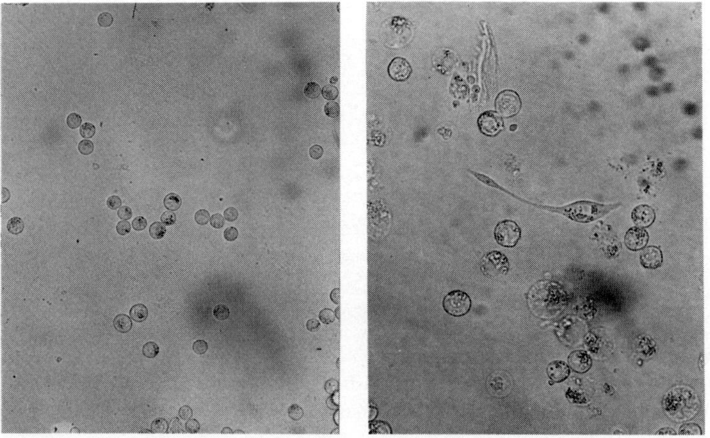

Fig. 7. Redifferentiation potential of Bestatin (2). Effect of the consecutive Bestatin-estradiol regimen on FM3A cells *in vitro*. Cellular enlargement and morphological differentiation into bizarre configurations were induced (Okuyama *et al.* 1985).

and Bestatin were capable of increasing the R.I. However, the greatest value was observed in the combined Bestatin-estradiol group.

Pharmacokinetic analysis of the redifferentiating effects of Bestatin and estradiol in combination   Using Bestatin and estradiol, pharmacokinetic studies were carried out by exposing the cells to a range of doses of one agent against a fixed dose of the other and measuring the resultant changes in the R.I. Bestatin was capable of inducing morphological changes indicative of redifferentiation in a dose-dependent manner (Fig. 8). With estradiol, however, the R.I. increased over a narrow range (Fig. 9). These findings indicated that there is

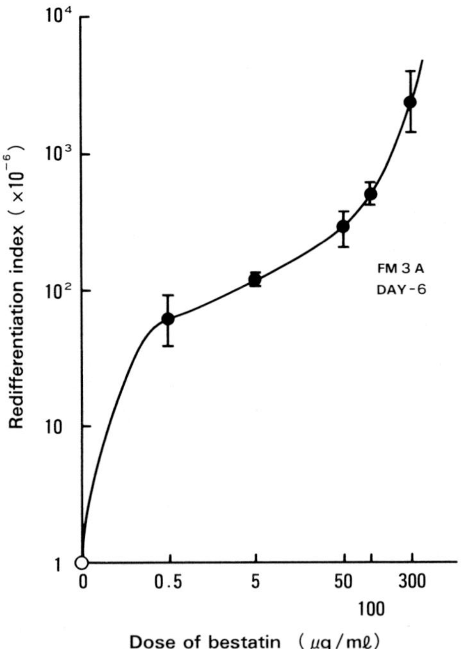

Fig. 8.   Redifferentiation potential of Bestatin (3). Dose response to Bestatin of a fixed dose of estradiol. The induction of redifferentiation was proportional to the dose of bestatin: the more bestatin, the greater the redifferentiation (Okuyama and Mishina 1985). From the clinical point of view, this observation indicates that as much Bestatin as possible should be dispensed against a particular range of sex hormone.

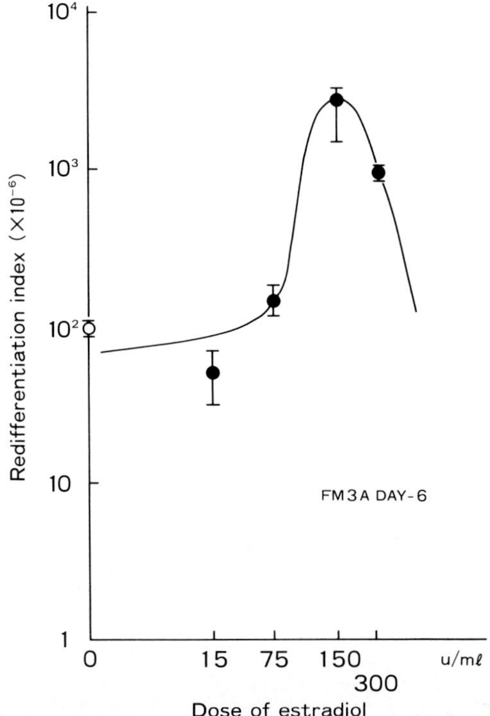

Fig. 9. Redifferentiation potential of Bestatin (4). Dose response to estradiol of a fixed dose of Bestatin. A narrow range of estradiol dosage induced maximal redifferentiation. This observation together with the data in Fig. 8 strongly suggest a potential clinical application of the Bestatin-hormone regimen (Okuyama and Mishina 1985; Okuyama *et al.* 1985).

good reason to believe that the dose of Bestatin can be increased as tolerated against an appropriate dose range of the sex hormones. This observation may be of some importance in terms of the clinical application of Bestatin and hormones.

Effects of Bestatin on negative cell membrane charge Prolonged exposure to 300 μg per ml of Bestatin was capable of reducing the negative cell membrane charge of FM3A experimental carcinoma cells.

Effects of Bestatin and/or estradiol on cell volume Prolonged exposure of cancer cells to Bestatin was shown to increase the cell volume, a change that proceeded with increasing length of exposure. Estradiol alone did not appear to affect the cell volume, however. Nor did it affect the volume of the Bestatin-treated cells.

Effects of Bestatin on proliferative parameters   Bestatin seemed to exert cytokinetic effects on cancer cells. It was seen to increase the fraction of cells in G_2 and M. However, cell uptake of tritium thymidine was shown to increase fourfold following prolonged exposure to Bestatin. As Bestatin has already been shown to saturate the cell culture, these findings indicate that the agent blocks the cells at G_2.

Redifferentiating potential of testosterone   The dose study using testosterone suggested that its effect on FM3A mam-

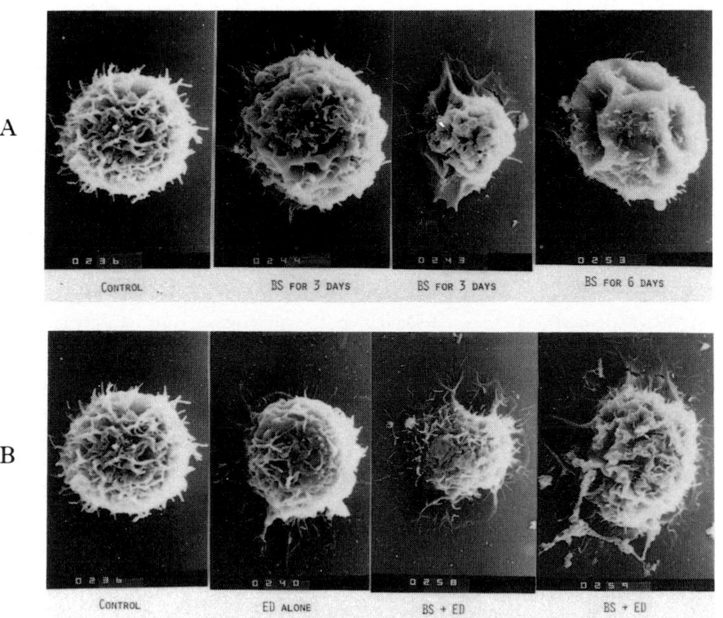

Fig. 10. Redifferentiation effect of Bestatin on FM3A cells *in vitro*: Scanning electron microscopic studies. (A) Bestatin alone was capable of inducing morphological changes that could be designated redifferentiation. Eventual disintegration seemed probable when exposure was prolonged. (B) The consecutive Bestatin-estradiol regimen resulted in pronounced development of neuron-like processes. Redifferentiation along the line of devolution has to be considered. The degree of devolution is greater with solid tumor cells than leukemic cells, and redifferentiation is apparently "normal" in the latter while it is bizarre in the former.

mary adenocarcinoma cells of the mouse is one of marginal cell killing. Its ability to induce redifferentiation was, however, limited.

Scanning electron microscopic changes in FM3A cells on exposure to Bestatin and estradiol, singly or in combination   Prolonged exposure to Bestatin alone led to morphological changes in the cells that were characterized by loss of the fine microvilli and eventual loss of rough processes (Fig. 10A). Added estradiol was seen to stimulate the growth of finer microvilli, further their arborization, and lead to their eventual disruption (Fig. 10B). Thus, the consecutive Bestatin-estradiol regimen induced phenotypic redifferentiation in the cancer cells, and probably led to their disintegration without further proliferation.

Redifferentiating potential of prostaglandin D_2 in FM3A and M1 cells   Prostaglandin D_2 was moderately cytotoxic against FM3A cells. When a dose of 5 μg per ml was added to the culture medium, whether in the presence or absence of Bestatin, cellular proliferation was arrested, resulting in reduc-

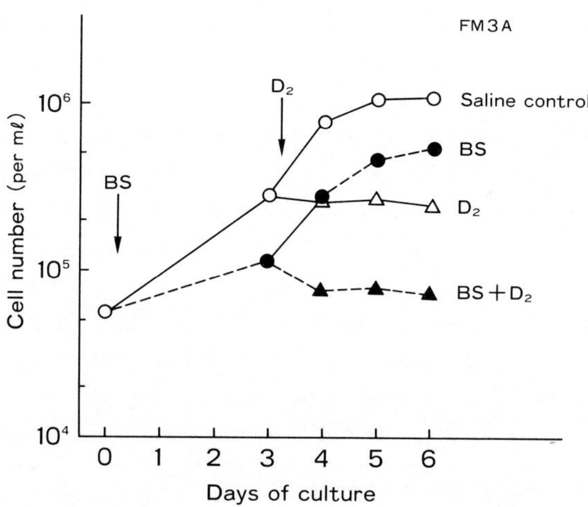

Fig. 11.   Temporal response to prostaglandin D_2 *in vitro* (1). FM 3A cells. Reduction of the culture's saturation density was attained with prostaglandin D_2. An additive response was observed with consecutive Bestatin-prostaglandin D_2 treatment. This agent is also thought to induce redifferentiation (Okuyama *et al.* 1985).

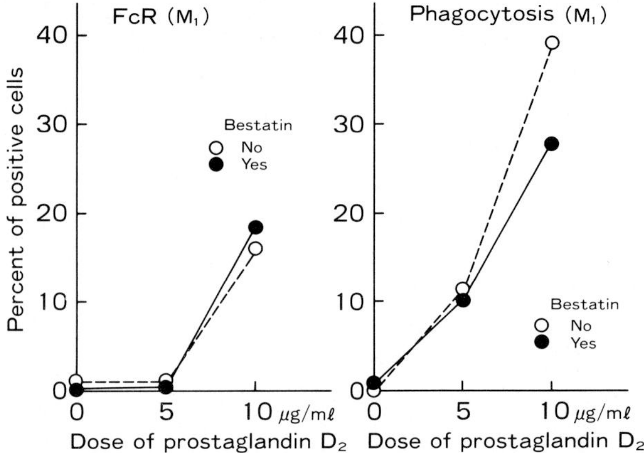

Fig. 12. Redifferentiating potential of prostaglandin D_2 *in vitro* (2). M1 leukemia cells. Differentiation of Fc receptors and phagocytic function was observed on exposure to the agent. Pretreatment with Bestatin did not appear to influence redifferentiation to any appreciable degree (Okuyama *et al.* 1985).

tion of the saturation density (Fig. 11). It induced sessile forms of redifferentiation. Pharmacokinetic analysis indicated that its redifferentiating capacity was in the dose range of 5–7.5 μg per ml.

This same agent, however, was less toxic against M1 leukemia cells. Temporal analysis showed that its cell killing effect became apparent rather precipitously, suggesting that the effect is brought about through the induction of redifferentiation. Phenotypic expression was characterized by cellular enlargement with Bestatin but not with prostaglandin D_2. Greater somal enlargement was achieved with prostaglandin D_2. The likelihood of functional redifferentiation was shown for FcR expression and phagocytosis (Fig. 12).

Comments on the Experimental Data

One of the scientific motivations for the present investigation was our studies on cancer redifferentiation with gallium element (Okuyama *et al.* 1978c; Okuyama *et al.* 1979c; Okuyama *et al.* 1984a). Because the magnitude of the cellular membrane negative charge seems proportional to the degree of malignancy (Yamada 1973; Okuyama *et al.* 1978b), we thought that coating cells with Bestatin, which binds to hydrolytic enzymes over the cell surface (Aoyagi *et al.* 1977), would induce redifferentiation of cancer cells, similar to trypsinized, monovalent concanavalin A for cultured tumorous fibroblasts (Burger and Noonan 1970). Bestatin triggers lymphocytes and T-cells to differentiate (Mueller *et al.* 1979). Prostaglandin D_2 is rich in the brain (Shimizu *et al.* 1979), and brain malignancies occur at a rate as low as 1.0 per 100,000 person-years among males in Miyagi, Japan (age-adjusted standard rate against the world population, 1973–1977) (Waterhous *et al.* 1982), while cancers of extracranial organs such as the stomach and prostate occur at rates of 88.0 and 4.9, respectively. We were also led to study prostaglandin D_2 by the report of its effect on the cellular membrane negative charge (Kondo *et al.* 1981), an effect that could well be related to the induction of cancer redifferentiation (Oku-yama *et al.* 1984a).

Do cell changes induced by Bestatin and sex hormones or prosta-glandin D_2 represent actual cancer redifferentiation? Needless to say, our reply to the question is yes. First of all, it is necessary to ask what "differentiated" cancer cells would look like. The cancer cells that were experimentally induced to differentiate appeared quite different from mature "normal" cells. In contrast, those leukemic cells that successfully differentiated seemed to retain the normal morphological properties of macrophages or granulocytes, but were never at all bizarre (Abe *et al.* 1981; Fibach *et al.* 1972; Fibach *et al.* 1973). The fact that these cells were not particularly different from those of their mother organ raises the possibility that their distance or deviation from the normal may be minimal. According to Nowell (1976), human leukemias can be considered to ensue with minimal chromosomal change and human solid tumors with high aneuploidy. In contemporary oncogene theory, that statement can be translated into single-step or "mono-oncogene" leukemogenesis, and multistep or "multi-oncogene" carcinogenesis. Most of the retroviral oncogenes known from the animal kingdom that serve as proto-oncogenes in humans are definitely leukemogenic and sarcomagenic only. In other words, leukemic cells may not be far deviated from the norm, and their induction of redifferentiation would certainly result in normal morphological and functional maturation. In contrast, in epithelial tumor or cancer cells, DNA changes leading to chromosomal aberration and overt carcinogenesis can be so great that their reversion or devolution would be likely to blur any tint of the original organ tissues. Thus, the induction of cancer redifferentiation per se can possibly be a measure of the extent of devolution.

Mechanisms of induction of cancer redifferentiation in vitro
The observed changes in Bestatin-treated FM3A murine mammary undifferentiated adenocarcinoma cells can be summarized as follows: (1) increased cell size; (2) reduced negative cell membrane charge; (3) threefold increase in tritiated thymidine uptake; (4) blocking of cells at the G_2+M phase as shown by flow fluorocytometry; and (5) roughening of the cell surface on scanning electron microscopy, as the cells apparently lost the fine villi, while cancer cells treated with estradiol developed much finer villi. On the consecutive Bestatin-estradiol regimen, the finer villi were accompanied by large processes on the one hand and degenerative changes to the surface structures, probably leading to the eventual death of such cells, on the other. We may, therefore, speculate that redifferentiation of undifferentiated mammary adenocarcinoma cells can be achieved, that these redifferentiated cells die off following a definite life span, and that Bestatin plays a preparatory role.

Prostaglandin D_2 kills cancer cells *in vitro* (Fukushima *et al.* 1982). It controls metastatic phenomena (Fitzpatrick and Stringfellow 1979; Stringfellow and Fitzpatrick 1979), probably through altering the negative cell membrane charge (Kondo *et al.* 1981). Induction of morphological change of redifferentiation was attained in both FM3A mammary adenocarcinoma and M1 leukemia cells. Somal and nuclear enlargement was thought probable in M1 cells, too. This effect was observed only when Bestatin was administered, singly or in combination, and was greater in the consecutive Bestatin-prostaglandin D_2 combination.

One of the principal dynamic changes may be cessation of cellular proliferation. It may not necessarily be an absolute change, as in the case of redifferentiation of leukemic cells along their programmed maturation into granulocytes, however. With advancing maturation, the magnitude of proliferative capacity in such cases obviously decreases until differentiation is completed. The production of melanin by the melanoma cells, therefore, does not necessarily imply "redifferentiation": the function was already in existence prior to therapy. Melanin production is an *a priori* property of the tumor. The mechanisms leading these neoplastic cells to cytostasis can be versatile (Ruddon 1981). With both Bestatin and prostaglandin D_2, the initiating effect following their binding to the cancer cell surface at leucine aminopeptidase sites or D_2 receptors may be the change in the negative cell membrane charge. Bestatin binding itself would certainly trigger DNA synthesis in both normal lymphocytes and tumor cells. In the former, subsequent cell propagation and functional maturation would lead to immunostimulation (Mueller *et al.* 1983). Neoplastic cells would stop advancing through the cell cycle at G_2+M. The accumulation of cells with somal (and nuclear) enlargement appears to support this assumption, together with the results of flow cytofluorometry. The reduction in negative cell membrane charge could result directly from binding to the Bestatin molecules, although we are not sure if this is a sequel to other intracellular events. A similar reduction in the negative cell membrane charge may result from prostaglandin D_2 binding (Kondo *et al.* 1981). That reduction may be closely related to proliferative capacity, as studied by irradiation (Sato *et al.* 1975).

G_2 block and sojourn as the probable mechanisms of "gene expression" of redifferentiation   Differentiation in normal cells takes place in the G_1 phase. Inhibitors of DNA synthesis allow cancer cells to accumulate in the G_1 phase, and may therefore induce differentiation of selected neoplastic cells such as in myeloid leukemia (Sachs 1978). Prostaglandin D_2 also blocks cancer cells at the G_1 phase (Bhuyan *et al.* 1984). Therefore, its redifferentiating potential is probably related to the function of the G_1 phase. The reported inhibition of both DNA polymerases α and β would thus be a sequel of blocking at the G_1 phase (Kawamura and Koshihara 1984). Studies using X-rays and serum-free medium have shown that the expression of differentiated phenotypes can also

occur in the G_2 phase of the cell cycle, and in polyploid cells as well (Prasad and Kumar 1975). Bestatin molecules preferentially bind to cells at the end of the S phase and in the G_2 phase (Mueller *et al.* 1982). We can thus surmise that duplication and triplication of the genetic information would entice untoward expression of the genes, resulting in bizarre configurations.

Immediate clinical implications of experimental results   Of course, one of the immediate applications of the above experiments is the induction of cancer cell redifferentiation, most likely of sex hormone-dependent cancers of the mammalian symbol organs, such as those of the breast and prostate. A possible second application would be to hematopoietic malignancies, especially granulocytic leukemias. In view of the well-known differentiating capacity of normal lymphoyctes, lymphocytic leukemias might respond satisfactorily to Bestatin. The Bestatin-induced $G_2 + M$ block of cancer cells could be used in cooperation with anticancer agents that interfere with the same cellular mechanisms.

Clinical Studies

However primitive, the morphological and cytokinetic data appear sufficient to justify clinical studies with Bestatin, which has been officially approved for clinical trials.

Bestatin and sex hormones for patients with skin metastases from breast cancer   Selected patients with skin metastases from surgically treated breast cancer were given Bestatin and fluoxymetholone. The subjects were patients at the Department of Radiology, Tohoku Rosai Hospital, Sendai. Skin biopsy was performed at least twice, prior to and in the middle of the consecutive Bestatin-hormone therapy, for histological studies.

First, Bestatin was administered for three to four weeks; then fluoxymetholone, a synthetic testosterone preparation, was given in combination. This plan was observed in principle throughout the study. Illustrative cases are described below.

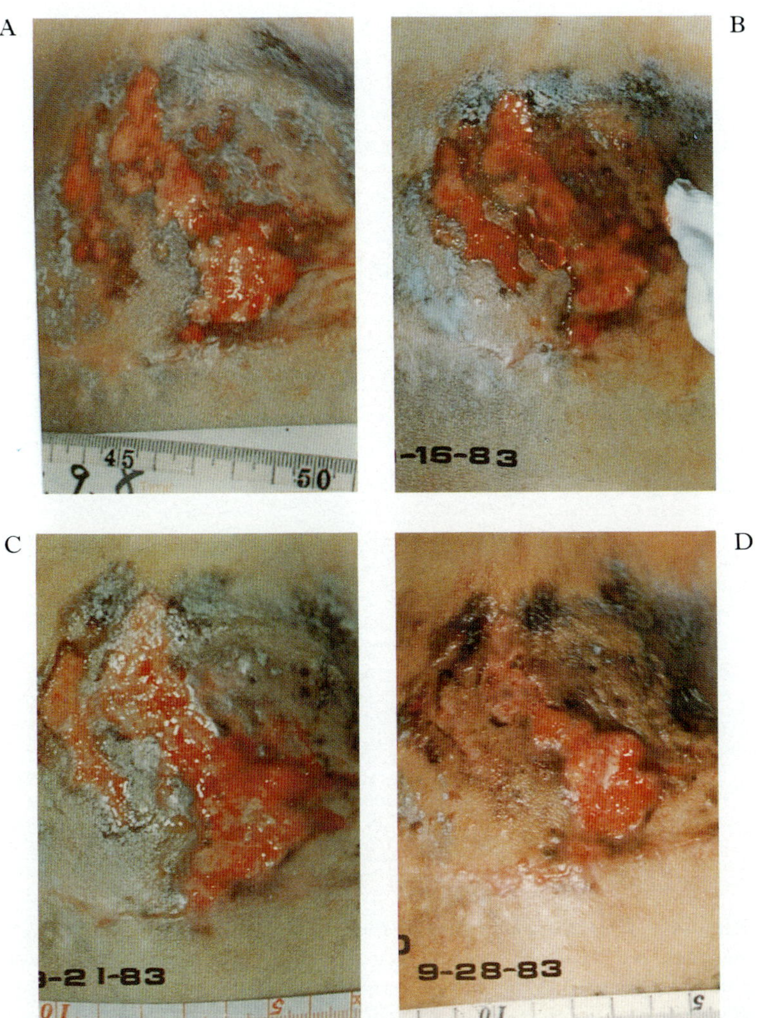

Fig. 13. Therapeutic effects of the consecutive Bestatin-hormone regimen on breast cancer (1). Case 1: Inflammatory breast cancer six months after surgery on the left breast. No post-operative radiotherapy was given. A. Before treatment. Bestatin was started on her after this photograph. B. Bestatin for 8 days. C. After 13 days of Bestatin. Fluoxymetholone (4 mg t.i.d.) was added to Bestatin. D. After seven days of the combined regimen. At first Bestatin did not appear to exert any anticancer effects; rather, it appeared to increase the tumor masses for the first two weeks (B and C). When fluoxymetholone was added, the tumors showed an abrupt decrease in size during the first week (D).

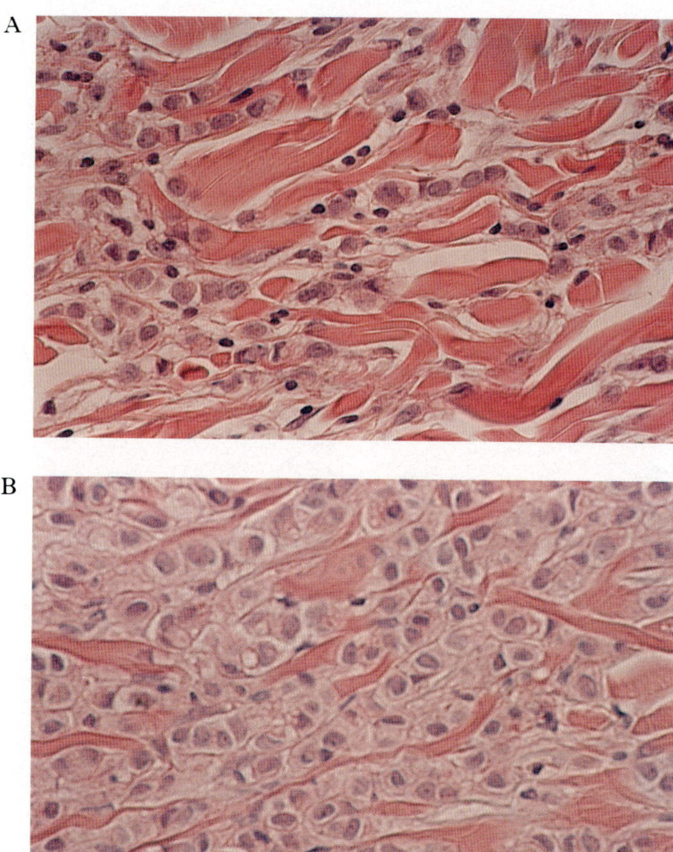

Fig. 14. Therapeutic effects of the consecutive Bestatin-hormone regimen on breast cancer (2). Case 2: Tumor sheet formation as histopathological evidence of cancer redifferentiation. A. Pre-Bestatin bioptic picture. B. After a course of consecutive Bestatin-hormone regimen. Cancer cells are known to pile up on each other because of the loss of contact inhibition. Lymphocytic infiltration is apparent (A). At the end of the fourth week of the combined regimen, the nodules started shrinking, and biopsy of one nodule revealed tumor sheet formation instead of the tumor cord formation typical of tumors. Here, the cancer cells do not pile up, but form trabeculae similar to hepatic cords. This was thought to represent the probable return of lost contact inhibition. This may be regarded as a sign of cancer redifferentiation. There was no definite lymphocytic infiltration in spite of claims of antitumor T-cell activation. (Hematoxylin-eosin stain, ×400) (Okuyama *et al.* 1985).

Clinical Results and Comments

The clinical results indicated that the regimen was moderately effective in reducing tumor size and could well lead to the disappearance of smaller nodular metastases. Histological studies indicated that the redifferentiation of cancer cells may be induced by this therapeutic regimen (see below).

Case Studies

Case 1   The patient was referred to us because of post-operative recurrence of inflammatory breast cancer and skin metastases (Fig. 13). The ulcerative tumors first became hemorrhagic after nine days of Bestatin (60 mg t.i.d.) (Fig. 13 B). The tumors had become less bloody by the fourteenth day of Bestatin administration. When 4 mg t.i.d. of fluoxymetholone was added to Bestatin, definite reduction in tumor size was observed during the following week (Fig. 13D). Skin biopsy was carried out four times (on each day of photography for Fig. 13). The inflammatory changes disappeared by the nineth day of Bestatin administration. Somal and nuclear enlargement was apparent, as was disappearance of inflammatory cell infiltrates. Sites of remaining cancer nodules following five days of combined fluoxymetholone revealed that the alveoli of cancer cells were less disorderly than previously, i.e., there was less piling up.

Case 2   In this patient, abrupt dissolution of skin metastases was observed during a consecutive Bestatin-hormone regimen. Sporadic, nodular skin metastases of about 6×6 mm in diameter remained unchanged during a year of treatment with cytostatic medication consisting of tegafur and cyclophosphamide. The Bestatin-hormone regimen was started by dispensing Bestatin at 60 mg t.i.d. for three weeks, then adding 40 mg t.i.d. of fluoxymetholone. The nodules remained unchanged during the first two weeks of the combined regimen, then became swollen, and started shrinking by the end of the fourth week. The upper nodule over the nuchal area was biopsied. During the subsequent two weeks, the nodules were reduced in size and ultimately disappeared. This lytic contraction of tumors following a period of incubation suggests a loss of cancer cells via redifferentiation, that is, the acquisition by the cancer cells of a limited life span. Figure 14A presents the histological picture prior to Bestatin administration. Cancer cells infiltrated the muscle, piling up on each other. Lymphocytic infiltration was also present. As shown in Fig. 14B, after the Bestatin-hormone regimen, the cancer cells formed trabeculae, creating a tumor sheet instead of a cord. The lymphocytic infiltration disappeared, and the expected somal and nuclear enlargement of cancer cells was apparent. In addition, the cells did not pile up on each other as they had previously. The sheet formation may represent the return of contact inhibition, implying the probable induction of redifferentiation among these cells and the acquisition of a limited life span.

Case 3   In this patient, the breast cancer spread over the entire right anterior chest, and numerous nodules had formed. While radiotherapy eradicated some of the nodules, patchy areas of cancerous ulcers developed. With the administration of Bestatin and fluoxymetholone, portions of the ulcers started healing. There seemed to be constant flux among the nodules: some were newly emerged while others underwent disintegration. A conspicuous feature was the flattening of the nodules, which measured about 10 mm in diameter. The flattened nodules decayed after a definite life span. Carmofur was concomitantly administered.

Histological study revealed the characteristic somal and nuclear enlargement accompanied by a tendency toward trabecular arrangement. Attempts to form glandular alveoli were also noted here and there.

Case 4   When referred to us, this patient had a large ulcerative skin metastasis of approximately 7×5 cm accompanied by nodules in the right anterior chest. Prior to the administration of Bestatin and fluoxymetholone, the cancer cells were seen to form primitive glandular alveoli. After three weeks of treatment, the glandular structures seemed to have "matured": circular alveolar structures were being formed here and there. This, however, could have been due to disintegration of the centrally seated cells. No secretory phenomena were suggested.

Case 5   This patient had long refused medical and surgical assistance, and visited our clinic only after strong persuasion by her friends. The left breast was fully expanded as a result of tumor growth and inflammation, and numerous nodular skin metastases were observed. To alleviate the tumor pain in the left breast, radiotherapy was carried out. The nodules were not included in the field of radiotherapy, however. Biopsy of one of the nodules revealed that the cancer cells had aggregated to form alveolar patterns, and abortive secretory sequelae were thought probable. Under the circumstances, this was the only biopsy obtainable.

Thus, however primitive or abortive it might be, cancer redifferentiation leading to eventual cancer cell death seems to be induced by the regimen of Bestatin and sex hormones.

Discussion

Redifferentiation as a technique of reversing devolution
Both leukemogenesis and carcinogenesis are sequelae of genetic changes leading to cellular devolution. Differentiation is the genetic expression of normal precursor cells, in principle gene expression without irreversible structural changes in the relevant DNA molecules. What then is the induction of redifferentiation of malignant cells? It is true that leukemia or cancer cells are genetically different from their normal counterparts. However, these malignant cells can be led to express relevant genes of their own, thereby acquiring a definite life span. This concept is schematically illustrated in Fig. 15.

As discussed earlier, there seems to be a different degree of devolution between leukemias and cancers. In his model of neoplastic evolution, Nowell suggested that this difference was one of early vs late malignant clonal evolution (1976): human leukemias resulting from minimal chromosome change may be early in clonal evolution, while the solid cancers resulting from much greater changes in aneuploidy are viewed as late in the developmental process. In this regard, Fanconi's anemia seems to be an evolutionary experiment. If we assume that DNA change as a result of chromosomal fragility due to Cu,ZnSOD deficiency and defective DNA repair is primarily homogeneous throughout the body, and throughout the chromosomes as well, the average time

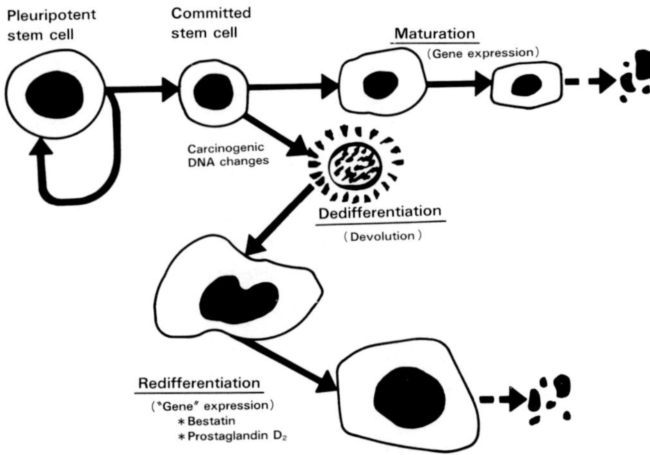

Fig. 15. Cancer redifferentiation vs maturation and dedifferentiation. Normal maturation and differentiation consists of gene expression in appropriate cells in appropriate locations at appropriate times. Cancer redifferentiation, however, is the expression of the inappropriate, disordered gene(s) of inappropriate cells in inappropriate locations at inappropriate times. Completely normal to quasinormal redifferentiation can be attained in leukemias and neurogenic tumors, but not in most epithelial cancers, presumably because of the greater deviation of the disordered genes or their greater degree of devolution. Carcinogenesis itself is an evolutionary phenomenon, and currently inducible cancer redifferentiation may also be better understood in terms of an evolutionary concept.

required for the establishment of a leukemogenic chromosomal setup is about 15 ± 7 years, while that required for the accumulation of chromosomal abnormalities for epithelial cancers is about 24 ± 7 years (Okuyama and Mishina 1987a). We can assume that this average difference of about 10 years approximates the minimal length of time during which the multiple carcinogenetic oncogenes are sequentially prepared, although the process per se is stochastic and the "quick evolution" of carcinogenesis probably proceeds along the lines of the selection principle of evolution (Cairns 1981). Needless to say, the entire process can also be modified by factors such as the surveillance mechanisms.

Spontaneous regression of tumors as an evolutionary experiment on carcinogenesis   The spontaneous regression of tumors can be regarded as one of nature's probable experiments on carcinogenesis, one of a different direction (Everson and Cole 1966). Although leukemias are not included there, nonepithelial tumors comprise the majority of cases, 60%. The ease of regression is reciprocally related to the number of carcinogenetic steps in the DNA, and the epithelial solid tumors may not regress easily because of the multitude of chromosomal changes.

Mechanisms of redifferentiation   We were not able to clarify the exact biochemical processes that led breast cancer cells towards differentiation. Nonetheless, a variety of agents may be efficient enough to halt cancer cell proliferation. The next step is to develop techniques that would expedite the redifferentiation of gene expression, as suggested elsewhere (Uehara *et al.* 1985). It is hoped that our hypothesis of the evolutionary stratification of carcinogenesis will cut further into the problem.

Potentiation of anticancer immunity with Bestatin   In spite of claims that Bestatin stimulates anticancer immunity, we could not confirm lymphocytic participation in any of our clinical materials. We reviewed the enlarged color microphotographs presented at three Bestatin research conferences (1978-1979), but were unable to find any lymphocytic infiltrations except in one case of esophageal cancer that had been effectively irradiated (Ishikawa *et al.* 1979). Thus, Bestatin probably activates immune reactions only when tumor cell reduction is sufficient for the agent to eradicate residual tumor cells, although other invisible immune reactions could have been involved.

Modification of metastatic potential with Bestatin   From a biological point of view, the probable alteration of metastatic potential should also be discussed here. The initial observation by Svanberg and Elisson (1983) was based on the clinical evolution of metastasis and autopsy materials. Experimental data have also been presented (Pimm and Baldwin 1985). Our clinical impression is that those patients treated with Bestatin appeared to develop fewer distant metastases but seemed more likely to develop local, infiltrative progression.

Therapeutic tactics expandable with Bestatin   One of the main limitations of radiotherapy and chemotherapy is the barrier of probabilistic cell killing (Withers and Peters 1980), or log kill (Salmon and Apple 1974). A host of techniques can help to overcome this limitation: (1) increasing tumoral accretion of anticancer agents (Okuyama *et al*. 1978a); (2) potentiation by inhibiting the repairable DNA damage of radiotherapy and chemotherapy (Okuyama and Matsuzawa 1979; Okuyama and Mishina 1980; 1985e); (3) rescue of the normal, intervening tissues in radiotherapy to permit augmentation of the therapeutic radiation dosage (Okuyama and Mishina 1982d); and (4) biological amplification of the radiotherapeutic and chemotherapeutic aftermath through emperipolesis (Okuyama *et al*. 1979b), immunopotentiation through common antigenization (Sasaki and Kunimatsu 1980), and exfoliation (Okuyama *et al*. 1984b). The present induction of cancer redifferentiation may fall into the category of biological techniques. The primary importance of the principle may be limited to combatting cells residual from radiotherapy and chemotherapy, and cells disseminated at the time of surgical manipulation, until satisfactorily potent redifferentiating agents are developed.

Thus, the problem of cancer redifferentiation is best approached via an evolutionary concept. This approach may provide a better understanding of the processes of redifferentiation, and may be fruitful in the development of more specific and/or more potent redifferentiating agents.

Chapter 13

Cytochrome *c* in the Treatment of Radiation Dermatitis and Ulcers

To our surprise, the intractable radiation ulcers of 23 years' history have healed with the use of ubiquinone ointment.
——*T. Sugai*, Dermatology, *1987*

Introduction

Radiation damage to the intervening normal tissues in the form of radiation dermatitis, ulcers, and eventual fibrosis frequently torments cancer patients who receive radiotherapy. Although the administration of corticosteroids has been effective in promptly alleviating pain and subduing the signs and symptoms of acute inflammation, their tendency to foster local and/or systemic infections is sometimes discouraging. Skin transplants may not always take, especially when doses of irradiation have already been administered. Previously, the most serious dermal complications of infected radiation ulcers resulting from radiotherapy with deep X-rays were eventually completely healed by use of hyperbaric oxygen therapy (Mishina *et al.* 1977). In addition to the successful control of infections through the production of activated oxygen molecules, improved local oxygenation was thought to be largely responsible for the results. We thus had a rationale for the clinical application of cytochrome *c* to patients with radiation dermatitis (Okuyama and Mishina 1982d). As soon as clinical evidence was obtained for the therapeutic effect of cytochrome *c*, we attempted to determine whether the same principle could be expanded to the use of ubiquinone for these dermopathies (Okuyama and Mishina 1983b). An integrated clinical and experimental demonstration of its use is described here.

One of the most conspicuous findings in the present investigation is that epithelization of the radiation ulcers was prompted by use of ubiquinone ointment as well as receding of signs and symptoms of inflammation such as pain and erythema. The process of wound healing consists of granulation formation and epithelization. The red granulation tissue which contains capillaries and therefore is well oxygenated fosters epithelization, while the white granulation tissue, which is poor in capillary content and therefore is poorly oxygenated, discourages it and leads to eventual fibrosis.

Thus, the system of wound healing can be considered to consist of two or three compartments: (1) fibrosing, (2) epithelizing, and (3) intermediating. The ultimate goal of covering the wound is achieved by either epithelization or scar formation. If ubiquinone restores the electron transport system, which is vulnerable to physical stress and is easily depleted of ubiquinone, the intermediating granulation tissue ignites the epithelizing system. Should the intermediating granulation tissue fails to restitute it for one reason or another, however the fibrosing system will be ignited.

This compartmentalization may indicate an evolutionary transition of the hypoxic and scar-forming to the oxic and epithelizing tissue. The cytochrome *c* effect using cytochrome *c* proper or ubiquinone preparation thus has an evolutionary significance.

Studies

A detailed description of experiments using cancer cell culture and on ultraviolet experimental model for radiation dermatitis in the rabbit is found elsewhere (Okuyama and Mishina 1985i; Okuyama *et al.* 1985a).

Clinical studies   Patients with a variety of malignant primary and metastatic tumors were treated with an initial peroral administration of cytochrome *c* following radiotherapy. However, as soon as its lack of interference with the anticancer effects of irradiation was confirmed experimentally, it was given from the outset.

Peroral and/or intravenous administration of cytochrome *c* of equine origin was carried out. Synthetic ubiquinone (ubidecarenone, Eisai Pharmaceutical, Tokyo) was incorporated to constitute 0.5% by weight of a hydrophilic ointment.

Histological studies on the cytochrome c rescue of radiation dermatitis   A 53-year-old woman with thyroid cancer was pre-operatively irradiated in the anterior neck to 4700 R. During the seven days before surgery, she was treated with 10 mg t.i.d. of peroral cytochrome *c*. At the time of surgery, a skin specimen was obtained from the field of irradiation. A 47-year-old man with recurrent maxillary carcinoma served as a control: a skin specimen was obtained from the field of radiotherapy (to 2250 R) two years after radical surgery. To provide semiquantitative evaluation of the effect of cytochrome *c* on fibrous changes, specimens of Masson's elastica stain from cases of post-radiotherapy surgery were reviewed. The amount of Masson-positive material was semiquantitated by scoring from $+1$ to $+5$. Figure 3B was scored $+5$, and Fig. 3D, $+3$. The surgical materials were a variety of malignancies: six were treated with cytochrome *c* and nine were untreated.

Results

Absence of cytochrome c interference with the anticancer effects of radiation   Cytochrome *c* was found not to interfere with the anticancer effects of irradiation even at the lower doses.

Reduction of radiation dermatitis in an ultraviolet model
In the ultraviolet system, cytochrome *c* was definitely effective in reducing palpable indurations (nine out of the 10 irradiated spots in the control and two out of the 10 irradiated skins in the treated group as of day 5). Microscopic examination revealed that the skin thickness was significantly reduced (Fig. 1).

Treatment of radiation dermatitis by peroral administration of cytochrome c in humans   The peroral dose of cytochrome *c* was effective in treating acute radiation dermatitis. Beneficial effects were also evident on chronic radiation dermatitis (Table 1). Representative cases are described below.

Table 1. Cytochrome c effect on radiation dermatitis (1): Rescue and prevention by peroral cytochrome c, and dose-responsiveness

Patient No.	Age/Sex	Primary cancer	Site of irradiation	Radiation skin dose	Concomitant chemotherapy	1) Time of start and 2) Response to Cy c	Remarks
1	18/F	Sarcoma botryoides, pelvis	Rt. inguinal metastases	4,000 R	BLM	1) Post-RT 2) Excellent	
2	53/F	Lung	Rt. chest metastases	4,000 R	BLM D-penicil-lamine	1) Post-RT 2) Excellent	
3	48/F	Lung	Metastases to lumbar vertebral bodies	11,000 R	BLM CDDP	1) Post-RT 2) Excellent	Fig. 2
4	57/F	Rt. breast	Rt. chest, postoperative	5,000 R	BLM	1) During RT and Post-RT 2) Excellent	Dose-responsive (+Cy c i.v.)
5	42/M	Lung	Metastases to rt. neck and upper mediastinum	9,500 R	BLM ACD	1) During RT 2) Excellent*	Esophagitis Dose-responsive (+Cy c i.v.)
6	75/F	Submandibular tumor	Lt. mouth	6,400 R	BLM CDDP D-penicil-lamine	1) During RT 2) Oral mucositis and ulceration demanded prednine	Exacerbated by drug eruption (+Cy c i.v.)
7	57/M	Spinal cord tumor	Lower thoracic vertebral bodies	10,600 R	BLM ACD	1) Pre-RT and post-RT 2) Excellent	Least atrophic, less fibrotic
8	68/F	Lt. breast	Recurrence by ulceration Lt. chest	4,000 R	BLM Carmofur	1) Post-RT 2) Excellent	Crushed the healing wound: then subjected to ubiquinone ointment
9	48 F	Rt. breast	Rt. chest, postoperative (intractable infection over the sutures of skin graft)	4,000 R	BLM	1) Post-RT 2) Excellent	

BLM=bleomycin in oil, 2-5 mg, im.   CDDP=cisplatin, i.v.   ACD=actinomycin-D, 25-50 μg.   RT=radiotherapy

* Esophageal pains necessitated additional i.v. Cytochrome c

Patient 3 was irradiated at the lumbar vertebral bodies for metastases from lung cancer. The total skin dose amounted to 11,000 R, and signs and symptoms of acute radiation dermatitis developed (Fig. 2). Peroral cytochrome *c* supplemented

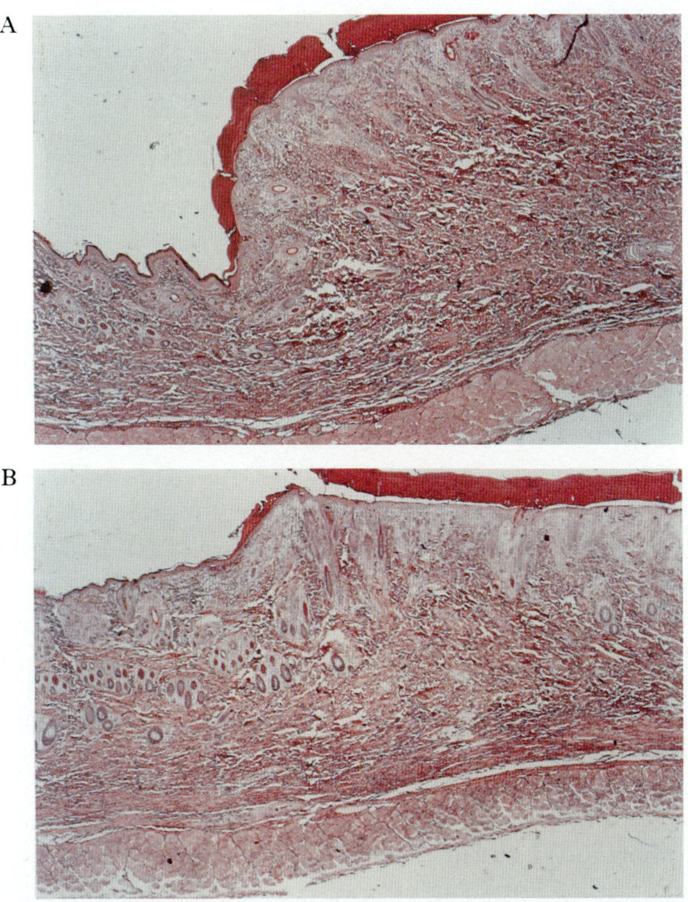

Fig. 1. Treatment of ultraviolet-induced dermatitis through cytochrome *c*. Rabbit skin was exposed to a fixed dose of ultraviolet irradiation (250 to 400 nm). Intravenous treatment with 30 mg of cytochrome *c* once a day for five consecutive days was effective in reducing inflammatory changes in the irradiated skin. Relative thickness was computed by dividing the thickness of the irradiated skin by that of the nonirradiated skin. The values were 1.70 ± 0.30 in the control and 1.31 ± 0.07 in the cytochrome *c*-treated group (statistically significant at $p < 0.05$) (Okuyama *et al.* 1985).

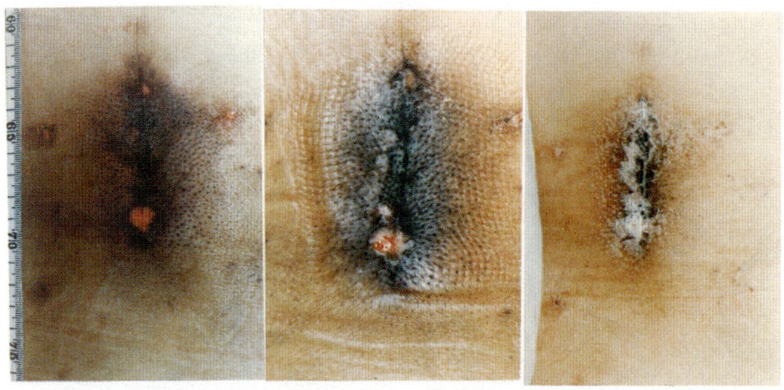

Berfore treatment   One week of cyto-chrome *c* treatment   Two weeks of cyto-chrome *c* treatment

Fig. 2. Therapeutic effect of cytochrome *c* on radiation dermatitis. Ten milligrams t.i.d. of cytochrome *c* was perorally administered after 11,000 R to 7×15 cm of skin. Chemotherapy with cisplatin and bleomycin could have contributed to worsening the dermatitis. Prompt improvement was observed.

with an intravenous infusion of 2400 mg of glutathione and 2000 mg of vitamin C cured the acute inflammation in two weeks, without resorting to corticosteroids. The patient is still alive and free of any symptoms of dermatitis or ulcers.

Patient 4 was irradiated postoperatively to 5000 R in the right anterior chest because of right breast cancer. She developed radiation dermatitis of erythema of moderate degree in spite of 10 mg t.i.d. of peroral cytochrome *c*. Additional daily infusions of 60 mg of cytochrome *c* administered intravenously resulted in prompt cure of the dermopathy.

Patient 7 was exposed to 10,600 R because of spinal cord tumor metastasis to the lower thoracic vertebral bodies. To reinforce the radiotherapeutic effect against the tumor, small doses of bleomycin and actinomycin D were administered just before each radiotherapy session. The peroral administration of cytochrome *c* began when the skin dose reached 3300 R. There was slight erythema over the field of radiotherapy at the time it was completed. The patient, however, did not have any aches or pains. The drug was administered for 15 months. The skin appeared slightly brownish but remained soft, although there was some resistance to palpation at depth.

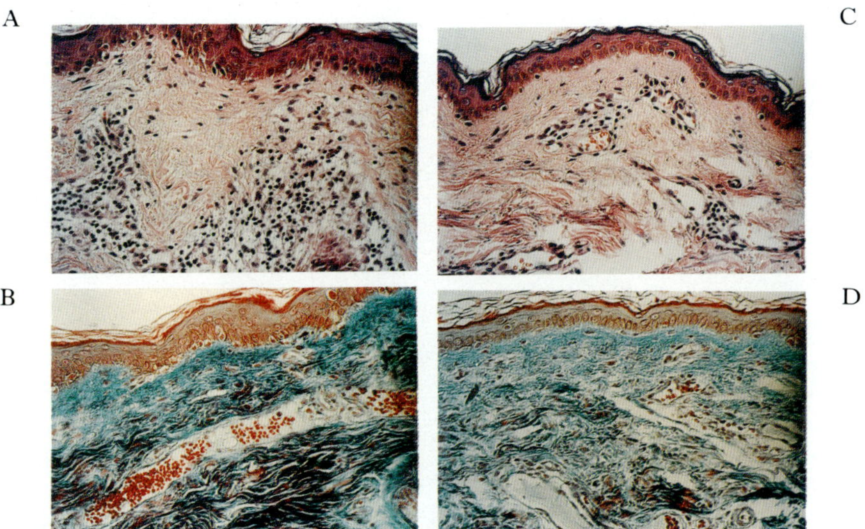

Fig. 3. Histological evaluation of the therapeutic effect of cytochrome *c*. I. Irradiation of 2250 R to the skin, but no treatment with
cytochrome *c*. A and B: Hyperemia, and venous engorgement,
and perivascular lymphocytic infiltration are noted. B: Deposition
of Masson's elastic positive material: grade +5. II. 4700 R to the
skin, and cytochrome *c* treatment. Much less hyperemia, venous
engorgement, and lymphocytic infiltration. D. Deposition of Masson-positive material: grade +3. (A, C, hematoxylin-eosin stain; B,
D, Masson's elastica stain).

*Histological evaluation of the effect of cytochrome c on radia-
tion dermatitis: Studies on the skin peritumorous tissues*
Skin specimens of patients irradiated but not treated with
cytochrome *c* showed signs of acute inflammation: hyperemia,
vascular dilation, pronounced lymphocytic infiltration, and
accumulation of Masson-positive material in the subcutis.
When patients were treated with cytochrome *c*, these signs
improved greatly (Fig. 3). A comparision of the scores between the cytochrome *c*-treated patient and controls revealed
a significant difference: 2.2±0.8 vs 4.4±0.5.
*Application of ubiquinone ointment to intractable radiation
dermatitis*   Because of the favorable clinical and experimental data, the peroral administration of cytochrome *c* was
used regularly for the prevention of radiation dermatitis as
well as for treatment. However, the dermatides in a minority

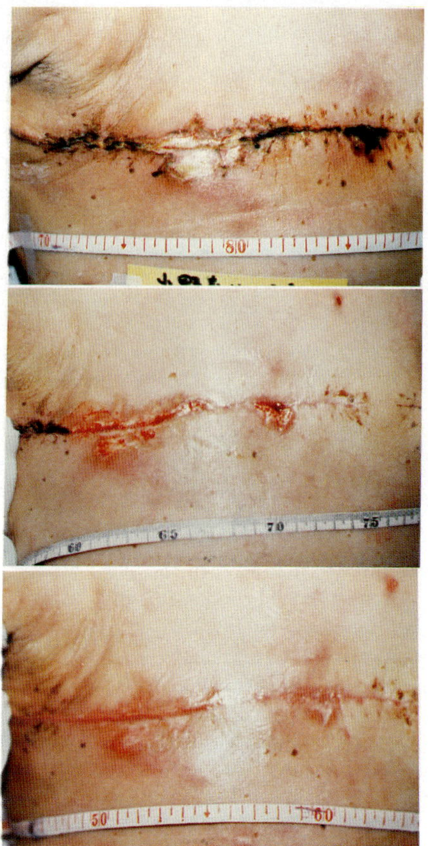

Fig. 4. Therapeutic effect of ubiquinone ointment on radiation dermatitis: Treatment of delayed healing of surgical wounds. Pre-surgically, 3000 R to the skin was administered because of bilateral breast cancer. Skin healing was delayed, presumably because of skin tension as well as irradiation. First, a course of hyperbaric oxygen therapy was tried in vain. The patient was then subjected to ubiquinone ointment. Her therapeutic response was excellent following debridement. Thus, such wounds may constitute a kind of radiation ulcer

of patients overwhelmed its effects. In such cases, we applied ubiquinone ointment and achieved satisfactory success. In addition, the ointment helped in the healing of surgical wounds among patients who had already been exposed to radiation prior to surgery (Table 2).

Table 2. Cytochrome *c* effect on radiation dermatitis (2): Expansion to ubiquinone ointment

Patient No.	Age/Sex	Primary cancer	Site of irradiation	Radiation skin dose	Concomitant chemotherapy	1) Cy *c* 2) Time of start, and response to CQ	Remarks
1	82/F	Rt. breast	Rt. side neck	5,000R	BLM	1) Cy *c* + 2) Post-RT Excellent	Fulminant dermatitis triggered by a traumatic erosion
2	59/F	Rt. breast	Rt. chest	5,700R	BLM carboquone	1) Cy *c* + 2) 1 yr post-RT Excellent	
3	73/F	Uterine cervical	Lower abdomen	Not known	Not known	2) 17 yrs post-RT Excellent	
4	68/F	Lt. breast	Lt. chest, ulcerated	4,000R	BLM HCFU	1) Cy *c* + 2) post-RT Excellent	Healing ulcer crushed and exacerbated, responded to CQ
5	56/F	Lt. breast	Lt. chest	3,000R	BLM FT	1) Cy *c* − 2) Post-RT and post-surgery, Excellent	Delayed healing of surgical wounds
6	47/F	Bilateral breast	Bilateral chest	3,000R	HCFU	1) Cy *c* − 2) Post-RT and post-surgery, Excellent	Delayed healing of surgical wounds (Fig. 4)
7	48/F	Lt. breast	Lt. chest	4,000R	BLM	1) Cy *c* − 2) Post-RT and post-surgery, Excellent	Delayed healing of surgical wounds

Cy c=Cytochrome c, 10 mg t.i.d. per os.
CQ=Ubiquinone ointment, 0.5%.

Patient 1 was irradiated on the right side of the neck for a large cancer metastasis. The skin dose was 5000 R. In spite of the peroral cytochrome *c* regimen, a scratch in the field of radiotherapy triggered the development of radiation dermatitis. Intravenous cytochrome *c* was not of much benefit. The patient was then subjected to ubiquinone ointment. Her response was remarkable, and the skin appeared normal even one year later.

Patient 6 was intriguing because of the ointment's effect on the delayed healing of surgical wounds. Following 3000 R to both breast cancers, bilateral radical mastectomy was carried out. The skin tension was so great that the sutures broke, and tension necrosis was present here and there. After a course of hyperbaric oxygen therapy proved ineffective, topical application of ubiquinone ointment was undertaken following appropriate debridement. The response was excellent (Fig. 4).

Discussion

We have no knowledge as to how van Bekkum's observation on the effect of cytochrome *c* has actually affected the medical world (1955). Nonetheless, it was gratifying to see how promptly patients with radiation dermatitis were relieved of pains, and how quickly signs of acute and chronic inflammation and ulcers receded without resort to corticosteroids when cytochrome *c* and ubiquinone were administered (Okuyama and Mishina 1982d; 1983b; Asoh and Sugai 1987). There appears to be a dose-responsive relationship in the effect of cytochrome *c*. The surgical wounds in the previously irradiated skin may have represented a kind of radiation ulcer whose healing was expedited by the use of ubiquinone ointment. Thus, the effectiveness of cytochrome *c* is now a clinical principle rather than an *in vitro* observation. Cytochrome *c* did not appear to interfere with the anticancer effect of radiotherapy, enabling it to be used even during periods of radiotherapy.

The electron transport system in the mitochondria of cells can be damaged by irradiation, and the oxidative phosphorylation depressed (Potter and Bethel 1952; van Bekkum 1955).

Whatever the biochemical pathology, direct inactivation or easy deletion of cytochrome *c* and ubiquinone in the mitochondria would certainly be amenable to the concept of reconstitution (van Bekkum 1956).

When perorally administered, exogenous radio-iodinated cytochrome *c* was absorbed through the intestine into the circulation, and accumulated in organs (Tajima *et al.* 1970). It localized in the perinuclear multivesicular bodies and helped restore the integrity of the endoplasmic reticulum and mitochondria (Ohnishi *et al.* 1972). When applied to the skin, ubiquinone is easily absorbed (Yokoi *et al.* 1983), arrives at the target cells, and reconstitutes the electron transport system, as evidenced by the increased ATP production observed with exogenous ubiquinone in experimental ischemia (Abe *et al.* 1980). The therapeutic effects of ubiquinone appeared greater than those of cytochrome *c*, presumably on account of drug concentrations at the sites of dermopathies and the additives to the ointment.

The prompt alleviation of the pain is remiscent of angina pectoris, whose pain is known to result from myocardial ischemia. This pain is relieved as soon as vasodilation secures sufficient oxygenation. Oxygenation enables the myocardial mitochondria to produce the ATP that is so urgently needed. The administration of cytochrome *c* and ubiquinone would abolish pain through ATP production. Improvement in other signs and symptoms of inflammation is also related to the recovered synthesis of ATP. The experimental model using ultraviolet irradiation may have simulated acute radiation dermatitis, and the therapeutic efficacy of cytochrome *c* in that model reiterated its effectiveness (Okuyama *et al.* 1985a).

Epithelial cells seem to be characterized by their sensitivity to oxygen concentrations, as evidenced by the way they line up and orient themselves according to their polarity: polarity may result because all substances entering and leaving the body must traverse the epithelium in a direction perpendicular to its surface (Bloom and Fawcett 1975). The same may be true with the skin, and its regeneration may be encouraged when the effect of oxygen, through eoxgenous cytochrome *c* and ubiquinone, comes into play. Intractable radiation ulcers and surgical wounds in skin previously subjected to radiotherapy were also healed. Because it is a sequel to acute radiation damage, the emergence of radiation fibrosis can also be reduced.

Whenever an attempt is made to rescue damage to normal tissues resulting from anticancer therapy, it is necessary to confront the possibility of neutralizing the anticancer effects. Our *in vitro* experiment seemed to suggest that this might not be the case with cytochrome c, the target of radiation cell kill is the nuclear DNA while that of rescue by cytochrome c is the electron transport system in the mitochondria. This difference may constitute biological selectiveness. Our clinical impression was also in accordance with the experiment.

Thus, van Bekkum's formulation of the effect of cytochrome c is now of clinical significance in the treatment of radiation dermatitis, ulcers, and related states, and the probable side effects of corticosteroids can be avoided. It is hoped that skin grafting can be avoided in selected cases. It would probably be helpful to increase the dosage tolerated by the patient to obtain better ultimate therapeutic results.

Current plan for prevention and treatment of radiation damage in normal tissues   The preceding clinical and experimental data served as the basis for the following therapeutic plan used in our department:

I.   Preventive measure: Peroral cytochrome c, 10 mg, t.i.d.

II.   Treatment of radiation dermatitis and esophagitis: When signs and symptoms are severe, an additional 60 mg of cytochrome c is adminstered intravenously. A test for possible hypersensitivity to cytochrome c is mandatory. When dermopathy is severer, ubiquinone ointment is applied. If the damage is located such that direct application of the ointment is impracticable or if the inflammation is too severe, corticosteroids are used. In one case, the administration of predonine was indicated because of drug sensitivity to bleomycin (case 6 in Table 1). If ulcers persist, treatment for hypozincemia is initiated (Okuyama *et al*. 1983b).

A tendency to constipation was seen in several cases when peroral cytochrome c was administered for some time, especially among the elderly. The individual merits of the peroral route and topical application deserve consideration.

The processes of inflammation can also be a replay of evolutionary history. The well-known participation of phagocytic cells, capillary endothelial cells, and fibroblasts may be symbolic (Bradley *et al.* 1978; Kan and Yamane 1983). All of these are prevertebral cells, not to mention pre-eukaryotic, and prosper under hypoxia rather than normal oxygen or hyperoxia. The human skin has been constructed to adapt itself to an oxygen-containing, homeothermic atmosphere, and the pronounced effects of cytochrome *c* on epithelial growth may be related to this preference for an oxygen-containing environment.

The principle of cytochrome *c* effect can be expanded to tissue damage other than radiation dermopathies, e.g., thermal wounds (Okuyama *et al.* 1987b).

Summary

Cancer status [is characterized by] an increase in the water content, a decrease in the SOD content, and defective excision repair of the DNA damage.
——*S. Okuyama and H. Mishina,*
Radiology, 1984

Cancer Therapy Strategies

This portion of the book described a search for efficient modes of cancer cell elimination based on evolutionary principles. As discussed above, most of the current therapeutic measures carry evolutionary significance. As mammalian life has been provided with a host of devices that help it to evade carcinogenesis, it has become capable of eliminating cancer cells in one way or another.

Exfoliation is one of the simplest mechanisms, especially among neoplasms in organs undergoing constant cell renewal. Starting with graft-versus-host reactions, immunological mechanisms for removing cancer cells may be of rather recent origin. Their anticancer efficacy resides in quasispecific immunity. Specific *B* immunity may not yet be of prime importance. Carcinogenesis through retroviral infections and chemical carcinogenesis may be the most recent from the evolutionary point of view, and tumors in these categories would be the most vulnerable to aggression from *B* immunity, as is true of most experimental mammalian carcinomas. Thus, quasispecific immunity against cancer, which can be activated by the use of most of the biological immunomodulators (BMR), seems, at the moment, practical as well as scientific.

The discrete concept of ascending (or antigenizing) and descending limbs (or actual effectuation on the target cells) of immune reactions is important (Schlager *et al.* 1978a, b). This concept appears sound from the clinical point of view as well, and led us to expanded studies involving Bestatin, an agent that was originally designed to affect the lymphocytes. Because we are radiotherapists, the entire therapeutic plan was reviewed according to radiotherapeutic principles, with other modalities of treatment considered as well. To overcome the limitations of each modality, strategic integration, symbolized in terms of *T-PR-B* and/or *S-PC-B*, was considered. The evolutionary analysis fitted more easily than expected at the outset, in light of the perpetuation of repair of DNA damage caused by radiotherapy and (alkylating) chemotherapy (*PR* and *PC*). A remarkable agent, herbimycin, was found to interfere with the processes of oncogene expression (Uehara *et al.* 1984).

At the moment, we have no appropriate means of activating tumor suppressor genes or anti-oncogenes (Klein 1987). However, the chromosomal manipulation experiments of Matsuya *et al.* (1978) seem to afford hope even in terms of anticancer therapy. Nevertheless, before we arrive at the ultimate anticancer therapy, we have much to learn from evolution.

Epilogue: The Evolutionary Concept as the Scientific Core of Oncology

> *We are at the threshold of a previously unknown world where oncogenes, antioncogenes and other cellular genes interact within complex regulatory circuits.*——*George Klein and Eva Klein,* Tumor Biology, *1985*

It is not the similarity between chickens and humans, but the differences that we are concerned with. Humans are differentiated from chickens by virtue of the breast and uterus in the female and the prostate in the male, the mammalian symbol organs. Chickens in turn can be differentiated from frogs and crocodiles by the presence of lungs and a thyroid gland, which enable the chickens to adapt to elevated atmospheric oxygen concentrations and lead a homeothermic life. The vertebrates are characterized not only by vertebral bones and a well-organized central nervous sytem, but also by immune systems ranging from the quasispecific to the specific. Prevertebral life is characterized by the fibrous and hematopoietic organs, whose constituent cells are at home in a hypoxic milieu (Bradley *et al.* 1978; Kan and Yamane 1983) and can be migratory and/or phagocytic. This discrimination seems well embodied in the respective neoplasms in terms of the aptitude for carcinogenesis and latitude of therapeutic responsiveness.

Cell biology used to be mainly descriptive, with real understanding largely limited to glycolysis and the TCA cycle. Even with elucidation of the electron transport system in the mitochondria, cell biology was far from the current recognition of the endosymbiotic evolution of eukaryotic cells (Margulis 1980).

As radiotherapists, we naturally began our evolutionary

conceptualization of cancer with the origin of radiosensitivity, and developed our concepts by arranging our observations along the line of evolution (Okuyama and Mishina 1980; 1981 a; 1984b). The evolutionary concept of cancer is concerned with cancer status, or what cancer is. In this regard, it is similar to Setala's devolutionary concept of cancer (1984). Two or three authors have used the term evolution in the domain of carcinogenesis: Cairns desribed it as "quick evolution" (1981), while Klein referred to it as "microevolution"(1987). Cairns held to Darwinism by describing the process of carcinogenesis as selection of fitter variants. Klein described "mobile and transposable" oncogenes. By "evolution," these scientists seem to have implied the stepwise progression of carcinogenesis. Another meaning of our evolutionary concept of cancer concerns the trend in cancer incidence from leukemias in childhood to solid epithelial tumors in the adulthood (the nonepithelial-epithelial tumor shift) (Okuyama and Mishina 1986b; 1987a). That trend may bear genetic implications in terms of the ease of carcinogenesis (Nowell 1976) or the number of oncogene changes required for leukemogenesis and carcinogenesis (Watson *et al.* 1987). However, it can be understood to express the age-related probability to developing leukemia or cancer. The same evolutionary rule was seen to apply to carcinogenesis in the population of Nagasaki following the atomic bombing, and possibly to that in Hiroshima as well (Okuyama and Mishina 1988a). Nonetheless, the trend represents an evolutionary orientation. The radiological and radioisotopic diagnosis of cancer was also found to be closely related to its evolutionary properties. The radiosensitivity of tumors from different organ systems differs, but the mode of variation was found to depend on the evolutionary history of each organ and to be closely related to evolutionary changes in the earth's physical and chemical environment (Okuyama and Mishina 1985h).

We began our studies on the sensitivity of cancer to tetracyclines, and eventually realized that that property of cancer cells may represent endosymbiotic fragility or *locus minoris resistentiae* (Okuyama *et al.* 1987a; Setala 1984). Further research into this fragility is likely to be fruitful.

Will the ultimate cancer therapy be solely dependent on

anti-oncogene/oncogene products (Uehara *et al.* 1985) and pro-tumor suppressor gene medication? Will there be problems of penetrability and the probabilistic barrier? Whatever the problems, the future is not without hope.

References

Abe, E., Miyaura, C., Sakagami, H., Takeda, M., Konno, K., Yamazaki, T., Yoshiki, S. and Suda, T. (1981). Differentiation of mouse myeloid leukemia cells induced by la, 25-hydroxyvitamine D_3. *Proc. Nat. Acad. Sci., USA*, **78**, 4990–4994.

Abe, S., Sekiguchi, N., Shimizu, K. and Suyama, I. (1969). Population exposure due to natural radiation in each prefecture of the Kyushuu district. In: *Radioactivity Survey Data in Japan*, National Institute of Radiological Sciences, Chiba, Japan, No. **25**. p. 4.

Abe, T., Okamoto, F., Karino, K., Ohori, K. and Komatsu, S. (1980). Myocardial protection with conenzyme Q_{10} during two hours of aortic cross-clamping—Evaluation from the aspects of high energy phosphates and lactate in the myocardium—. In: *Biomedical and Clinical Aspects of Coenzyme Q*, **2**, ed. by Yamamura, Y., Folkers, F. and Ito, Y. Elsevier/North Holland, Amsterdam. pp. 77–87.

Abels, D. and Reed, W. B. (1973). Fanconi-like syndrome. Immunologic deficiency, pancytopenia, and cutaneous malignancies. *Arch. Derm.*, **107**, 419–423.

Abrams, H. D., Rohrschneider, L. R. and Eisenman, R. N. (1982). Nuclear localization of the putative transforming protein of myelocytomatosis virus. *Cell*, **29**, 427–439.

Ahmed, .F. E. and Setlow, R. B. (1978). Excision repair in ataxia telangeictasia, Fanconi's anemia, Cockayne syndrome, and Bloom's syndrome after treatment with ultraviolet radiation and N–acetoxyl–2–acetylaminofluorene. *Biochem. Biophys. Acta*, **521**, 805–817.

Alberts, B., Bray, D., Lewis, J., Raff, M., Roberts, K. and Watson, J. D. (1983). *Molecular Biology of the Cell*, Garland, New York.

Alexander, J. W. and Good. R. A. (1977). *Fundamentals of Clinical Immunology*, Saunders, Philadelphia.

Algire, G. H. and Chalkley, H. W. (1945). Vascular reactions of normal and malignant tissue *in vivo*. I. Vascular reactions of mice to wounds and to normal and neplastic transplants. *J. Nat. Cancer Inst.*, **6**, 73–85.

Alimena, G., Billistrom, R., Casalone, R., Gallo, E., Mitelman, F. and Pasquali, F. (1985). Cytogenetic pattern in leukemic cells of patients with constitutional chromosome anomalies. *Cancer Genet. Cytogenet.*, **16**, 207–218.

Allard, C., DeLamirande, G. and Cantero, A. (1953). Mitochondrial population in mammalian cells. IV. Preliminary results on the variation in the mitochondrial population of the average rat liver cell during azo dyes carcinogenesis. *Canad. J. Med. Sci.*, **30**, 543–548.

Ando, Y., Nakano, S., Saito, K., Shimamoto, I. and Ichijo, M. (1986). Prevention of adult T–cell leukemia virus infection from mother to child. *Proc. Jpn. Cancer Assoc.*, 45th. Ann. Mtg., Sapporo, Oct. 21–23, 1986. p. 491. (Abstract)

Aoki, T. (1984). Lentinan. In: *Immunology Ser.* 25: *Immune Modulating Agents and Their Mechanisms*, ed. by Fenichel, R. L. and Chirigos, M. A. Dekker. New York. pp. 63–77.

Aoyagi, T., Ishizuka, M., Takeuchi, T. and Umezawa, H. (1977). Enzyme inhibitors in relation to cancer therapy. *Jpn. J. Antibiot.*, **30 (Suppl.)** , 121–132.

Arakawa, E. T. (1968). Residual radiation in Hiroshima and Nagasaki. *Hiroshima Igaku*, **21** 930–948. (English and Japanese)

Archambeau, J. O., Bennett, G. W. Levine G. S., Cowen, R. and Bond, V. P. (1974). Proton radiation therapy. *Radiology*, **110,** 445–457.

Arimizu, N., Inoue, S., Murata, T. and Saegusa, T. (1972). RI diagnosis of malignancy. Bone tumors, *Nihon Rinsho*, **30,** 606–614. (Japanese)

Asada, K. (1976). Oxygen toxicity. *Seikagaku*, **48,** 226–257. (Japanese)

Asakawa, H., Otawa, H., Yamada, H. and Matsumoto, K. (1982). Combination therapy of gastric carcinoma with radiation and chemotherapy. *Tohoku J. Exp. Med.*, **137,** 445–452.

Asoh, S. and Sugai, T. (1987). Topical coenzyme Q_{10} (CQ_{10}) in a patient with radiation ulcers. *Hifu*, **29,** 326–329. (Japanese with an English summary)

Awano, T. and Matsuzawa, T. (1977). Accumulation and biological effects of gallium in malignant cell lines *in vitro. Kakuigaku*, **14,** 73–81. (Japanese)

Baba, T. (1966). Parenchymo-stromal interrelation in the infiltrative growth of malignant tumors. *Gan no Rinsho*, **12,** 438–442. (Japanese)

Baird, P. (1983). Serological evidence for the association of papillomavirus and cervical neoplasia. *Lancet.* **ii,** 17–18.

Baker, T. G. (1971). Comparative aspects of the effects of radiation during oogenesis. *Mutat. Res.*, **11,** 9–22.

Baldwin, E. (1957). *Dynamic Aspects of Biochemistry*, 3rd ed., University Press, Cambridge.

Baserga, (1965). The relationship of the cell cycle to tumor growth and control of cell division: a review. *Cancer Res.*, **25,** 581–595.

Bellanti, J. A. (1971) *Immunology*, Asian ed., Saunders-Igaku Shoin, Tokyo.

Benedict, W. F., Lange, M., Greene, J., Derencseny, A. and Alfi, O. S. (1979). Correlation between prognosis and bone marrow chromosomal patterns in children with acute nonlymphocytic leukemia: Similarities and differences compared to adults. *Blood,*

54, 818–823.

Bennegard K., Eden, E., Ekman, L., Schersten, T. and Lundholm, K. (1982). Metabolic balance across the leg in weightlosing cancer patients compared to depleted patients without cancer. *Cancer Res.,* **42,** 4293–4299.

Berkner, L. V. and Marshall, L. C. (1965). History of major atmospheric components. *Proc. Nat. Acad. Sci., USA,* **53,** 1215–1225.

Bhuyan, B. K., Adams, E. G., Li, L. H., Timmins, L., Badiner, G. J. and Barden, K. (1984). Cytotoxicity and cell cycle effects of prostaglandins (PGS) on human and murine melanoma cells. *Proc. Am. Assoc. Cancer Res.,* **25,** 354. (Abstract)

Bierman, E. L. and Glomset, J. A. (1981). Disorders of lipid metabolism. In: *Textbook of Endocrinology,* 6th ed., ed. by Williams, R. H., Saunders, Philadelphia. pp. 876–906.

Birbeck, M.S.C. and Wheatley, D. N. (1965). An electron microscopic study of the invasion of ascites tumor cells into the abdominal wall. *Cancer Res.,* **25,** 490–492.

Bloom, W. and Fawcett, D. W. (1975). *A Textbook of Histology,* 10th ed., Saunders, Philadelphia.

Bond, V. P., Fliedner, T. M., Cronkite, E. P., Rubini, J. R. and Robertson, T. S. (1959). Cell turnover in blood and blood-forming tissues studied with tritiated thymidine. In: *Kinetics of Cellular Proliferation,* ed. by Stohlman, F. Jr., Grune and Stratton, New York. pp. 188–200.

Bracken, M. B., Brinton, L. A. and Hayashi, K. (1984). Epidemiology of hydatidiform mole and choriocarcinoma. *Epidemiol. Rev.,* **6,** 52–75.

Bradley, T. R., Hodgson, G. S. and Rosendaal, M. (1978). The effect of oxygen tension on haemopoietic and fibroblast cell proliferation *in vitro. J. Cell Phys.,* **97,** 517–522.

Brookes, M. (1971) *The Blood Supply of Bone. An Approach to Bone Biology,* Butterwoths, London.

Buick, R. N. and Pollak, M. N. (1984). Perspectives on clonogenic tumor cells, stem cells, and oncogenes. *Cancer Res.,* **44,** 4909–4918.

Burger, M. M. and Noonan, K. D. (1970). Restoration of normal growth by covering of agglutinin sites on tumor cell surface. *Nature (Lond.),* **228,** 512–515.

Burns, T. W. (1979). Endocrinology. In: *Sodeman's Pathologic Physiology. Mechanisms of Disease,* ed. by Sodeman, W. A. Jr. and Sodeman, T. M., Saunders, Philadelphia. pp. 1002–1058.

Burton, M. A., Gray, B. N. Self, G. W. Heggle, J. C. and Twonsend, P. S. (1985). Manipulation of experimental rat and rabbit liver tumor blood flow with angiotensin II. *Cancer Res.,* **45,** 5390–5393.

Cairns, J. (1975). Mutation selection and the natural history of cancer. *Nature (Lond.)*, **255**, 197–200.

Cairns, J. (1981). The origin of human cancers. *Nature (Lond.)*, **289**, 353–357.

Carswell, E. A., Old, L. J., Kassel, R. L., Green, S., Fiore, N. and Williamson, B. (1975). An endotoxin-induced serum factor that causes necrosis of tumors. *Proc. Nat. Acad. Sci., USA*, **72**, 3666–3670.

Casarett, A. P. (1968). *Radiation Biology*, Prentice-Hall, Englwood-Cliff,New Jersey.

Chapvil, M., Ryan, J. N. and Zukoski, C. F. (1972). The effect on zinc on lipid peroxidation in liver microsomes and mitochondria. *Proc. Soc. Exp. Biol. Med.*, **141**, 150–153.

Chaudhuri, P. K., Thomas, P. A., Walker, M. J., Briele, H. A., Das Gupta, T. K. and Beattie, C. W. (1982). Steroid receptors in human lung cancer cytosols. *Cancer Lett.*, **16**, 327–332.

Chiyoda, S., Mizoguchi, H., Kosaka, K., Takaku, F. and Miura, Y. (1975). Influence of leukaemic cells on the colony formation of human bone marrow cells *in vitro. Br. J. Cancer*, **31**, 355–358.

Cole, M. A., Crawford, D. W., Warner, N. F. and Puffer, H. W. (1972). Correlation of regional disease and *in vivo* PO_2 in rat mammary adenocarcinoma. *Am. J. Pathol.*, **112**, 61–67.

Cooper, E. H., Bedford, A. J. and Kenny, T. E. (1972). Cell death in normal and malignant tissues. *Year Book of Cancer*, pp. 59–119.

Craig, A. B., Jr. and Waterhouse, C. (1957). Body-composition changes in patients with advanced cancer. *Cancer*, **10**, 1106–1109.

Cronkite, E. P. (1967). Extracorporeal irradiation of the blood and lymph in the treatment of leukemia and for immunosuppression. *Ann. Int. Med.*, **67**, 415–423.

Cronkite, E. P. (1974). Radiation injury. In: *Harrison's Principles of Internal Medicine*, 7th ed., ed. Wintrobe, M. M., Thorn, G. W., Adams, R. D., Isselbacher, K. J. and Petersdorf, R. G. Int. Student ed., McGraw-Hill Kogakusha, Tokyo. pp. 712–718.

Damadian, R. (1971). Tumor detection by nuclear magnetic resonance. *Science*, **171**, 1151–1153.

David, J-C., Bassez, T., Bonhomme, M. and Rusquet, R. (1985). Inhibition of DNA ligase from human thymocytes and normal or leukemic lymphocytes by antileukemic drugs. *Cancer Res.*, **45**, 2177–2183.

Debiec-Rychter, M., Kaluzewski, B., Zajackzkowska, D. and Pokuszynska, K. (1982). Mosaicism 48, XX, $+8$, $+21/47$, XX, $+21$ in Down syndrome and rapid progression from preleukaemia to acute leukaemia. *Lancet*, **ii**, 448–449.

Denekampf, J., Hill, S. A. and Hobson, B. (1983). Vascular occlusion and tumor cell death. *Eur. J. Cancer Clin. Oncol.*, **19**, 271–275.

Dillman, R. O. and Koziol, J. A. (1983). Statistical approach to immunosuppression: classification using lymphocyte surface markers and functional assays. *Cancer Res.*, **43**, 417–421.

Donner, P., Greiser-Wilke, I. and Moelling, K. (1982). Nuclear localization and DNA binding of the transforming gene product of avian myelocytomatosis virus. *Nature (Lond.)*, **296**, 262–266.

Dosik, H., Hsu, L. Y., Todaro, G. J., Lee, S. L., Hirschhorn, K., Seliro, E. S. and Alter, A. A. (1970). Leukemia in Fanconi's anemia: Cytogenetic and tumor virus susceptibility studies. *Blood*, **36**, 341–352.

Edmonds, D. K., Lindsay, K. S., Miller, J. F., Williamson, E. and Wood, P. J. (1982). Early embryonic mortality in women. *Fertil. Steril.*, **38**, 447–453.

Edwards, C. L. and Hayes, R. L. (1969). Tumor scanning with 67 Ga citrate. *J. Nucl. Med.*, **10**, 103–105.

El-Hefnawi, H., El-Hefnawi, M. and Rashed, A. (1962). Xeroderma pigmentosum. I: A clinical study of 12 Egyptian cases. *Br. J. Dermatol.*, **74**, 201–213.

Everson, T. C. and Cole, W. H. (1966). *Spontaneous Regression of Cancer. A study and abstract of reports in the world medical literature and of personal communications concerning spontaneous regression of malignant disease.*, Saunders, Philadelphia.

Farr, L. E., Sweet, W. H., Robertson, J. S., Foster, C. G., Locksley, H. B., Sutherland, D. L., Mendesohn, M. L. and Stickley, E. E. (1954). Neutron capture therapy with boron in the treatment of glioblastoma multiforme. *Am. J. Roentgenol. Rad. Ther.*, **71**, 279–293.

Fauci, A. S. and Dale, D. C. (1975). The effect of hydrocortisone on the kinetics of normal human lymphocytes. *Blood*, **46**, 235–243.

Fett, J. W., Strydom, D. J., Lobb, R. R., Alderman, E. M., Bethune, J. L., Riodan, J. R. and Vallee, B. L. (1985). Isolation and characterization of angiogenin, an angiogenic protein from human carcinoma cells. *Biochemistry*, **24**, 5480–5486.

Fibach, E., Hayashi, M. and Sachs, L. (1973). Control of normal differentiation of myeloid leukemic cells to macrophages and granulocytes. *Proc. Nat. Acad. Sci., USA*, **70**, 343–346.

Fibach, E., Landau, T. and Sachs, L. (1972). Normal differentiation of myeloid leukaemic cells induced by a differentiation-inducing protein. *Nature: New Biology*, **237**, 276–278.

Fingerhut, B. and Veenema, R. J. (1977). An animal model for the study of prostatic adenocarcinoma. *Invest. Urol.*, **15**, 42–48.

Fitzpatrick, F. A. and Stringfellow, D. A. (1979). Prostaglandin D_2 formation by malignant melanoma cells correlates inversely with cellular metastatic potential. *Proc. Nat. Acad. Sci., USA*, **76**,

232   REFERENCES

1765–1769.

Fletcher, G. H. (1973). *Textbook of Radiotherapy*, 2nd ed., Lea and Febiger, Philadelphia.

Fletcher, J. W., Herbig, F. K. and Donati, R. M. (1975). ^{67}Ga citrate distribution following whole-body irradiation or chemotherapy. *Radiology*, **117**, 709–712.

Folkman, J., Merler, E., Abernathy, C. and Williams, G.(1971). Isolation of a tumor factor responsible for angiogenesis. *J. Exp. Med.*, **133**, 275–288.

Fujii, S. and Okuda, H. (1979). Studies on toxohormone. In: *Progress in Cancer Biochemistry. In memory of Dr. Nakahara, Gann Monogr. on Cancer Res.*, 24, Jpn. Sci. Soc., Tokyo, pp. 215–222.

Fujimura, T., Katano, M., Sakata, M. and Torisu, M. (1983). New clinical management of malignant ascites: The mechanism of neutrophil accumulation in ascitic fluid. *Fed. Proc.*, **42**, 680. (Absract)

Fujita, S. (1983). Natural history of human gastric carcinomas in terms of their genesis and progression. *Asian Med. J.*, **26**, 787–805.

Fukuda, H., Matsuzawa, T., Abe, Y., Endo, S., Yamada, K., Kubota, K., Hatazawa, J., Sato, T., Ito, M., Takahashi, T., Iwata, R. and Ido, T. (1982) Experimental study for cancer diagnosis with positron-labeled fluorinated glucose analogs: (^{18}F)-2–fluoro-2-deoxy-D–mannose: A new tracer for cancer detection. *Eur. J. nucl. Med.*, **7**, 294–297.

Fukuda, H., Matsuzawa, T., Tada, M., Takahashi, T., Ishiwata, K., Yamada, K., Abe, Y., Yoshioka, S., Sato, T. and Ido, T. (1986). 2–Deoxy-2(^{18}F) fluoro–D–galactose: A new tracer for the measurement of galactose metabolism in the liver by positron emission tomography. *Eur. J. nucl. Med.*, **11**, 444–448.

Fukushi, K. (1983). To strike cancers with Salmonellae. *J. Tohoku Soc. Microbiol.*, **24**, 25–27. (Japanese)

Fukushi, K., Kamiya, S., Asano, H., Sasaki, J., Nishikawa, Y. and Katori, T. (1986). Tumor regression induced by synthetic cord factor analogues combined with endotoxin. *Immunochemotherapy of Cancer*, ed. by Tohno, S., Yoshida, Y., Fukushi, M., Fukushima, M., Kudo, H., Sato K. and Yokoyama, M. Hirosaki Univ. Sch. Med., Hirosaki, pp. 15–26.

Fukushima, M., Kato, T., Ueda, R., Ota, K., Narumiya, S. and Hayaishi, O. (1982). Prostaglandin D$_2$, a potential antineoplastic agent. *Biochim. Biphys. Res. Commun.*, **105**, 956–964.

Furue, H. (1987). Biological characteristic and clinical effect of sizofilan (SPG). *Drugs of Today*, **23**, 335–346.

Gallo, R. C., Saxinger, W. C., Gallagher, R. E., Gillespie, D. H., Aulakh, G. S. and Won-Staal, F. (1977). Some ideas on the origin of leukemia in man and recent evidence for the presence of type C viral related information. In: *Origin of Human Cancer*, ed. by Hiatt, H. H., Watson, J. D. and Winsten, J. A. Cold Spring Harbor Lab., Univ. of Tokyo Press, Tokyo, pp. 1253–1285.

Gatti, R. A. and Good, R. A. (1971). Occurrence of malignancy in immunodeficiency diseases. A literature review. *Cancer*, **28**, 89–98.

Generoso, W. M., Cain, K. T., Krishna, M. and Huff, S. W. (1979). Genetic lesions induced by chemicals in spermatozoa and spermatids of mice are repaired in the egg. *Proc. Nat. Acad. Sci., USA*, **76**, 435–437.

German, J., Bloom, D. and Passarge, E. (1977). Bloom's syndrome. V. Surveillance for cancer in affected families. *Clin. Genet.*, **12**, 162–168.

Gibson, N. W., Zlotogorski, C. and Erickson, L. C. (1985). Specific DNA interstrand crosslinking by chlorethylnitrosoureas but not from crosslinking by other anti-tumor alkylating agents. *Carcinogenesis*, **6**, 445–450.

Goldman, J. M. (1986). The chronic myeloid leukemias. In: *Comprehensive Textbook of Oncology*, ed. by Moosa, A. R., Robson, M. C., Schimpf, S. C. Williams and Wilkins, Baltimore, pp. 541–546.

Gold, J. (1968). Proposed treatment of cancer by inhibition of gluconeogenesis. *Oncology*, **22**, 185–207.

Goldstein, A., Aronow, L. and Kalman, S. M. (1974). *Principles of Drug Action: The Basis of Pharmacology*, Wiley, New York, pp. 227-300.

Golub, E. S. (1987). *Immunology: A synthesis*, Sinauer, Sunderland, Mass.

Good, R. A. (1971). Disorders of the immune system. *Immunobiology. Current Knowledge of Basic Concepts in Immunology and Their Clinical Applications*, ed. by Good, R. A. and Fisher, Y.D.W. Sinauer, Stamford, pp. 3–16.

Good, R. A., Petersen, R.D.A., Finstad, J. and Gabrielsen, A. E. (1965). Morphologic studies of the development of the lymphoid tissues. *Ser. Haemat.*, **8**, 1–28.

Goodman, L. S. and Gilman, A. (1975). *The Pharmacological Basis of Therapeutics*, 4th ed., Macmillan, New York. pp. 1248–1307.

Goseki, N., Onodera, T., Kasaki, G., Tsuruta, K., Mori, S. and Tsukada, K. (1984). Methionine- and cystine-free amino acid imbalance by total parenteral nutrition as an adjunct to cancer chemotherapy. In: *Parenteral and Enteral Hyper-Alimentation*, ed. by Ogoshi, S., and Okada, A. Elsevier Sci., Tokyo, pp. 343–355.

Goseki, N., Onodera, T., Koike, M. and Kosaki, G. (1987). Inhibitory effect of L-methionine-deprived amino acid imbalance using total parenteral nutrition on growth of ascites hepatoma in rats. *Tohoku J. Exp. Med.*, **151**, 191–200.

Grisham, M. B., Bernstein, L. H. and Everse, J. (1983). The cytoplasmic maleate dehydrogenase in neoplastic tissues; Presence for a novel isozyme? *Br. J. Cancer*, **47**, 727–731.

Gruffs, B., Rogers, W. and Cameron, I. (1979). Total parenteral nutrition and inhibition of gluconeogenesis on tumor-host responses. *Oncology*, **36**, 216–223.

Hagemeijer, A., Haehlen, K. and Abels, J. (1981). Cytogenetic follow-up of patients with nonlymphocytic leukemia. II. Acute nonlymphocytic leukemia. *Cancer Genet. Cytogenet.*, **3**, 109–124.

Hamilton, W. J., Boyd, J. D. and Mossman, H. W. (1959). *Human Embryology (Prenatal Development of Form and Function)*, Heffer, Cambridge.

Hamuro, J. and Chihara, G. (1984). Lentinan, a T–cell–oriented immunostimulator. Its experimental and clinical applications and possible mechanism of immune modulation. In: *Immune Modulation Agents and Their Mechanisms*, ed. by Feinchel, R. L. and Chirigas, M. A. Marcel Dekker, New York, pp. 409–435.

Hanafusa, H., Halpern, C. C., Buchanan, D. L. and Kawai, S. (1977). Recovery of avian sarcoma virus from tumors induced by transformation-defective mutants. *J. Exp. Med.*, **146**, 1735–1747.

Harada, Y. (1973). Studies on the blood flow in brain tumors. *Nippon Acta Radiol.*, **33**, 740–756.

Harris, G. and Lawley, P. D. (1985). Defective DNA repair in RA families. Evidence for a possible environmental factor. *Br. J. Cancer*, **51**, 607–608. (Abstract)

Harrison, M. W. (1975). Apoptosis in rapidly proliferating normal cell populations. Thesis presented for degree of Bachelor of Medical Science, Univ. Queensland, as cited in: Kerr and Searle (1980)

Hashizume, T., Maruyama, T., Nishikawa, K. and Nishimura, A. (1974). Estimation of absorbed dose in thyroids and gonads of survivors in Hiroshima and Nagasaki. *Acta Radiol.*, **13**, 411–424.

Hauschka, T. S. (1961). The chromosomes in ontogeny and oncogeny. *Cancer Res.*, **21**, 957–974.

Hayashi, I. and Konno, K. (1983). Local therapeutic effect of aclacinomycin against carcinomatous pleurisy and pericarditis. In: *Proc. 13th Int. Congr. Chemother.*, Vienna, Aug. 28–Sep. 2, 1983. Tom **16**. pp. 260/32–33.

Heaton, D. C., Fitzgerald, P. H., Jan Fraser, G. and Abbott. G. D. (1981). Transient leukemoid proliferation of the cytogenetically unbalanced +21 cell line of a constitutional mosaic boy. *Blood*, **57**, 883–887.

Hellstein, S., Axelsson, B. and Eksborg, S. (1983). Absorption of adriamycin after intravesical administration. Experimental studies in the rat. In: *Proc. 13th Int. Congr. Chemother.*, Vienna,

Aug. 28–Sep. **2**, 1983. Tom **16**, pp. 285/5-7.

Hersey, P., Edwards, A., Lewis, R., Kemp, A. and Mcinnes, J. (1982). Deficent natural killer activity in a patient with Fanconi's anemia and squamous cell carcinoma. Association with defect in interferon release. *Clini. Exp. Immunol.*, **48**, 205–212.

Higashi, T., Wako, H., Yamaguchi, M. and Suga, K. (1988). The relationship between Ga-67 accumulation and cell cycle in malignant tumor cells in vitro. *Eur. J. nucl. Med.*, **14**, 153–158.

Himori, T., Ohnuma, T. and Wakui, A. (1983). Chemotherapeutic susceptibility of human CFU-c and established human acute myelogenous leukemia cells (HL-60) in culture. *Gan to Kagaku Ryoho*, **10**, 1170–1178. (Japanese with an English summary)

Hirayama, T. (1986). Personal communication.

Hisada, K., Hiraki, T., Mishima, T., Watanabe, R., Yokoyama, K., Kato, S. and Wakabayashi, T. (1968). Tumor scanning with ^{131}I-human fibrinogen. *J. Nucl. Med.*, **9**, 324. (Abstract)

Hochachka, P. W. (1980). *Living without Oxygen. Closed and open systems in hypoxia tolerance*, Harvard Univ. Press, Cambridge, Mass.

Holrodye, C. P., Gabuzda, T. G., Putnam, R. C., Paul, P. and Reichard, G. A. (1979). Altered glucose metabolism in metastatic carcinoma. *Cancer Res.*, **35**, 3710–3714.

Hood, L. E., Weissman, I. L. and Wood, W. B. (1978). *Immunology*, Benjamin/Cummings, Menlo Park, Calif.

Horowitz, N. H. (1945). On the evolution of biochemical synthesis. *Proc. Nat. Acad. Sci.*, *USA*, **31**, 153–155.

Housset, M., Daniel, M. T. and Degos, L. (1982). Small doses of ARA-C in the treatment of acute myeloid leukaemia: differentiation of myeloid leukaemia cells? *Br. J. Haemat.*, **51**, 125–129.

Huret, J. L., Tanzer, J. and Henry-Amar, M. (1986). Aberrant breakpoints in chronic myelogenous luekemia; oncogenes and fragile sites. *Hum. Genet.*, **74**, 447–448.

Ibrahin, G. A., Zweker, B. A. and Theologides, A. (1981). Remote tumor effects on lactic dehydrogenase of mouse muscle fibers with different glycolytic oxidative metabolic potentials. *Proc. Soc. Exp. Biol. Med.*, **168**, 119–122.

Ichikawa, Y. (1969). Differentiation of a cell line of myeloid leukemia. *J. Cell Physiol.*, **74**, 223–234.

Ichimaru, M., Ohkita, T. and Ishimaru, T. (1986). Leukemia, multiple myeloma, and malignant lymphoma. In: *Cancer in Atomic Bomb Survivors*, ed. by Shigematsu, I. and Kagan, A. Jpn. Cancer Assoc. *Gann Monogr. on Cancer Res.*, Jpn. Sci. Soc., Tokyo, **32**, 113–127.

Ichimura, O., Suzuki, S., Sugawara, Y. and Osawa, T. (1983). Lymphokines induction by streptococcal preparation OK–432 (Picibanil) in mice: Characterization of interleukin 1 (IL–1), interleukin 2 (IL-2) and natural killer cell activating factor (NKAF). *OK-432. Proc. Int. Symposium, 13th Int. Congr. Chemother.*, Vienna, Aug. 28–Sep. 2, 1983. Tom **17**. pp. 287/19–22.

Ido, T. (1986). Personal communication.

Iizuka, S., Taniguchi, N. and Makita, A. (1984). Enzyme-linked immunoadsorbent assay for human manganese-containing superoxide dismutase and its content in lung cancer. *J. Nat. Cancer Inst.*, **72**, 1043–1049.

Ikeda, T., Hayashi, I., Matsuo, T., Maeda, H. and Shimokawa, I. (1986). The cancer registry in Nagasaki City, with atomic bomb survivor data, 1973–1977. In: *Cancer in Atomic Bomb Survivors*, ed. by Shigematsu, I. and Kagan, A. Jpn. Cancer Assoc. Gann Monogr. **32**, 41–52.

Ipsen, J. and Feigl, P. (1970). Comparison of rate tables. In: *Bancroft's Introduction to Biostatics*, 2nd ed., Harper and Row, New York, pp. 130–141.

Ishikawa, T., Sato, H., Isono, Y., Onoda, S. and Koide, Y. (1979). Experience of use of bestatin on patients with esophageal cancers. 2nd report. *Bestatin Kenkyukaishi*, **3**, 66–69. (Japanese)

Ishimaru, Y., Kurano, R. and Hayashi, H. (1980). A cell surface-associated adhesive glycoprotein from cancer cell. *Cancer Cell Biology*, ed. by Nagao, T. and Mori, W. *Jpn. Cancer Assoc. Gann Monogr. on Cancer Res.*, Jpn. Sci. Soc., **25**, 9–27.

Ishiwata, K., Ido, T., Abe, Y., Matsuzawa, T. and Iwata, R. (1988). Tumor uptake studies of S-adenosyl-L(methyl-^{11}C) methionine and L-(methyl-^{11}C) methionine. *Nucl. Med. Biol.*, **15**, 123–126.

Israel, L. (1982). Results of continuous bleomycin and cisplatinum in squamous cell carcinoma of the lung. In: *Proc. 3rd Bleomycin Conference*, Tokyo, May 19, 1982, pp. 29–46.

Israel, L., Penot, J. C., Aguilera, J., Breau, J. L., Soudant, J. and Morer, J. F. (1983) Bleomycin and *cis*-platinum with or without mitomycin C in 110 previously untreated patients with head and neck cancer. *Am. J. Clin. Oncol.*, **5**, 305–311.

Ito, Y., Okuyama, S., Awano, T., Takahashi, K., Sato, T. and Kanno, I. (1971). Diagnostic evaluation of ^{67}Ga scanning of lung cancer and other diseases. *Radiology*, **101**, 355–362.

Ito, Y. and Muranaka, A. (1982). Factors influencing the localization of radiotracers in tumors. In: *General Processes of Radiotracer Localization*, Vol. I, ed. by Anghileril, L. J. CRC Press, Boca Raton, Florida, pp. 95–151.

Itoga, T. (1967). Hematological diseases. b) General aspects of leukemia. *Hiroshima Igaku*, 20 (Suppl.): Proc. Res. Soc. for the Late Effects of the Atomic Bombs, 7th Mtg, Hiroshima, Oct. 16–17, 1965, pp. 40–42.

Iwama, N. and Takahashi, T. (1983). Histological reconstruction of colonic adenoma and adenocarcinoma. 81st Conference of the

Research Institute for Tuberculosis and Cancer, Tohoku Univ., Sendai, Dec. 1983.

Izakovic, V., Strbbakova, E., Kaiserova, E. and Krizan, P. (1985). Bovine superoxide dismutase in Fanconi anaemia. Therapeutic trial in two patients. *Hum. Genet.*, **70**, 181–182.

Joenje, H., Frants, R. R., Arwort, F., de Bruin, G.J.M., Koslense, P. J., van de Kamp, J.J.P., de Koning, J. and Eriksson, A. W. (1979). Erythrocyte superoxide dismutase deficiency in Fanconi's anemia established by two independent methods of assay. *Scand. J. Clin. Lab. Invest.*, **39**, 759–764.

Johansson, J., Cederlung, E., Moodbidri, S. B., Sheth, A. and Jorvall, H. (1986). Superoxide dismutase in human testis preparations. *Biosci. Rep.*, 6, 535–541.

Jong, E. C. and Klebanoff, S.J. (1980). Eosinophil-mediated mammalian tumor cell cytotoxicity: Role of the peroxidase system. *J. Immunol.*, **124**, 1949–1953.

Joyce, R. M. and Vincent, P.C. (1983). Advantage of reduced oxygen tension in growth of human melanomas in semi-solid cultures: Quantitative analysis. *Br. J. Cancer*, **48**, 385–393.

Kan, M. and Yamane, I. (1983). Oxygen-dependent growth declining and effect of vitamin E for human diploid fibroblasts in serum-free, BSA-containing culture. *Tohoku J. Exp. Med.*, **139**, 389–398.

Kaneko, Y., Rowley, J. D., Mauer, H. S., Varakajis, D. and Moohr, J. W. (1982). Chromosome pattern in childhood acute nonlymphocytic leukemia. *Blood*, **60**, 389–399.

Kaplan, M. H., Susin, M., Pahwa, S. G., Fetten, J., Allen, S. L., Lichtman, S., Sarngadharan, M. G. and Gallo, R. C. (1987). Neoplastic complications of HTLV–III infection. Lymphomas and solid tumors. *Am. J. Med.*, **82**, 389–396.

Kasai, H. Crain, P. F., Kuchino, Y., Nishimura, S., Ootsuyama, A. and Tonooka, H. (1986). Formation of 8–hydroxyguanine in cellular DNA by agents producing oxygen radicals, radiation and H2O2. *Proc. Jpn. Cancer Assoc.*, 45th Ann. Mtg. Sapporo, Oct. 1986, p. 34 (Abstract)

Kato, H. (1986). Cancer mortality. In: *Cancer in Atomic Bomb Survivors*, ed. by Shigematsu, I. and Kagan, A. Jpn. Cancer Assoc. Gann Monogr. on Cancer Res., Jpn. Sci. Soc., Tokyo, **32**, 53–74.

Kawai, S., Duesber, P. H. and Hanafusa, H. (1977). Transformation-defective mutants of RSV with src gene deletions of varying lengths. *J. Virol.*, **24**, 910–914.

Kawamura, M. and Koshihara, Y. (1984). Prostaglandin D_2 lowers nuclear DNA polymerase activity in cultured mastocytoma cells. *Prostaglandins*, **27**, 517–524.

Kerr, J.F.R. and Searle, J. (1980). Apoptosis: Its nature and kinetic role. In: *Radiation Biology in Cancer Research*, ed. by Meyn, R. E. and Withers, H. R. Raven Press, New York. pp. 367–384.

Kersey, J. H., Spector, B. D. and Good, R. A. (1973). Primary immunodeficiency diseases and cancer: The immunodeficiency-cancer registry. *Int. J. Cancer*, **12**, 333–347.

Kersey, J. H., Spector, B. D. and Good, R. A. (1974). Cancer in children with primary immunodeficiency diseases. *J. Pediat.*, **84**, 263–264.

Kimball, R. E., Reddy, K., Pierce, T. H., Schwartz, L. W., Mustafa, M. G. and Cross, C. E. (1976). Oxygen toxicity: augmentation of anti-oxidation defense mechanisms in rat lung. *Am. J. Physiol.*, **230**, 1425–1431.

Klatzman, D., Cavaille-Coll, M., Brunet, J. B., Rozenbaum, W., Kernbaum, S., Barre-Sinoussi, F., Chermann, J. C., Montagnier, L. and Gluckman, J. C. (1984). Immune status of AIDS patients in France: Relationship with lymphadenopathy associated virus tropism. *Ann. New York Acad. Sci.*, 437: *Acquired Immune Deficiency Syndrome*, 228–237.

Klein, G. and Klein, E. (1985). Evolution of tumours and the impact of molecular oncology. *Nature (Lond.)*, **315**, 190–195.

Klein, G. (1987). The approaching era of the tumor suppressor genes. *Science*, **238**, 1539–1545.

Kobayashi, H. (1975). *Kiso Seibutsugaku Kouza 5. Naibunpitsu Gensho*, ed. by Honjo, I., Ishida, J. Kimura, Y. and Sato, J. Shokabo, Tokyo. (Japanese)

Kobayashi, H. (1980). Evolution of the metabolic endocrine system: Its phylogenetic significance. In: *Hormones, Adaptation and Evolution*, ed. by Ishii, S., Hirano, T. and Wada, M. Jpn. Sci. Soc. Press, Tokyo, pp. 15–21.

Kobayashi, M. (1986). Experimental study on Ga–67 uptake and ATP metabolism in cultured tumor cells. *Kanagawa Shigaku*, **20**, 439–448. (Japanese)

Kohne, D. E. (1970). Evolution of high-organism DNA. *Quart. Rev. Biophys.*, **3**, 327–375.

Komuro, Y., Yoshida, S., Homma, T., Yoneda, S. and Ebihara, Y. (1982). Histological studies on changes of rabbit pleura induced by immunostimulants and anticancer agents with immunostimulants. *Haigan*, **22**, 389–395. (Japanese)

Kondo, K., Shimizu, T. and Hayaishi, O. (1981). Effects of prostaglandin D_2 on membrane potential in neuroblastoma x glioma hybrid cells as determined with a cyanine dye. *Biochem. Biophys. Res. Commun.*, **98**, 648–655.

Kondo, S. (1973). *Molecular Radiation Biology*, Univ. of Tokyo Press, Tokyo. (Japanese)

Kraemer, K. H., Lee, M. M. and Scotto, J. (1984). DNA repair protects against cutaneous and internal neoplasia: evidence from xeroderma pigmentosum. *Carcinogenesis*, **5**, 511–514.

Krishan, A. (1973). Bleomycin-induced fine structural alterations in cultured mouse fibroblasts and human lymphocytes of neoplastic origin. *Cancer Res.*, **33**, 777–785.

Kroon, A. M. and van den Bogert, C. (1985). The mitochondrial genome as a target for chemotherapy of cancer. In: *Achievements and Perspectives of Mitochondrial Research*, Vol. II: *Biogenesis*, ed. by Quagliariello, E. *et al.*, Elsevier, Amsterdam, pp. 21–33.

Kubota, K., Yamaguchi, T., Abe, Y., Fujiwara, T., Hatazawa, J. and Matsuzawa, T. (1983). Effects of smoking on regional cerebral blood flow in neurologically normal subjects. *Stroke*, **4**, 720–724.

Kubota, K., Yamada, K., Fukuda, H., Endo, S., Ito, M., Abe, Y., Yamaguchi, K., Fujiwara, T., Sato, T., Ito, K., Yoshioka, S., Hatazawa, J., Matsuzawa, T., Iwata, R. and Ido, T. (1984). Tumor detection with carbon–11–labeled amino acids. *Eur. J. Nucl. Med.*, **9**, 136–140.

Kubota, K., Ishiwata, K., Fujiwara, T., Sato, T., Kubota, R. and Matsuzawa, T. (1988). Development of metabolic cancer diagnosis with positron emission tomography. II. Radiotherapeutic effects on the tumor uptake of ^{11}C-L-methionine. *Proc. Jpn. Cancer Assoc.*, 47th Ann. Mtg., Tokyo, Sep. 1988, p. 380. (Abstract)

Kudo, T., Abo, S., Itabashi, T., Onodera, K., Shikama, T., Hashimoto, M., Kawamura, Y., Tsuji, K., Watanabe, K., Ikeda, T. and Izumi, I. (1985). Enhancing activity of bacterial preparation on blood flow in tumor tissue, with reference to cancer chemotherapy.—Experimental and clinical studies—. *Gan to Kagaku Ryoho*, **12**, 2166–2171. (Japanese)

Kumagai, K. (1985). Novel development of NK cell sciences. In: *Macrophages and Their Surroundings.—Differentiation, Mobilization, and Versatility of Their Function and Regulation—*, ed. by Kojima, M., Saito., K. and Hanaoka, M. Yodosha, Tokyo, pp. 342–357. (Japanese)

Kumano, N., Suzuki, S., Oizumi, K., Konno, K., Himori, T., Mitachi, T. and Wakui, A. (1985). Imbalance of T cell subsets in cancer patients and its modification with bestatin, a small molecular immunomodulator.*Tohoku J. Exp. Med.*, **147**, 125–133.

Kurachi, K., Davie, E. W., Strydom, D.J., Riodan, J. F. and Vallee, B. L. (1985). Sequence of the cDNA and gene for angiogenin, human angiogenesis factor. *Biochemistry*, **24**, 5494–5499.

Kuroki, T. (1981). Induction by cholera toxin of synchronous divisions *in vivo* epidermis resulting in hyperplasia. *Proc. Nat. Acad. Sci., USA*, **78**, 6958–6962.

Kuroki, T., Ito, T., Hosomi, J., Munakata, K., Uchida, T. and Nagai, Y. (1982). Cyclic AMP as a mitotic signal for epidermal keratocytes, but not for dermal fibroblasts. *Cell Struct. Funct.*, **7**,

295–305.

Land, H., Parada, L.F. and Weinberg, R. A. (1983a). Cellular oncogenes and multistep carcinogenesis. *Science*, **222**, 771–778.

Land, H., Parada, L. F. and Weinberg, R. A. (1983b). Tumorigenic conversion of primary embryo fibroblasts requires at least two cooperative oncogenes. *Nature (Lond.)*, **304**, 596–602.

Langer, R., Conn, H., Vacanti, J., Haudenschild, C. and Folkman, J. (1980). Control of tumor growth in animals by infusion of an angiogenesis inhibitor. *Proc. Nat. Acad. Sci., USA*, **77**, 4331–4335.

Laurence, J., Gottlieb, A. B. and Kunkel, H. G. (1984). Soluble factors inhibitory for T–cell–dependent immune responses in patients with the acquired immune deficiency syndrome and its prodromes. *Ann. New York Acad. Sci.*, **437**: *Acquired Immune Deficiency Syndrome*, pp. 518–525.

Lawley, P. D. and Brookes, P. (1965). Molecular mechanisms of the cytotoxic action of difunctional alkylating agents and of resistance to this action. *Nature (Lond.)*, **206**, 480–483.

Lennox, B. and Lennox, M. E. (1986). *Heinemann Medical Dictionary*, Heinemann Medical, London.

Leuthauser, S.W.C., Oberley, L. W., Oberley, T. D. and Loven, D. P. (1984). Lowered superoxide dismutase activity in distant organs of tumor-bearing mice. *J. Nat. Cancer Inst.*, **72**, 1065–1074.

Lindmark, L., Bennegard, K., Eden, D., Ekman, L., Schersten, T., Svaniger, G. and Lundholm, K. (1984). Resting energy expenditure in malnourished patients with and without cancer. *Gastroenterology*, **87**, 402–408.

Liotta, L. (1986). Induction of the metastatic phenotype by DNA transfection. Abbott–UCLS Symposium: Cellular and Molecular Biology of Tumors and Potential Clinical Applications, Steamboat Springs, Co., Jpn. 20–25, 1986.

Lipkin, M., Sherlock, P. and Bell, B.M. (1959). Generation time of epithelial cells in the human colon. *Nature (Lond.)*, **195**, 175–177.

Little, C. and Longo, D. L. (1986). Non-Hodgkin's lymphomas: Epidemiology, etiology, pathology, natural history, and disease evolution. In: *Comprehensive Textbook of Oncology*, ed. by Moosa, A. R., Robson, M. C. and Schimpff, S. C. Williams and Wilkins, Baltimore, pp. 574–580.

Loven, D. P., Guernsey, B. L. and Oberley, L. W. (1984). Transformation affects superoxide dismutase activity. *Int. J. Cancer*, **33**, 783–786.

Lundholm, K., Edstrom, S., Ekman, L., Karlberg, I., Walker, P. and Schersten, T. (1981). Protein degradation in human skeletal muscle tissue: the effect of insulin, leucine, amino acids and ions. *Clin. Sci.*, **60**, 319–326.

Lundholm, K., Edstrom, S., Karlberg, I., Ekman, L. and Schersten, T. (1982). Glucose turnover, gluconeogenesis from glycerol, and estimation of net glucose cycling in cancer patients. *Cancer*, **50,** 1142–1150.

Maki, T., Yoshida, K., Koizumi, A. and Takahashi, T. (1963a). Recurrence due to intraluminally exfoliated gastric cancer cells. *Tohoku J. Exp. Med.*, **79,** 309–318.

Maki, T., Majima, S., Yoshida, K. and Takahashi, T. (1963b). Cancer cell dissemination during surgical manipulation. *Tohoku J. Exp. Med.*, **79,** 319–333.

Makinodan, T. (1977). Immunity and aging. In: *Handbook of the Biology of Aging*, ed. by Finch C. E. and Hayflick, L. van Nostrand Reinhold, New York, pp. 379–408.

Margulis, L. (1981). *Symbiosis in Cell Evolution*, Freeman, San Francisco.

Maruyama, T. (1986). Atomic bomb dosimetry for epidemiological studies of survivors in Hiroshima and Nagasaki. In: *Cancer in Atomic Bomb Survivors*, ed. by Shigematsu, I. and Kagan, A. Jpn. Cancer Assoc. *Gann Monogr. on Cancer Res.*, Jpn. Sci. Soc., Tokyo, **32,** 9–28.

Masaoka, T. and Inoue, T. (1986). Indication and results of bone marrow transplantation for acute leukemia. *Gan to Kagaku Ryoho*, **13,** 1811–1815. (Japanese)

Mathé, G., Amel, J. L., Schwartzenberg, L., Schneider, M., Cattan, A., Schlumberger, J. R. and De Vassal, F. (1969). Active immunotherapy for acute lymphoblastic leukaemia. *Lancet*, **i,** 697–699.

Mattern, J., Klinga, K., Runnebaum, B. and Volm, M. (1985). Influence of hormone therapy on human lung tumors transplanted into nude mice. *Oncology*, **42,** 388–390.

Matthews, R.E.F. (1983). The origin of viruses from cells. *Aspects of Cell Regulation*, ed. by Daniellie, J. F. Academic Press, New York. pp. 245–280.

Matsubara, S., Suzuki, M., Nakamura, M., Edo, K. and Ishida, N. (1980). Isolation of an inhibitor of type II interferon induction from tumor ascitic fluids. *Cancer Res.*, **40,** 2534–2538.

Matsuya, Y., Kusano, T., Endo, S., Takahashi, N. and Yamane, I. (1978). Reduced tumorigenicity by addition *in vitro* of Sendai virus. *Eur. J. Cancer*, **14,** 837–850.

Matsuzawa, T., Okuyama, S., Awano, T. and Takazawa, K. (1976). Combined effects of X-ray and bleomycin in cancer cell survival. *Panminerv. Med.*, 18, 103–104.

Matsuzawa, T., Onozawa, M., Morita, K. and Kakehi, M. (1972). Radiosensitization of bleomycin on lethal effect of mouse cancer cell *in vitro*. *Strahlenther.*, **144,** 614–617.

Matsuzawa, T. (1981). The attempt for changing cancer cell to normal terminal cell. *Gan-to-Kagaku Ryoho*, **8**, 47–53. (Japanese with an English summary)

Mehard, C. W., Packer, L. and Abraham, S. (1971). Activity and ultrastructure of mitochondria from mouse mammary gland and mammary adenocarcinoma. *Cancer Res.*, **31**, 2148–2160.

Metzler, D. E. (1977). *Biochemistry. The chemical reactions of living cells*, Int. ed., Academic Press, New York.

Minna, J. D. and Bunn, Jr., P. A. (1982). Paraneoplastic syndromes. In: *Cancer. Principles and Practice of Oncology*, ed. by DeVita, Jr. V. T., Hellman S. and Rosenberg, S. A. Lippincott, Philadelphia. pp. 1476–1517.

Mishina, H., Hariu, T., Shiojima, S., Imaizumi, A. and Sato, T. (1977). Hyperbaric oxygen therapy of roentgen ulcers. *Yakuri to Chiryo*, **5**, 1437–1442. (Japanese)

Mishina, H., Okuyama, S., Lin, I.S., Yamagata, R., Taima, T., Ogasawara, T. and Yamamoto, K. (1982) Esophageal cancer treated by low dose irradiation, crescendo cisplatin and bleomycin polyacrylate pasta. *Sci. Rep. Res. Inst. Tohoku Univ.-C*, **29**, 9–16.

Mishina, H., Okuyama, S., Yuasa, R., Saijo, S. and Kaneko, Y. (1985). Radiochemotherapy of head and neck cancers: Dose reduction through the combination of cisplatin, bleomycin and tegafur. *Gan to Kagaku Ryoho*, **12**, 947–950. (Japanese)

Mishina, H. and Okuyama, S. (1987a). Picibanil inhalation therapy for reinforcement of anti-cancer immunity. In: *Proc. 15th Int. Congr. Chemother.*, Istanbul, July 19–24, 1987, p. 254.

Mishina, H. and Okuyama, S. (1987b). Principia of cancer therapy. XIX. Effects of per rectum carmofur on radiotherapeutic efficacy of rectal carcinomas. *Sci. Rep. Res. Inst. Tohoku Univ.-C*, **34**, 1–5.

Mishina, H., Okuyama, S. and Kimura, H. (1989). Picibanil may expedite exfoliation of cancer cells. *Tohoku J. Exp. Med.* (submitted).

Mitelman, F. (1985). *Catalog of Chromosome Aberrations in Cancer*, Liss, New York.

Möller, G. and Möller, E. (1978). Immunologic surveillance against neoplasia. In: *Immunological Aspects of Cancer*, ed. by Castro, J. E. Univ. Park Press, Baltimore, pp. 205–217.

Montesano, R., Becker, R., Hall, J., Likhachev, A., Lu, S. H., Umbenhauer, D. and Wild, C. P. (1985). Repair of DNA alkylating adducts in mammalian cells. *Biochemie*, **67**, 919–928.

Monzen, T. and Wakabayashi, T. (1986). Tumor and tissue registries in Hiroshima and Nagasaki. In: *Cancer in Atomic Bomb Survivors*, ed. by Shigematsu, I. and Kagan, A. Jpn. Cancer Assoc. *Gann Monogr. on Cancer Res.*, Jpn. Sci. Soc., Tokyo, **32**, 29–40.

Moore, R. A. and Melchionna, R. H. (1937). Production of tumors of the prostate of the white rat with 1,2–benzpyrene. *Am. J.*

Cancer, **30**, 731–741.

Moreadith, R. W. and Lehninger, A. L. (1984). The pathways of glutamate and glutamine oxidation by tumor cell mitochondria. Role of mitochondrial NAD (P+)-dependent malic enzyme. *J. Biol. Chem.*, **259**, 6215–6221.

Morikawa, K., Hosokawa, M., Hamada, J., Sugawara, M. and Kobayashi, H. (1985). Host-mediated therapeutic effects produced by appropriate timed administration of bleomycin on a rat fibrosarcoma. *Cancer Res.*, **45**, 1502–1506.

Mueller, W.E.G., Maidof, A., Arendez, J. Geurtsen, W., Zahn, R. K. and Schmidseder, R. (1979a). Additive effects of bleomycin and neocarzinostatin on degradation of DNA, inhibition of DNA polymerase, and cell growth. *Cancer Res.*, **39**, 3768–3773.

Mueller, W.E.G., Zahn, R. K., Arendez, J., Munsch, N. and Umezawa, H. (1979b). Activation of DNA metabolism in T–cells by bestatin. *Biochem. Pharmacol.*, **28**, 3131–3137.

Mueller, W.E.G., Leyhausen, G., Zahn, R. K., Schuster, D. K. and Gramzow, M. (1983). Biochemical and biological studies on bestatin. In: *Proc. 13th Int. Congr. Chemother.*, Vienna, 28 Aug.– 2 Sep., 1983. Symposium 67. Chemo-immunotherapy (Bestatin). Tom **11**, Part 204/15–20.

Muranaka, A., Ito, Y., Hashimoto, M., Namba, M., Nishitani, K., Otsuka, N., Nagai, K., Narabayashi, I. and Kaji, T. (1980). Uptake and excretion of ^{67}Ga-citrate in malignant tumors and normal cells. *Eur. J. Nucl. Med.*, **5**, 31–37.

Naganuma, A., Satoh, M., Koyama, Y. and Imura, N. (1985). Protective effect of metallothionen inducing metals on lethal toxicity of *cis-diamminedichloroplatinum* in mice. *Tox. Lett.*, **24**, 203–207.

Nagashima, K., Yoshida, M. and Seiki, M. (1986). Expression mechanism of the three pX gene products of HTLV–I. *Proc. Jpn. Cancer Assoc.*, 45th Ann. Mtg, Sapporo, Oct. 1986 (Abstract)

Nakahara, W. and Fukuoka, F. (1961). *Chemistry of Cancer Toxin: Toxohormone*, Springfield, Ill.

Nakamura, H. (1983). *Biseibutu kara mita Seibutsu Shinkagaku*, Baifukan, Tokyo. (Japanese)

Nakamura, T. (1985). Control of cell proliferation *in vivo* and *in vitro*. *Igaku no Ayumi*, **133**, 931–936. (Japanese)

Nakano, N. (1966). Establishment of cell lines *in vitro* from a mammary ascites tumor of mouse and biological properties of the established lines in a serum containing medium. *Tohoku J. Exp. Med.*, **88**, 69–84.

Nakatsugawa, S. and Sugawara. T. (1982). Inhibition of X–ray-induced potentially lethal damage (PLD) repair by cordycepin (3′deoxyadenosine) and enhancement of its action by 2′–deoxyformycin in Chinese hamster *hai* cells in the stationary phase *in vitro. Radiation Res.*, **84**, 265–275.

Narisawa, T., Sano, M., Sato, M., Takahashi, T. and Arakawa, H. (1983). Relationship between cholecystectomy and colonic cancer in low-risk Japanese population. *Dis. Colon Rect.*, **26**, 512–515.

Naumovski, L. and Friedberg, E. C. (1983). A DNA gene required for the incision of damaged DNA is essential for viability in *Saccharomyces cerevisiae. Proc. Nat. Acad. Sci.*, *USA*, **80**, 4818–4821.

Nauts, H. C., Fowler, G. A. and Bogatko, F. H. (1953). A review of the influence of bacterial infection and of bacterial products (Coley's toxin) on malignant tumors in man. *Acta Med. Scand. Accompanies*, **145**: 1–103.

Neel, J. V., Satoh, C., Goriki, K., Fujita, M., Takahashi, N., Asakawa, J. and Hazama, R. (1986). The rate with which spontaneous mutation alters the electrophoretic mobility of polypeptides. *Proc. Nat. Acad. Sci.*, *USA*, **83**, 389–393.

Newbold, R. F. and Overell, R. W. (1983). Fibroblast immortality is a prerequisite for transformation by EJ c–H–*ras* oncogene. *Nature (Lond.)*, **304**, 648–651.

Newburger, P. E., Chovaniec, M. E. and Cohen, H. J. (1989). Activity and activation of the granulocyte superoxide-generating system. *Blood*, **55**, 85–92.

Noma, A., Nezu-Nakayama, K., Kita, M. and Okabe, H. (1978). Simultaneous determination of serum cholesterol in high- and low-density lipoproteins with use of heparin, Ca^+2, and anion exchange resin. *Clin. Chem.*, **29**, 1504–1508.

Nowell, P. C. (1976). The clonal evolution of tumor cell populations. *Science*, **194**, 23–28.

Oberley, L. W. and Buettner, G. R. (1979). Role of superoxide dismutase in cancer: A review. *Cancer Res.*, **39**, 1141–1149.

Oberley, L. W. and Oberley, T. D. (1984). The role of superoxide dismutase and gene amplification in carcinogenesis. *J. Theor. Biol.*, **106**, 403–422.

Ogawa, H., Hiraoka, Y. and Kawai, H. (1983). Intracavitary instillation for bladder tumor with antitumor agent. 5th report: Difference of the action of mitomycin C on normal bladder and tumor of the bladder (Experimental and clinical study). *J. Jpn. Soc. Urol.*, **74**, 596–607. (Japanese)

Ohnishi, H., Tsukada, S., Hayashi, Y. Ogawa, N., Yajima, G., Masugi, Y., Aihara, K. and Suzuki, K. (1972). Effects of cytochrome c on liver functions of old rats. *Nature: New Biology*, **239**, 84–86.

Ohno, S. (1971). Genetic implications of karyological instability of malignant somatic cells. *Physiol. Rev.*, **51**, 496–526.

Okamoto, H., Koshimura, S., Shin, S. and Shimizu, R. (1972). *Beta-Hemolytic Streptococcus as a Cancer Controller. A com-*

mentary on PC–B–45, Chugai Pharmaceut., Tokyo.

Okuyama, S. (1973). Accumulation of Ga and Sr radionuclides in the bone. 4th Conference of Northern Japan Society of Nuclear Medicine, Morioka, Feb. 2, 1973; *Med. Postgrad.*, **11**, 249–250.

Okuyama, S., Fukuda, H., Shishido, F. and Matsuzawa, T. (1975). Treatment of lung cancer by radiation followed by bleomycin. *Proc. 2nd Symposium on the Combination Radiotherapy of Bleomycin*, Tokyo, March 1, 1975, pp. 26–29. (Japanese)

Okuyama, S., Sato, T. and Matsuzawa, T. (1977). Proliferative and necrotic tissue labeling in tumor imaging: Studies with ^{67}Ga citrate and ^{131}I-iodo-deoxyuridine in experimental soft-tissue and bone carcinomas. *Sci. Rep. Res. Inst. Tohoku Univ.–C*, **24**, 73–78.

Okuyama, S., Mishina, H. and Matsuzawa, T. (1978a). Does OK–432 selectively increase bleomycin concentration in tumor? *Gann*, **70**, 385–386.

Okuyama, S., Sano, M., Yokoyama, K. and Matsuzawa, T. (1978b). Histopathological discrimination of ^{67}Ga deposition in experimental tumors. *Sci. Rep. Res. Inst. Tohoku Univ.–C*, **25**, 5–9.

Okuyama, S., Sato, T., Takahashi, K. and Matsuzawa, T. (1978c). Gallium modification of cancer biology: Experimental studies on V2 rabbit carcinoma. *Sci. Rep. Res. Inst. Tohoku Univ.–C*, **25**, 58–64.

Okuyama, S., Mishina, H., Sera, K. and Matsuzawa, T. (1979a). Compton soft-tissue imaging and its capability expanded by direct magnification and shinozaki color TV system. *Radiology*, **131**, 215–220.

Okuyama, S. and Matsuzawa, T. (1979). Consecutive radiation-bleomycin therapy of cancer: A perpetuation principle of radiation damage. *Sci. Rep. Res. Inst. Tohoku Univ.–C*, **26**, 1–10.

Okuyama, S., Mishina, H., Yamamoto, K. and Matsuzawa, T. (1979b). Emperipolesis as a cancer antagonist: Report of 2 cases. *Scil Rep. Res. Inst. Tohoku Univ.–C*, **26**, 11–17.

Okuyama, S., Takeda, S., Sato, T., Awano, T., Takusakawa, K. and Matsuzawa, T. (1979c). Biological mechanisms of gallium–67 tumor deposition. *Sci. Rep. Res. Inst. Tohoku Univ.–C*, **26**, 22–29.

Okuyama, S. and Mishina, H. (1980). Consecutive therapy of cancer aimed at perpetuation of repairable damage: A hypothesis unifying radiotherapy and chemotherapy. *J. Clin. Hematol. Oncol.*, 10, 83–93.

Okuyama, S. and Mishina, H.(1981a). Probable superoxide therapy of experimental cancer with D-penicillamine. *Tohoku J. Exp. Med.*, **135**, 215–216.

Okuyama, S. and Mishina, H. (1981b). Consecutive, multimodal therapy of cancer: Selective biological initiation (OK–432), cytoplasmic and nuclear damage (FT–207 and cyclophosphamide), inhibition of repair (bleomycin), and activation of cleansing and surveillance mechanisms. *Sci. Rep. Res. Inst. Tohoku Univ.–C*,

28, 7–14.

Okuyama, S. and Mishina, H. (1982a) Principles of anti-cancer prescription—Consecutive, multimodal therapy of cancer—. *Med. Postgrad.*, **20**, 17–28. (Japanese)

Okuyama, S. and Mishina, H. (1982b). Forced suicide as a new mode of cancer cell elimination. 11th Ann. UCLA Symposium: Rational basis for chemotherapy, Keystone, Co., Apr. 18–23, 1982. *J. Cell. Biochem. Suppl.*, **6**, Liss, New York. p. 370.

Okuyama, S. and Mishina, H. (1982c). Consecutive integration of multiple principia of cancer therapy: A hypothesis (A pamphlet circulated at the 11th UCLA Symposium: Rational basis for chemotherapy, Keystone, Co., Apr. 18–23, 1982).

Okuyama, S. and Mishina, H. (1982d). Principia of cancer therapy. I. Rescue of radiation damage. *Sci. Rep. Res. Inst. Tohoku Univ.-C*, **29**, 1–3.

Okuyama, S., Mishina, H., Oshida, M., Ojima, T., Imaizumi, A. and Yokoyama, A.(1983a). Principia of cancer therapy. II. Treatment of undermining ulcers complicating radiotherapy: Role of correction of hypozincemia. *Sci. Rep. Res. Inst. Tohoku Univ.-C*, **30**, 1–4.

Okuyama, S. and Mishina, H. (1983a). Principia of cancer therapy. III. Perpetuation principle of repairable chemotherapeutic damage: Cisplatin-bleomycin *in vitro. Sci. Rep. Res. Inst. Tohoku Univ.-C*, **30**, 5–7.

Okuyama, S., Mishina, H., Ito, Y. and Matsuzawa, T. (1983b). Principia of cancer therapy. IV. Induction of hemoconcentration for phlebotomy in polycythemia vera. *Sci. Rep. Res. Inst. Tohoku Univ.-C*, **30**, 29–30.

Okuyama, S., Mishina, H. and Maki, T. (1983c). Principia of cancer therapy. V. Clinical and histopathological criteria for cancer redifferentiaton. *Sci. Rep. Res. Inst. Tohoku Univ.-C*, **30**, 31–35.

Okuyama, S. and Mishina, H. (1983b). Principia of cancer therapy. VI. Application of ubiquinone ointment for intractable radition ulcers: An expanded cytochrome c effect? *Sci. Rep. Res. Inst. Tohoku Univ.-C*, **30**, 36–39.

Okuyama, S., Sano, M., Awano, T., Takeda, S., Yamada-Yokoyama, K., Takahashi, K. and Matsuzawa, T. (1984a). Gallium induces reduction of negative charge of the cell membrane and redifferentiation of cancer cells. *Tohoku J. Exp. Med.*, **142**, 347–348.

Okuyama, S. and Mishina, H. (1984a). Decrease in saturation density of mammalian carcinoma cell culture during exposure to *Bestatin*, a clinically applicable agent. *Tohoku J. Exp. Med.*, **142**, 349–350.

Okuyama, S. and Mishina, H. (1984b). Evolutionary concepts of cancer and its evidence observable in the radiological sciences.

Eizo Joho Medical, **16**, 865–871. (Japanese)

Okuyama, S. and Mishina, H. (1984c). Consecutive *bestatin-hormone* regimen induces redifferentiation of cancer cells *in vitro*. *Tohoku J. Exp. Med.*, **143**, 501–502.

Okuyama, S., Mishina, H., Hariu, T., Yamamoto, K., Matsushiro, T., Yamagata, R. and Taima, T. (1984b). Exfoliation as a novel mode of cancer cell elimination. *Tohoku J. Exp. Med.*, **143**, 503–504.

Okuyama, S., Mishina, H. and Takahashi, K. (1984c). Principia of cancer therapy. VII. Tetracyclines as cancer antagonists. *Sci. Rep. Res. Inst. Tohoku Univ.-C*, **31**, 27–29.

Okuyama, S. and Mishina, H. (1985a). Cancer biology and logical construction of anticancer strategies. *Med. Postgrad.*, **23**, 213–231. (Japanese)

Okuyama, S. and Mishina, H. (1985b). Bestatin-treated breast cancer cells redifferentiate dose-dependently in vitro as triggered by sex hormone. *J. Clin. Hemato. Oncol.*, **15**, 43–52.

Okuyama, S. and Mishina, H. (1985c). Evolutionary concept of cancer: A hypothesis. In: *Recent Advances in Chemotherapy. Anti-Cancer Section*, ed. by Ishigami, J. Univ. of Tokyo Press, Tokyo, pp. 217–218.

Okuyama, S. and Mishina, H. (1985d). Evolutionary concept of cancer in the development of tumor imaging agents. *Proc. Int. Symposium on Current and Future Aspects of Cancer Diagnosis with Positron Emission Tomography (PET 85)*, Sendai, Oct. 14–18, 1985, pp. 102–106.

Okuyama, S., Mishina, H. and Takahashi, M. (1985a). Histological evidence for rescue of radiation dermatitis in an ultraviolet model system. *Tohoku J. Exp. Med.*, **147**, 217–218.

Okuyama, S. and Mishina, H. (1985e). Principia of cancer therapy. IX. Categorization, symbolization and consecutive integration of principia of cancer radiotherapy. *Sci. Rep. Res. Inst. Tohoku Univ.-C*, **32**, 20–30.

Okuyama, S. and Mishina, H. (1985f). Principia of cancer therapy. X. Prostaglandin D_2 triggers redifferentiation of the bestatin-treated breast cancer cells *in vitro*. *Sci. Rep. Res. Inst. Tohoku Univ.-C*, **32**, 31–34.

Okuyama, S. and Mishina, H. (1985g). Principia of cancer therapy. XI. Prostaglandin D_2 induces redifferentiation of M1 leukemia cells in vitro irrespective of bestatin. *Sci. Rep. Res. Inst. Tohoku Univ.-C*, **32**, 35–38.

Okuyama, S. and Mishina, H. (1985h). Evolutionary concept of cancer in radiotherapy. *Kokenshi*, **37**, 125–131. (Japanese)

Okuyama, S., Mishina, H. and Maki, T. (1985b). Redifferentiation of cancer cells: Bestatin, estradiol, and prostaglandin D_2. *Ann. New York Acad. Sci.*, 459: *Hemoatopoietic Cellular Proliferation*, pp. 293–307.

Okuyama, S. and Mishina, H. (1986a). Control of myelophthisis carcinomatosa through reinforcement of chemotherapy by a course of Picibanil In: *Clinical Application of OK-432 for Control of Cancer*, ed. by Ota, K. Excerpta Medica, Tokyo, pp. 245–254.

Okuyama, S. and Mishina, H. (1986b). Hypothesis: Evolutionary concept of cancer. *Proc. Jpn. Cancer Assoc.*, 45th Ann. Mtg, Sapporo, Oct. 21–23, 1986, p. 596. (Abstract)

Okuyama, S. and Mishina, H. (1987a). Fanconi's anemia as a Nature's evolutionary experiment on carcinogenesis. *Tohoku J. Exp. Med.*, **153,** 87–102.

Okuyama, S., Mishina, H., Yoshizumi, A., Usuba, Y. and Takahashi, M. (1987a). Intratumoral doxycycline for skin metastases of human malignancies. *Tohoku J. Exp. Med.*, **151,** 241–244.

Okuyama, S. (1987). Kinetic mechanisms of deposition of the bone-seeking radiopharmaceuticals. In: *Houshasen Igaku Taikei*, Vol. **40A,** Nakayama Shoten, Tokyo. pp. 109–127. (Japanese)

Okuyama, S. and Mishina, H. (1987b). Lentinan for malignant lymphoma: Report of a case. *Kiso to Rinsho*, **21,** 4802–4804. (Japanese)

Okuyama, S., Okuyama, J. and Mishina, H. (1987b). Cytochrome c effect on thermal wounds. *Kokenshi*, **39,** 93–97. (Japanese with an English summary)

Okuyama, S. and Mishina, H. (1988a). Cancer incidence in the population of Nagasaki City 30 years after atomic bombing. *Tohoku J. Exp. Med.*, **155,** 23–39.

Okuyama, S. and Mishina, H. (1988b). Evolutionary cancer epidemiology. *Sci. Rep. Res. Inst. Tohoku Univ.-C*, submitted.

Okuyama, S., Mishina, H., Mita, M. and Funaki, K. (1988). Principia of cancer therapy. XIV. Can hypoxic milieau be a key of clonal selection in carcinogenesis? *Sci. Rep. Res. Inst. Tohoku. Univ.-C*, submitted.

Okuyama, S. and Mishina, H. (1988c). Principia of cancer therapy. XVII. Evolutionary concept of cancer: A biological, and radiological hypothesis. *Sci. Rep. Res. Inst. Tohoku Univ.-C*, submitted.

Okuyama, S. and Mishina, H. (1988d). Medroxyprogesterone acetate lung cancer. *Tohoku J. Exp. Med.*, submitted.

Okuyama, S., Mishina, H., Nakayama, H. and Ando, N. (1989a). Principia of cancer therapy. XX. Nuclear changes following radiochemotherapy with bleomycin. *Sci. Rep. Res. Inst. Tohoku Univ.-C*, to be submitted.

Okuyama, S., Mishina, H., Sato, K. and Okuyama, J. (1989b). Lysozymal ointment for an intractable radiation ulcer. *Sci. Rep. Res. Inst. Tohoku Univ.-C*, to be submitted.

Old, L. J., Clarke, D. A. and Benacerraf, B. (1959). Effect of bacillus Calmette-Guerin infection on transplanted tumors in the mouse. *Nature (Lond.)*, 184, 291–292.

Olofsson, T. and Olsson, I. (1980). Biochemical characterization of a leukemia-associated inhibitor (LAI) suppressing normal granulopoiesis *in vitro*. *Blood*, **55**, 983–991.

Pace, N. and Smith, R. E. (1946). Measurement of the residual radiation intensity at the Hiroshima and Nagasaki atomic bomb sites. *USAEC NMRI* 106A as cited in Arakawa 1969.

Pathak, M. A. and Epstein, J. H. (1971). Normal and abnormal reactions of man to light. In: *Dermatology in General Medicine*, ed. by Fitzpatrick, T. B., Arndt, K. A., Clark, W. H., Eisen, A. Z., van Scott, E. J. and Vaughan, J. H. McGraw-Hill, New York, pp. 977–1036.

Patterson, C. (1978). *Evolution*, British Museum, London.

Pedersen, P. L., Greenwalt, J. W., Chan, T. L. and Morris, H.P. (1970). A comparison of some ultrastructural and biochemical properties of mitochondria from Morris hepatomas 9618A, 7800, and 3924A. *Cancer Res.*, **30**, 2620–2626.

Pedersen, F. K., Hertz, H., Lundsteen, G., Platz, P. and Thomsen, M. (1977). Indication of primary immune deficiency in Fanconi's anemia. *Acta Paediat. Scand.*, **66**, 745–751.

Peeters-Joris, C., Vandevoorde, A. and Baudhuin, P. (1975). Subcellular localization of superoxide dismutase in rat liver. *Biochem. J.*, **150**, 31–39.

Persson, H., Henninghausen, L., Taub, R., DeGrado, W. and Leder, P. (1984). Antibodies to human c-*myc* oncogene product: Evidence of an evolutionarily conserved protein induced during cell proliferation. *Science*, **225**, 687–693.

Peskin, A. V., Koen, Ya. M., Zbarsky, I. B. and Konstatntinov, A. A. (1977). Superoxide dismutase and glutathione peroxidase activities in tumor. *FEBS Lett.*, **78**, 41–45.

Pimm, M. V. and Baldwin, R. W. (1985). Influence of bestatin, poly I: C, PPD and a pyrimidinone on growth and metastasis of rat mammary carcinoma. *Br. J. Cancer*, **51**, 595. (Abstract)

Potter, R. L. and Bethel, F. N. (1952). Oxidative phosphorylation in spleen mitochondria. *Federation Proc.*, **11**, 270. (Abstract)

Porvaznik, M. (1979). Tight junction disruption and recovery after sublethal gamma irradiation. *Radiation Res.*, **78**, 233–250.

Prasad, K. N. (1974). *Human Radiation Biology*, Harper and Row, Hagerstown.

Prasad, K. N. and Kumar, S. (1975). Expression of differentiated function in neuroblastoma cell culture. In: *The Cell Cycle in Malignancy and Immunity*, ERDA Symp. Ser., Energy Research and Development Administration Technical Information Center, Oak Ridge, Tenn., **33**, 132–155.

Purtillo, D. T. (1977). Opportunistic non-Hodgkin's lymphoma in X–linked recessive immunodeficiency and lymphoproliferative syndrome. *Semin. Oncol.*, **4**, 335–343.

Rassoulzadegan, M., Cowie, A., Carr, A., Glaichenhaus, N., Kamen, R. and Cuzin, F. (1982). The roles of indicidual polyoma virus early proteins in oncogenic transformation. *Nature (Lond.)*, **300**, 713–718.

Rassoulzadegan, M., Naghashfar, Z., Cowie, A., Carr, A., Grisoni, M., Kamen, R. and Guzin, F. (1983). Expression of the large T protein of polyoma virus promotes the establishment in culture of "normal" rodent fibroblast cell line. *Proc. Nat. Acad. Sci., USA*, **80**, 4354–4358.

Reed, K., Ravikumar, K. H., Gifford, R. R. and Grage, T. B. (1983). The association of Fanconi's anemia and squamous cell carcinoma. *Cancer*, **52**, 926–928.

Reiman, R. E., Rosen, G., Gelbard, A.S., Benua, R. S., Yeh, S.D.J. and Laughlin, J. S. (1984). Diagnostic demands in clinical and experimental oncology: application of substrates labelled with positron-emitting radionuclides. In: *Current Topics in Tumor Cell Physiology and positron-emission Tomography*, ed. by Knapp, W. H. and Vyska, K., Springer-Verlag, Berlin.

Reincke, U., Burlington, H., Carsten, A. L., Cronkite, E. P. and Laissue, J. A. (1978). Hematopoietic effects in mice of a transplanted, granulocytosis-inducing tumor. *Exp. Hemat.*, **6**, 421–430.

Reinherz, E. L. and Schlossman, S. F. (1980). The differentiation and function of human T lymphocytes. *Cell*, **19**, 821–827.

Reitzer, L. J., Wice, B. M. and Kennell, D. (1979). Evidence that glutamine, not sugar, is the major energy source for cultured HeLa cells. *J. Biol. Chem.*, **254**, 2669–2676.

Ribi, E., Grander, D. L., Milner, K. C. and Strain, S. (1975). Brief communication: Tumor regression caused by endotoxins and mycobacterial fractions. *J. Nat. Cancer Inst.*, **55**, 1253–1257.

Robbins, J. H., Kraemer, K. H., Luzner, M. A., Festoff, B. W. and Coon, H. G. (1974). Xeroderma pigmentosum: An inherited disease with sun sensitivity, multiple cutaneous neoplasms, and abnormal DNA repair. *Ann. Int. Med.*, **80**, 221–248.

Robbins, S. L. and Angell, M. (1976). *Basic Pathology*, 2nd ed., Asian ed., Saunders-Igaku Shoin, Tokyo.

Robbins, S. L. and Cortran, R. S. (1979). *Pathologic Basis of Disease*, 2nd ed., W. B. Saunders.

Rosner, F. and Lee, S. L. (1972). Down's syndrome and acute leukemia: Myeloblastic or lymphoblastic? Report of fortythree cases and review of the literature. *Am. J. Med.*, **53**, 203–218.

Roussel, M., Saule, S., Lagrou, C., Rommens, C., Beug, H., Graf, T. and Stehelin, D. (1979). Three new types of viral oncogene of cellular origin specific for haematopoietic cell transformation. *Nature (Lond.)*, **281**, 452–455.

Rubin, P. and Casarette, G.W. (1968). *Clinical Radiation Pathology*, Saunders, Philadelphia. pp. 1–37.

Rubinson, R. M. and Bolooki, H. (1972). Intrapelural tetracycline for control of malignant pleural effusion: A preliminary report. *Sth. med. J.*, **65**, 847–849.

Ruddon, R. W. (1981). *Cancer Biology*, Oxford Univ. Press, New York.

Ruley, H. E. (1983). Adenovirus early region 1A enables viral and cellular transforming genes to transform primary cells in culture. *Nature (Lond.)*, **304**, 602–606.

Rowley, J. D. (1984). Biological implications of consistent chromosome rearrangements in leukemia and lymphoma. *Cancer Res.*, **44**, 3159–3168.

Sachs, L. (1978). The differentiation of myeloid leukaemia cells: New possibilities for therapy. *Br. J. Haemat.*, **40**, 509–517.

Saijo, S., Satake, M., Shirato, M., Tomioka, S., Yuasa, R., Kaneko, Y., Mishina, H. and Okuyama, S. (1987). Clinical evaluation of treatment of cases of maxillary cancer. *Tokeibu Shuyo (Head and Neck Cancer)*, **14**, 281. (Abstract)

Saito, M., Ebina, T., Koi, M., Yamaguchi, T., Kawade, Y. and Ishida, N. (1982). Induction of interferon-gamma in mouse spleen cells by OK–432, a preparation of *Streptococcus pyogenes*. *Cell. Immunol.*, **68**, 187–192.

Saito, T., Ohira, S., Wakui, A., Yokoyama, M., Takahashi, H., Himori, T., Asamura, M., Kaneko, T., Kobayashi, Y., Sugawara, K. and Hashimoto, K. (1967). Pathophysiological studies on the effect of prednisolone on tumor-bearing rats. *Kokenshi*, **19**, 260–287. (Japanese)

Saito, T., Wakui, A. and Takahashi, H. (1973). Clinical studies of metastasis in advanced stomach cancer treated with anti-cancer drugs and prednisolone. *Gan to Kagaku Ryoho*, **19**, 935–940. (Japanese)

Salmon, S. and Apple, M. (1974). Cancer chemotherapy. In: *Review of Medical Pharmacology*, 4th ed., ed. by Meyers, F. H., Jawetz, E. and Goldfin, A. Maruzen Asian ed., Lange Medical-Maruzen, Tokyo, pp. 462–493.

Sarkar, S., Kacinski, B. M. and Kohorn, E. I. (1986). Demonstration of *myc* and *ras* oncogene expression by hybridization *in situ* in hydatidiform mole in the BeWo choriocarcinoma cell line. *Am. J. Obstet. Gynecol.*, **154**, 390–393.

Sasaki, M. and Kunimatsu, M. (1980). Immunological evidence of a surface structure commone to *Streptococcus pyogenes* preparation OK–432 and mouse ascites tumor cells. *Microbiol. Immunol.*, **24**, 259–264.

Sasaki, M. S. and Tonomura, A. (1973). A high susceptibility of Fanconi's anemia to chromosome breakage by DNA cross-linking agents. *Cancer Res.*, **33**, 1829–1836.

Sasaki, T., Yamamoto, M. and Sakka, M. (1981). Implications of thymidine labeling index in the growth kinetics of human solid tumors. *Gann*, **72**, 181–188.

Sato, C., Kojima, K., Matsuzawa, T. and Hinuma, Y. (1975). Relationship between loss of negative charge on nuclear membrane and loss of colony-forming ability in X–irradiated cells. *Radiation Res.*, **62**, , 250–257.

Sato, H., Sato, K., Sato, Y., Asamura, M., Kanamaru, R., Sugiyama, Z., Kaihara, T., Mimata, Y., Wakui, A., Suzuki, M., Hori, K., Abe, I., Saito, S. and Sato, H. (1981). Induced hypertension chemotherapy of cancer patients by selective enhancement of drug delivery to tumor tissue with angiotensin II. *Sci. Rep. Res. Inst. Tohoku Univ.-C*, **28**, 32–44.

Sato, H. (1987). Induced hypertension chemotherapy based on the functional characteristics of tumor vessels. *Igaku no Ayumi*, **141**, 594–598. (Japanese)

Sato, K. and Tsuiki, S. (1968). Fructose 1,6–diphosphatase of mouse Ehrlich Ascites tumor and its comparison with the enzymes of liver and skeletal muscle of the mouse. *Biochim. Biophys. Acta*, **159**, 130–140.

Sato, K., Takaya, S., Imai, F., Hatayama, I. and Ito, N. (1978). Different deviation patterns of carbohydrate-metabolizing enzymes in primary rat hepatomas induced by different chemical carcinogens. *Cancer Res.*, **38**, 3086–3093.

Sawamura, D. (1986). Analysis of antitumor action of *Mycobacterium bovis* (BCG).—Using an experimental tumor which shares common antigens with BCG—. *Hirosaki Igaku*, **38**, 751–759. (Japanese)

Scarpa, M., Rigo, A., Momo, F., Isacchi, G., Novelli, G. and Dallapiccola, B. (1985). Increased rate of superoxide ion generation in Fanconi anemia erythrocytes. *Biochem. Biophys. Res. Commun.*, **130**, 127–132.

Schersten, T., Lundholm, K., Eden, E., Edstrom, S., Ekman, L., Karlberg, I. and Warnold, I. (1979). Energy metabolism in cancer. *Acta Chir. Scand. Suppl.*, **498**, 130–136.

Schiffer, L. M. (1968). Kinetics of chronic lymphocytic leukemia. *Ser. Haematol.*, **1**, 2–23.

Schimpff, S. C. (1986). Acute leukemia. In: *Comprehensive Textbook of Oncology*, ed. by Moosa, A. R., Robson, M. C. and Schimpff, S. C. Williams and Wilkins, Baltimore, pp. 530–540.

Schlager, S. I., Ohanian, S. H. and Borsos, T. (1978a). Correlation between the ability of tumor cells to resist humoral immune attack and their ability to synthesize lipid. *J. Immunol.*, **120**, 463–471.

Schlager, S. I., Ohanian, S. H. and Borsos, T. (1978b). Identification of lipids associated with the ability of tumor cells to resist humoral immune attack. *J. Immunol.*, **120**, 472–480.

Schwartz, A. D. (1986). Cancer in children: An overview. *Comprehensive Textbook of Oncology*, ed. by Moosa, A. R., Robson, M. C. and Schimpff, S. C. Williams and Wilkins, Baltimore, pp. 1143–1148.

Segi, M. (1977). Graphic presentation of cancer incidence by site and by area and population. Compiled from *Cancer Incidence in Five Continents*, Vol. **3**, 1976.

Segi, M., Tominaga, S., Aoki, K. and Fujimoto, I. (1981). *Cancer Mortality and Morbidity Statistics*, Jpn. Cancer Assoc. *Gann Monogr. on Cancer Res.*, 26, Jpn. Sci. Soc. Press, Tokyo.

Setala, K. (1984). Carcinogenesis—Devolution towards an ancient nucleated pre-eukarytoic level. *Med. Hypotheses.* **15**, 209–230.

Setlow, R. B. (1985). Saturation of repair. *Basic Life Sci.*, **33**, 251–260.

Shatton, J. B., Morris, H. P. and Weinhouse, S. (1969). Kinetic, electrophoretic studies on glucose-ATP phosphotransferase in rat hepatomas. *Cancer Res.*, **29**, 1161–1172.

Sheiness, D. and Bishop, J. M. (1979). DNA and RNA from uninfected vertebrate cells contain nucleotide sequences related to the putative transforming gene of avian myelocytomatosis virus. *J. Virol.*, **31**, 514–521.

Sheppard, D. M., Fisher, R. A. and Lawler, S. D. (1985). Karyotypic analysis and chromosome polymorphisms in four choriocarcinoma cell lines. *Cancer Genet. Cytogenet.*, **16**, 251–258.

Shigematsu, I. and Kagan, A. (1986). *Cancer in Atomic Bomb Survivors, Jpn. Cancer Assoc. Gann Monogr. on Cancer Res.*, **32**, Jpn. Sci. Soc., Tokyo.

Shimizu, T., Mizuno, N., Amano, T. and Hayaishi, O. (1979). Prostaglandin D_2, a neuromodulator. *Proc. Nat. Acad. Sci.*, *USA*, **76**, 6231–6234.

Siegfried, J., Mass, M. and Hozier, J. (1986). Genes for tumor markers are clustered near cellular oncogenes. *J. cell. Biochem.*, *Suppl.*, 10A: UCLA symposium on Molecular and Cellular Biology, 15th Ann. Mtg.: "Cellular and Molecular Biology of Tumors and Potential Clinical Applications," Steamboat Springs, Co., Jan. 20–25, 1986, p. 43.

Singer, B. (1985). *In vivo* formation and persistence of modified nucleosides resulting from alkylating agents. *Environ. Health Perspect.*, 62, 41–48.

Slater, J. P., Mildvan, A. S. and Loeb, L. A. (1971). Zinc in DNA polymerases. *Biochem. biophys. Res. Commun.*, **44**, 37–43.

Smith, N. R., Sparks, R. L., Pool, T. B. and Cameron, I. L. (1978). Differences in the intracellular concentration of elements in normal and cancerous liver cells as determined by X–ray microanalysis. *Cancer Res.*, **38**, 1952–1959.

Sogawa, K. (1986). Recent progress in studies of the drug metabolizing enzyme P-450. *Gan to Kagaku Ryoho*, **13**, 2487–2494. (Japanese)

Srere, P. A. (1980). The intrastructure of the mitochondrial matrix. *Trends Biochem. Sci.*, **5**, 120–121.

Stacey, D. W., Smith, M. R. and DeGudicibus, S. J. (1986). Microinjection studies of cellular oncogene function. *J. Cell. Biochem.*, **Suppl. 10A,** p. 5. (Abstract)

Steel, G. G., Hodgett, J. and Janik, P. (1971). Cell population kinetics of a spontaneous rat tumor during serial transplantation. *Br. J. Cancer*, **20**, 784–800.

Steel, G. G. (1977). *Growth Kinetics of Tumours. Cell population kinetics in relation to the growth and treatment of cancer*, Clarendon Press, Oxford.

Stocco, D. M. and Hutson, J.C. (1980). Characteristics of mitochondria isolated by rate zonal centrifugation from normal liver and Novikoff hepatomas. *Cancer Res.*, **40**, 1486–1492.

Stoker, M. G. and Sussman, M. (1965). Studies on the action of feeder layers in cell culture. *Exp. Cell Res.*, **38**, 645–653.

Stringfellow, D. A. and Fitzpatrick, F. A. (1979). Prostaglandin D_2 controls pulmonary metastasis of malignant melanoma cells. *Nature (Lond.)*, **282**, 76–78.

Strydom, D. J., Fett, J. W., Lobb, R. R., Alderman, E. M., Bethune, J. L., Riodan, J. R. and Vallee, B. L. (1985). Amino acid sequence of human tumor derived angiogenin. *Biochemistry*, **24**, 5486–5494.

Sugano, H. (1980). Natural history of human cancers. *Tr. Soc. Pathol. Jpn.*, **69**, 27–57. (Japanese)

Sugimori, H., Kashimura, Y., Kashimura, M. and Taki, I. (1978). Nuclear DNA content of trophoblastic tumors. *Acta Cytologia*, **22**, 542–545.

Sugimura, T., Matsushima, T., Kawachi, T., Kogure, K., Tanaka, N., Miyake, S., Hozumi, M., Sato, S. and Sato, H. (1972). Disdifferentiation and decarcinogenesis. The isozyme patterns in malignant tumors and membrane changes of cultured tumor cells. *Gann Monogr. on Cancer Res.*, **13**, 31–45.

Sugiyama, T., Takahashi, R., Yamaguchi, T. and Aoyama, S. (1985). Human chromosomes and oncogenes. *Gendai Kagaku.* Suppl. 2: *Perspectives of Research on Oncogenes*, Tokyo Kagaku Dojin, Tokyo, pp. 47–58. (Japanese)

Sulitzeanu, D. (1985). Human cancer-associated antigens: Present status and implications for immunodiagnosis. *Adv. Cancer Res.*, **44**, 1–42.

Suwa, N., Niwa, T., Fukasawa, H. and Sasaki, Y. (1963). Estimation of intravascular blood pressure gradient by mathematical analysis of arterial casts. *Tohoku J. Exp. Med.*, **79**, 168–198.

Suzuki, J. and Komatsu, S. (1981). New embolization method using estrogen for dural arteriovenous malformation and meningioma. *Surg. Neuro.*, **16**, 438–442.

Suzuki, M., Hori, K., Abe, I., Saito, S. and Sato, H. (1981). A new approach to cancer chemotherapy: Selective enhancement of tumor blood flow with angiotensin II. *J. Nat. Cancer Inst.*, **67**, 663–669.

Suzuki, M., Takahashi, T. and Sato, T. (1987). Medial regression and its functional significance in tumor-supplying host arterioles. A morphometric study of hepatic arteries in human livers with hepatocellular carcinomas. *Cancer*, **59**, 444–450.

Suzuki, T., Kubomura, O., Takahashi, K., Hara, T. and Iio, M. (1985). Tumor study with C–11 pyruvate. *Proc. Int. Symposium on Current and Future Aspects of Cancer Diagnosis with Positron Emission Tomography (PET 85)*, Oct. 14–18, 1985, pp. 43–47.

Svanberg, L. E. and Elisson, O. (1983). Application of bestatin to the treatment of lung cancer. *Proc. 13th Int. Congr. Chemother.*, Vienna, 28 Aug.–2 Sep. 1983. Symposium 67. Chemo-immuno-therapy (Bestatin), Tom **11**, 204/36–41.

Sykes, A. J., McCormack, F. X. and O'Brien, T. J. (1978). A pre-liminary study of the superoxide dismutase content of some human tumors. *Cancer Res.*, **38**, 2759–2762.

Tachibana, T. (1974). Expression of surface antigens of tumor cells and irradiation—A clue of radiation therapy to cancer. *Gan no Rinsho*, **20**, 84–89. (Japanese)

Tajima, H., Ishiguro, J. and Ogawa, N. (1970). ^{131}I-cytochrome c: Its intestinal absorption and distribution in the rat. *Clinical Report 1970*, Mochida Pharmaceut., Tokyo, **4**, 597–604. (Japanese)

Takahashi, M. and Seiji, M. (1983). Acral melanoma in Japan. *Pigment Cell*, **6**, 150–165.

Takebe, H., Miki, Y., Kozuka, T., Furuyama, J., Tanaka, K., Sasaki, M. S., Fujiwara, Y. and Akiba, H. (1977). DNA repair characteristics and skin cancers of xeroderma pigmentosum patients in Japan. *Cancer Res.*, **37**, 490–495.

Takeda, S. and Takusagawa, K. (1978). Unpublished data.

Takeda, S., Okuyama, S., Takusagawa, K. and Matsuzawa, T. (1978). Lysosomal accumulation of gallium–67 in Morris hepatoma–7316A and Shionogi mammary adenocarcinoma–115. *Gann*, **69**, 267–271.

Tamemasa, O., Goto, R. and Suzuki, T. (1978). Preferential in-corporation of some ^{14}C-labeled D-amino acids into tumor-bering animals. *Gann*, **69**, 517–523.

Tamura, K., Shibata, Y., Matsuda, Y. and Ishida, N. (1981). Isola-tion and characterization of an immunosuppressive acidic protein from ascitic fluids of cancer patients. *Cancer Res.*, **41**, 3244–3252.

Tanaka, K., Numata, M., Umezu, Y., Kawamura, H., Marumo, T. and Hayashi, S. (1983). On the changes in urinary beta-D-Nacetylglucosaminidase (NAG) activity during cisplatin administration. *Tokeibu Shuyo*, 10, 99. (Abstract) (Japanese)

Tanaka, K., Umezu, Y., Sayama, S., Komatsu, T., Satoh, R. and Hayashi, S. (1985). Protective effects of fosfomycin on cisplatin-induced renal toxicity in the mouse. In: *Recent Adv. Chemother.*, Antimicrobial section 3, *Proc. 14th Int. Congr. Chemother.*, Kyoto, 1985, pp. 2626–2627.

Tanaka, N. (1972). *Action Mechanisms of Antibiotics. Molecular biology of their antibacterial and anti-cancer activities.*, Univ. of Tokyo Press, Tokyo.

Tannock, L.F. (1968). The relation between cell proliferation and the vascular system in a transplanted mouse mammary tumor. *Br. J. Cancer*, **22**, 258–273.

Temin, H. M. (1982). Viruses, protoviruses, development, and evolution. *J. Cell. Biochem.*, **19**, 105–118.

Terasima, T., Yasukawa, M. and Umezawa, H. (1970). Breaks and rejoining of DNA in cultured mammalian cells treated with bleomycin. *Gann*, **61**, 513–516.

Testa, J. R., Miz, U., Rowley, J.D., Vardiman, J.W. and Golombo, H.M. (1979). Evolution of karyotypes in acute nonlymphocytic leukemia. *Cancer Res.*, **39**, 490–495.

Theologides, A. (1982). Asthenia in cancer. *Am. J. Med.*, **73**, 1–3.

Thomas, Y., Rogozinski, L., Irigoyen, O. H., Friedman, S. M., Kung, P. C., Goldstein, G. and Chess, L. (1982a). Functional analysis of human T cell subsets defined by monoclonal antibodies. IV. Induction of suppressor cells with the OKT4+ population. *J. Exp. Med.*, **154**, 459–467.

Thomas, Y., Rogozinski, L., Irigoyen, O. H., Shen, H. H., Tallee, M. A., Goldstein, G. and Chess, L. (1982b). Functional analysis of human T cell subsets defined by monoclonal antibodies. V. Suppressor cells within the activated OKT4+ population belong to a distinct subset. *J. Immunol.*, **128**, 1386–1390.

Thorsrud, G. K. (1965). Reaction of the pleura to achromycin. *Acta Chir. Scand.*, **355**, Suppl. **1**, 48–50.

Thrasher, J. C., Clark, F. I. and Clarke, D.R. (1967). Changes in the vaginal epithelial cell cycle in relation to events of the estrus cycle. *Exp. Cell Res.*, **45**, 232–236.

Todaro, G. J., Green, H. and Swift, M.R. (1966). Susceptibility of human diploid fibroblast strains to transformation by SV40 virus. *Science*, **153**, 1252–1254.

Toge, T., Fujita, T., Yanagawa, E. and Hattori, T. (1987). Scanning electron microscopic studies on the surface structure of OK-432 activated macrophage. 15th Int. Congr. Chemother., Istanbul, Jul. 19–24, 1987, p. 218 (Abstract); *OK-432, Collected Papers*, pp. 98–99 (Japanese)

Tokuoka, S. (1986). Ovarian neoplasms in atomic bomb survivors. In: *Cancer in Atomic Bomb Survivors. Jpn. Cancer Assoc. Gann*

Monogr. on Cancer Res., **32,** ed. by Shigematsu, I. and Kagan, A. Jpn. Sci. Soc., Tokyo, pp. 179–189.

Tomiie, F., Yamamoto, A., Murakami, K. and Hamaoka, K. (1982). Bone changes in infants induced by prostaglandin E_1 as secondary hypertrophic osteoarthropathy. *Nipp. Acta Radiol.*, **42,** 1127–1136.

Tomioka, H. and Saito, H. (1979). Enhanced hydrogen peroxide release from macrophages stimulated with streptococcal preparation OK–432. *Infect. Immunity*, **26,** 779–782.

Torisu, M. and Katano, M. (1980). Treatment of terminal stage ascites with NSC–B116209 (Picibanil) *Proc. 11th Conf. on Immunotherapy of Cancer*, Tokyo, Nov. 8, 1980.

Torisu, M., Sakata, M., Fujimura, T., Itoh, H., Kimura, Y., Takesue, M., Yoshida, T. and Katano, M. (1985). Successful treatment of malignant ascites: Clinical evaluation and role of host's inflammatory cells in tumor cell destruction in ascites. In: *Basic Mechanisms and Clinical Treatment of Tumor Metastases*, ed. by Torisu, M. and Yoshida, T. Academic Press, Orlando, pp. 593–615.

Travis, E. L. (1975). *Primer of Medical Radiobiology*, Year Book Med., Chicago. pp. 133–149.

Tricott, G., Broeckaert-van Orshoven, A., Casteers-van Dele, M. and van den Berghe, H. (1981). 8/21 Translocation in acute myeloid leukaemia. *Scand. J. Haemat.*, **26,** 168–176.

Truitt, R. L. and Pollard, M. (1976). Allogeneic bone marrow chimerism in germ-free mice. IV. Therapy of "Hodgkin's-like reticulum cell sarcoma in SJL mice. *Transplantation*, **21,** 12–16.

Tsuiki, S. (1973). Alterations of isozymes in tumors. In: *Progress Cancer Biochemistry*, ed. by Sugimura, T., Endo, H., Ono T. and Sugano, H. *Jpn. Cancer Assoc. Gann Monogr. on Cancer Res.*, Jpn. Sci. Soc. Press, Tokyo, **24,** 223–243.

Uchida, T., Narabayashi, K., Takeda, S. and Matsuzawa, T. (1976). A study on accumulation mechanism of ^{111}In in malignant tumor. *Nipp. Act. Radiol.*, **36,** 1107–1112. (Japanese)

Uehara, Y. Hori, M., Takeuchi, T. and Umezawa, H. (1985). Screening of agents which convert "transformed morphology" of Rous sarcoma virus-induced rat kidney cells to "normal morphology": Identification of an active agent as herbimycin and its inhibition by intracellular *src* kinase. *Jpn. J. Cancer Res. (Gann)*, **76,** 672–675.

Ujeno, Y. (1985). Epidemiological studies on disturbances of human fetal development in areas with various doses of natural background radiation. II. Relationship between incidences of hydatidiform mole, malignant hydatidiform mole, and chorioepithelioma and gonad dose equivalent rate of natural background radiation. *Arch. Environ. Health*, **40,** 181–184.

Umezawa, H. (1978). Recent advances in bioactive microbial secondary metabolities. *J. Antibiot.*, **30** (**Suppl.**), 138–163.

Urbach, F. (1956). Pathophysiology of malignancy: I. Tissue oxygen tension of benign and malignant tumors of the skin. *Proc. Soc. Exp. Biol. Med.*, **92,** 644–649.

van Bekkum, D. W. (1955). The distubance of oxidative phosphorylation and the breakdown of ATP in spleen tissue after irradiation. *Biochim. Biophys. Acta,* **16,** 437–438.

van Bekkum, D. W. (1956). Oxidative phosphorylation in some radiosensitive tissues after irradiation. In: *Ciba Foundation Symposium on Ionizing Radiations and Cell Metabolism,* ed. by Wohlstenholme, G.E.W. and O'Conner, Y.C.M. Little and Brown, Boston, pp. 77–89.

van den Bogert, C., Dontje, B.H.J., Holtrop, M., Melis, T. E., Romijin, J. C., van Dongen, J.W. and Kroon, A.M. (1986). Arrest of the proliferation of renal and prostate carcinomas of human origin by inhibition of mitochondrial protein synthesis. *Cancer Res.,* **46,** 3283–3289.

van Duin, M., de Wit, J., Odijk, H. Westerveld, A., Yasui, A., Koken, M.H.M., Hoeijmakers, J.H.J. and Bootsma, D. (1986). Molecular characterization of the human excision repair gene *ERCC-1*: cDNA cloning and amino acid homology with the yeast DNA repair gene *RAD10*. *Cell,* **44,** 913–923.

Watanabe, M. (1982). Chromatin. In: *Mechanism of radiation Injury.—Physical Initial Step to Cell-Molecular Damages,* ed. by Yamamoto, O. Gakkai Shuppan Center, Tokyo, pp. 304–346. (Japanese)

Waterfield, M. D. (1986). The role of growth factors in cancer. In: *Introduction to the Cellular and Molecular Biology of Cancer,* ed. by Franks, L. M. and Teich, N. M. Oxford Univ. Press, Oxford, pp. 251–276.

Waterhous, J., Muir, C., Shanmugaratnam, K. and Powell, J. (1982). *WHO Cancer Incidence in Five Continents,* Vol. 4, Int. Agency Res. Cancer, Lyon.

Watson, J. D., Hopkins, N. H., Roberts, J. W., Steitz, J. A. and Weiner, A. M. (1987). *Molecular Biology of the Gene,* 4th ed., Benjamin/Cummings, Menlo Park, Calif., pp. 1058–1096.

Weber, G. (1977). Enzymology of cancer cells. (Second of two parts). *New Engl. J. Med.,* **296,** 541–551.

Weiden, P. L., Sullivan, K. M., Flurnoy, N., Storb, R., Thomas, E. D. and The Seattle Marrow Transplantation Team (1981). Antileukemic effect of chronic graft-versus-host disease. Contribution to improved survival after allogeneic marrow transplantation. *New Engl. J. Med.,* **304,** 1529–1533.

Weiser, R. S., Myrvik, Q. N. and Pearsall, N. N. (1969). *Fundamen-*

tals of Immunology for Students of Medicine and related Sciences, Lea and Febiger, Philadelphia.

Weiss, S. J. and LoBuglio, A. F. (1980). An oxygen-dependent mechanism of neutrophil-mediated cytotoxicity. *Blood*, **55**, 1020–1024.

Werner, D., Meier, G. and Lommel, R. (1973). A factor reducing protein synthesis from Ehrlich Ascites cells. *Eur. J. Cancer*, **9**, 819–824.

Westerveled, A. and Freeke, M. A. (1971). Cell cycle of multinucleate cells after cell fusion. *Exp. Cell Res.*, **65**, 140–144.

Willingham, M. C., Pastan, I., Shih, T. Y. and Scolnick, E. M. (1980). Localization of the *src* gene product of the Harvey strain of MSV to plasma membrane of transformed cells by electron microscopic immunocytochemistry. *Cell*, **19**, 1005–1014.

Weissman, I. L., Hood, L. E. and Wood, W. B. (1978). *Essential Concepts in Immunology*, Benjamin/Cummings. Menlo Park, Calif.

Withers, H. R. and Peters, L. J. (1980). Basic principles of radiotherapy. Biologic aspects of radiation therapy. In: *Textbook of Radiotherapy*, 3rd ed., ed. by Fletcher, G. H. Lea and Febiger, Philadelphia. pp. 103–180.

Yamada, T. (1973). Changes of cell surface negative charge of mammalian cells accompanying pathological transformation. In: *Saibo Denki Eido Jikkenho*, ed. by Yamada, T. Bunkodo, Tokyo, pp. 130–155. (Japanese)

Yamaguchi, K., Fukuda, H., Matsuzawa, T., Abe, Y., Itoh, M., Takahashi, H., Wakui, A., Tada, M., Ishiwata, K., Oowada, Y. and Ido, T. (1987). Differential diagnosis between hepatocellular carcinoma and metastatic liver tumor using 2–deoxy-2-(^{18}F) fluoro-D-galactose with positron emission tomography. In: *CYRIC Ann. Report 1986*, Cyclotron and Radioisotope Ctr., Tohoku Univ., Sendai, pp. 303–311.

Yamanaka, N., Nishida, K. and Ota, K. (1979). Increase of superoxide dismutase activity in various human leukemia cells. *Physiol. Chem. Physics.*, **11**, 253–256.

Yamaura, H. (1971). Experimental studies on the morphology and functions of blood vessels in tumor. *Kokenshi*, **23**, 100–120. (Japanese)

Yamaura, H. and Sato, H. (1973). Experimental studies on angiogenesis in AH109A ascites tumor tissue transplanted to a transparent chamber in rats. In: *Chemotherapy of Cancer Dissemination and Metastasis*, ed. by Garantthini S. and Franchi, G. Raven, New York, pp. 149–175.

Yatani, R., Soga, T., Yabana, T., Shiraishi, T., Noda, M. and Takeda, S. (1982). DNA excision repair of colone cancer cells and their repair patch sizes *in vitro. Photomed. Photobiol.*, **5**, 21–

22.
Yokoi, T., Nakajima, K., Tomita, K., Okuda, T. and Nakamura, T. (1983). *Japan Patent* No. **58**-180410.

Yoshimitsu, K., Kobayashi, Y. and Usui, T. (1984). Decreased superoxide dismutase activity of erythrocytes and leukocytes in Fanconi's anemia. *Acta Haemat.*, **72**, 208–210.

Yuasa, Y. (1985). transforming genes—Detection and mechanism of activation. *Igaku-no-Ayumi*, 133, 1153–1159. (in Japanese)

Zielke, H. R., Ozand, P. T., Tildon, J. T., Sevdalian, D. A. and Cornblath, M. (1976). Growth of human diploid fibroblasts in the absence of glucose utilization. *Proc. Nat. Acad. Sci.*, *USA*, **73**, 4111–4114.

Zosimovskaya, A. I. and Ljapunova, N.A. (1966). The duration of mitosis and mitotic cycle periods in the primary culture of human embryonic fibroblasts. *Tistologiya*, **8**, 208–215.

zur Hausen, H. (1982). Human genital cancer: Synergism between two virus infections or synergism between a virus infection and initiating events? *Lancet*, **ii**, 1370–1372.

Index